NEURONAL PLASTICITY

Neuronal Plasticity

Edited by

Carl W. Cotman, Ph.D.
Department of Psychobiology
University of California
Irvine, California

Raven Press ▪ New York

Raven Press, 1140 Avenue of the Americas, New York, New York 10036

Made in the United States of America

Library of Congress Cataloging in Publication Data

Main entry under title:

Neuronal Plasticity

  Includes bibliographies and index.
  1. Neural circuitry-Adaptation. I. Cotman, Carl W.
QP363.3.N48   599'.01'88   77-72807
ISBN 0-89004-210-1

Preface

Only a few years ago it was a commonly held belief that the nervous system could be "wired" in only one way during development and, once formed, the only changes in its circuitry were those due to neuronal loss. The concept of a highly static and immutable nervous system posed a serious limitation for understanding behavioral plasticity and phenomena such as the recovery of function after injury. Recent findings, however, clearly show that neuronal circuitry is highly adaptable at a structural level even in the mature nervous system. In response to internal perturbations such as lesions or external perturbations such as altered environments during development, neuronal circuitry often actively reorganizes by forming new synapses. It is the analysis of the structural plasticity of neuronal circuitry elicited by various perturbations that is the focus of this book.

The chapters in this volume describe the current state of knowledge on the types of changes which occur as a result of these perturbations, what factors provoke them, their significance, and the mechanisms that underly them. In general, the book is organized according to systems along the neuraxis so that close comparisons can be made between systems with similar structures and function. Many of the responses are similar among systems , but the uniqueness of these responses must not be overlooked. Each response must be considered in light of the function, structure, and chemistry of the system in which it occurs. The most dramatic structural changes, and the most universal, are those which occur in response to partial denervation. After partial denervation the remaining undamaged inputs will often grow and form new functional synapses in place of those lost. This process, commonly called axon sprouting or reactive synaptogenesis, appears to be widespread and occurs at all levels of the neuraxis. One key problem is the elucidation of a set of general principles describing what changes do and do not occur in response to the various types of perturbations. At present the changes appear to be highly dependent on the system; however, a few selection rules do exist and they appear to be generally applicable. Remodeling of neuronal circuitry in the mature CNS is a delicate interplay between plasticity and rigidity.

In many ways problems of circuit remodeling in the mature nervous system are analogous to those seen in the development of neuronal circuitry during ontogeny. What initiates growth? And what events determine which connections form and how many? Answers to these and related questions are particularly evasive at present, but many investigations are focusing on these issues and are discovering a key role for initiation factors, trophic materials, and glial responses, to name just a few.

A number of chapters deal with the significance of reactive synaptogenesis.

v

After lesions it may either promote or partially prevent recovery. In some cases recovery depends on experience. What are the underlying mechanisms? The overall changes brought on by denervation are really quite complex, and not all functional changes need involve the formation of new synapses. All types of changes need to be considered in elucidating the final outcome. It is now clear that, following damage to the nervous system, responses may include axon sprouting and synaptogenesis, the switching of functional activity, general depressed functioning (diaschisis), supersensitivity, the shedding of synapses from disturbed neurons and the regeneration of damaged axons. Each of these is discussed in one or more chapters.

The nervous system is not particularly susceptible to injury in the normal course of events, but still injury does occur and when it does it has serious consequences. Reactive synaptogenesis and other underlying adjustments may aid in recovery but they are unlikely to ever be as satisfactory as the original design. Perhaps ultimately we will see the time when neurons can be induced to regenerate their connections or even be replaced. Some neurons, even in the CNS, will regenerate, but others clearly will not. Why? A host of factors appear to be involved including the mobilization of synthesis in the cell body, axoplasmic flow of materials, environment, and a proper complement of trophic materials. In fact there is evidence showing that regeneration and sprouting may be two incompatible processes.

It appears that reactive synaptogenesis and other forms of plasticity provoked by denervation are not simply capacities reserved for repair, but may represent a display of an inherent brain plasticity. There are instances where it appears as if synapse formation can take place in the adult brain without denervation. It may turn out that synaptogenesis in the adult brain is an ongoing process which can be externally influenced by specific factors which mimic the effects of denervation. At present the influences of external perturbations are most dramatic during development. During early development neuronal circuitry appears to be highly modifiable and can respond to various environmental changes. In the visual system, for example, abnormal experience during a critical period in development can dramatically alter the functional capacity of the system. The nature of the changes, their significance, and a perspective on why this plasticity exists is given for the reader to consider.

The authors of this volume bring into focus many of the major issues in neuronal plasticity and provide at least tentative answers. The volume is not intended to tell a story, but it is intended to bring a message. This message is that neuronal circuitry at all levels of the neuraxis is modifiable and at least somewhat repairable. It appears as if the structural plasticity of neuronal circuitry is a very powerful capability which we are only beginning to appreciate. We are experiencing a quiet but almost revolutionary change in thinking from a few years ago. The type of vision which comes to mind reminds me of Sherrington's enchanted loom. Viewed over hours or perhaps days, the threads will break, sometimes by accident, sometimes intentionally. When they break new threads grow and branch and weave a new pattern—"a shifting but always meaningful pattern." Hopefully the material and arguments presented in this book will provide new perspectives and serve as a stimulus for new investigations toward understanding the adaptive capacities and functions of *Neuronal Plasticity.*

Acknowledgments

I am grateful to Ms. Julene Mueller for secretarial assistance in the preparation of this volume and also to Dr. J. V. Nadler, Dr. J. Rostas, Ms. Ellen Lewis, and Mr. John Ryan for their helpful discussion and assistance.

Carl W. Cotman
Irvine, California

Contents

xi

Contributors

Jerald J. Bernstein
Department of Neuroscience
University of Florida
College of Medicine
Box J-244
Gainesville, Florida 32601

Mary E. Bernstein
Department of Ophthalmology
University of Florida
College of Medicine
Box J-244
Gainesville, Florida 32601

Carl W. Cotman
Department of Psychobiology
University of California
Irvine, California 92717

Michael E. Goldberger
Department of Anatomy
The Medical College of Pennsylvania
3350 Henry Avenue
Philadelphia, Pennsylvania 19129

Patricia S. Goldman
Laboratory of Neuropsychology
National Institute of Mental Health
Building 9, Room 1N107
Bethesda, Maryland 20014

Bernice Grafstein
Department of Physiology
Cornell University Medical College
New York, New York 10021

G. A. Monti Graziadei
Department of Biological Science
Florida State University
Tallahassee, Florida 32306

P. P. C. Graziadei
Department of Biological Science
Florida State University
Tallahassee, Florida 32306

Tong Hyub Joh
Department of Neurology
Laboratory of Neurobiology
Cornell University Medical College
1300 York Avenue
New York, New York 10021

C. -P. Ko
Department of Physiology
University of Colorado Medical Center
4200 East Ninth Avenue
Denver, Colorado 80262

Michael E. Lewis
The Psychological Laboratory
University of Cambridge
Cambridge, England

Irvine G. McQuarrie
Department of Surgery (Neurosurgery)
Cornell University Medical College
New York, New York 10021

E. G. Merrill
Department of Anatomy
Cerebral Functions Research Group
University College London
Gower Street
London WC1E 6BT England

Marion Murray
Department of Anatomy
The Medical College of Pennsylvania
3350 Henry Avenue
Philadelphia, Pennsylvania 19129

J. Victor Nadler
Department of Psychobiology
University of California
Irvine, California 92717

Arild Njå
Department of Physiology and Biophysics
Washington University
School of Medicine
660 South Euclid Avenue
St. Louis, Missouri 63110

John D. Pettigrew
Beckman Laboratories of Behavioral Biology
California Institute of Technology
Pasadena, California 91125

Dale Purves
Department of Physiology and Biophysics
Washington University
School of Medicine
660 South Euclid Avenue
St. Louis, Missouri 63110

Donald J. Reis
Department of Neurology
Laboratory of Neurobiology
Cornell University Medical College
1300 York Avenue
New York, New York 10021

Stephen D. Roper
Department of Anatomy
University of Colorado Medical Center
4200 East Ninth Avenue
Denver, Colorado 80262

Robert A. Ross
Department of Neurology
Laboratory of Neurobiology
Cornell University Medical College
1300 York Avenue
New York, New York 10021

L. T. Rutledge
Department of Physiology
University of Michigan Medical
School
Ann Arbor, Michigan 48104

Nakaakira Tsukahara
Department of Biophysical Engineering
Faculty of Engineering Science
Osaka University
Toyonaka, Osaka, Japan

P. D. Wall
Department of Anatomy
Cerebral Functions Research Group
University College London
Gower Street
London WC1E 6BT England

Michael R. Wells
Department of Neuroscience
University of Florida
College of Medicine
Box J-244
Gainesville, Florida 32601

Neuronal Plasticity, edited by
Carl W. Cotman.
Raven Press, New York © 1978.

Synaptic Remodeling in the Partially Denervated Parasympathetic Ganglion in the Heart of the Frog

S. Roper and C. -P. Ko

Departments of Anatomy and Physiology, University of Colorado Medical Center, Denver, Colorado 80262

INTRODUCTION

When nervous tissue is damaged, remaining intact axons in the affected area often sprout collateral branches and establish new connections. For several decades sprouting has been recognized to be a widespread phenomenon, occurring in the central, peripheral, and autonomic nervous systems (5,8,13,16,18,21). To date, however, its significance has eluded even the most trenchant research efforts, and we still do not know whether collateral sprouting represents an attempt by the nervous system to restore function to the damaged tissue, or whether it is random, uncontrolled growth resulting in nonspecific and perhaps quite inappropriate interconnections among nerve cells. We do not know whether axonal sprouting is initiated only by trauma or whether it is an ongoing process that we detect most readily in denervated regions. Nevertheless, investigations have demonstrated that collateral sprouting does result in functional synaptic connections (5,9,15,19), and there is little doubt that novel axonal pathways

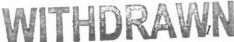

1

are created after damage to nervous tissue. Thus, an understanding of neuronal sprouting is critical both to neurologists treating disorders resulting from lesions in the nervous system and to investigators studying basic mechanisms of synapse formation, maintenance, and plasticity.

Our studies, summarized below, fall into the latter category, namely the investigation of the cellular mechanisms underlying sprouting. We have been examining neuronal sprouting in the parasympathetic cardiac ganglion in the interatrial septum of the frog heart. This preparation has several advantages for investigating synaptic transmission between nerve cells and for studying axonal sprouting. The most salient feature of the ganglion is that the interatrial septum is very thin so that individual neurons, their processes, and even some synapses can be seen in the living, isolated preparation. Furthermore, the organization of synapses here is less complex than in other preparations, and it is possible to detect subtle changes in neuronal interconnections after experimental manipulations.

Using the amphibian cardiac ganglion as a model, we have focused on three questions. Do sprouting nerve terminals release transmitter normally? What are some of the factors initiating and controlling sprouting? And what is the relationship between collateral sprouting and axonal regeneration? This basic information is essential before the real significance of neuronal sprouting in the nervous system can be assessed.

INNERVATION OF THE FROG CARDIAC GANGLION

The right and left cardiac branches of the vagus nerves enter the heart at the sinus venosus. Before continuing into the heart, some of the axons cross to the opposite side via a chiasm. Distal to the chiasm and embedded in the thin, interatrial septum are two nerve bundles, a ventral and a dorsal one, with most of the axons from the left cardiac branch travelling in the dorsal and most right axons travelling in the ventral bundle. When the interatrial septum is pinned out flat, it is convenient to refer to a left/right branch of the ganglion rather than *dorsal/ventral,* respectively, and henceforth this convention will be used. The parasympathetic neurons which comprise the cardiac ganglion in the frog lie along the nerve bundles traversing the interatrial septum (Fig. 1).

Preganglionic vagal axons form synapses *en passant* with the cardiac ganglion cells. These parasympathetic neurons, in turn, send their postganglionic axons back into the interatrial bundles to reach cardiac muscle fibers in the walls of the atria and ventricle.

Initially, experiments were conducted on both branches of the cardiac ganglion, but it soon became evident that data collection would be simplified and variability reduced by concentrating on one branch only and standardizing the operative and recording procedures. Thus, even though the results apply equally to either half, the following electrophysiological and morphological data were

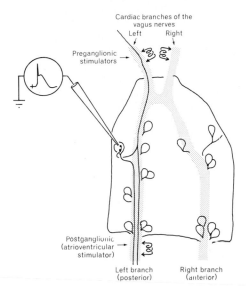

Fig. 1. Schematic drawing of the parasympathetic ganglion in the interatrial septum of the frog heart. Shown here is the interatrial septum, viewed as if pinned out flat, with the walls of the atria and ventricle dissected away. The cardiac branches of the vagus nerves enter the heart and form a chiasm near the top. Ganglion cells innervate and inhibit cardiac muscle fibers in the walls of the atria and ventricle, and they receive synaptic contacts from preganglionic (vagal) axons. Neurons on the *left* (posterior) branch traversing the interatrial septum were impaled with microelectrodes and responses evoked by stimulating the preganglionic or postganglionic (atrioventricular) nerve bundles were recorded. Postganglionic stimulation would often excite neurons both antidromically as well as synaptically, as shown in this drawing.

collected from the left branch only. As will be shown below in greater detail, the parasympathetic neurons on either branch receive their predominant synaptic input from the ipsilateral vagus nerve; for example, the ganglion cells on the left branch are primarily innervated by the left vagus nerve.

Physiological and Histological Techniques

Our experiments consisted of mapping vagal connections to the cardiac ganglion in partially denervated frogs, using intracellular recordings of synaptic potentials and employing histological techniques (cf. 6,17) (Fig. 1). By using Zeiss Nomarski optics we were able to position microelectrodes under direct visual control and to impale selected parasympathetic neurons (Fig. 2). The solution bathing ganglia during intracellular recordings was a Ringer solution of the following composition: 112 mM NaCl, 5 mM KCl, 5 mM Hepes buffer (pH 7.2), and 5 mM $CaCl_2$. The slightly elevated Ca^{2+} concentration improved the microelectrode penetrations and enhanced synaptic transmission. Higher concentrations were avoided to prevent impulse conduction failure.

Mapping the innervation pattern of the cardiac ganglion electrophysiologically

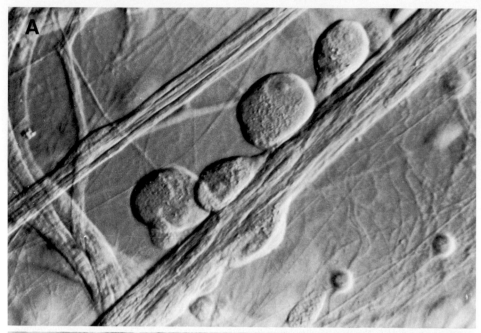

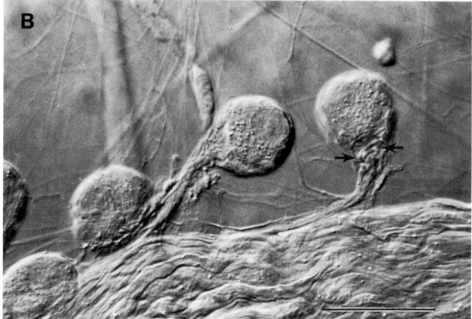

FIG. 2. Microphotographs of living parasympathetic ganglion cells from the frog heart as viewed with Nomarski differential interference contrast optics (with a X40 water immersion objective). **A:** A cluster of ganglion cells lies along a small nerve bundle on the interatrial septum. Nuclei and nucleoli are seen in some of the neurons. A small band of striated cardiac muscle fibers can be seen crossing the field in the lower left. **B:** Ganglion cells from another preparation. The cell bodies and short length of postganglionic axons are visible. The preganglionic nerve terminal often coils around the axon hillock before it deposits boutons on the cell surface (see McMahan and Kuffler, 1971), and this can be seen in the neuron on the right *(arrows)*. Calibration, 40 microns.

required that we establish rigid criteria for accepting the results from each microelectrode impalement; inadequate penetrations would decrease the amplitude of all intracellular responses and make it likely that small synaptic potentials be overlooked. Thus, we accepted only those cells whose resting potentials were greater than 35mV and in which action potentials could be elicited, since experience showed us that spontaneous excitatory postsynaptic potentials (and hence single-quantum evoked responses) could be detected with confidence if these criteria were met. Accordingly, after the vagal innervation to a ganglion cell was recorded, the excitability was tested and the resting potential was measured upon withdrawing the electrode. Most recordings (greater than 80%) were taken from neurons having resting potentials between 40 to 60 mV and action potentials which overshot resting potential. The average proportion of cells from control frogs in which no evoked synaptic responses could be detected was only 0.5%, thereby increasing our confidence in the reliability of the dissection and recording procedures.

Parasympathetic neurons for electrophysiological studies were selected at random along the left branch of the ganglion, although it was inevitable that larger cells probably gave the most stable recordings. About 20 to 40 cells were successfully impaled in a typical experiment, and this sample was used to estimate the innervation pattern of the ganglion cell population along the left branch. The total number of ganglion cells along this branch is about 300.

Innervation of ganglion cells was examined histologically by staining synaptic boutons with one of two methods, either zinc iodide-osmium or methylene blue diluted 1:50,000 g/ml in 80% Leibovitz culture medium (17). Stained ganglia were viewed in whole-mount preparations. The zinc iodide-osmium technique was highly capricious and did not stain synaptic boutons in every ganglion equally well. Methylene blue staining was more consistent, but the stained boutons faded after about 30 to 60 min in the staining solution and no permanent slide of the tissue could be obtained.

PREGANGLIONIC INNERVATION OF UNOPERATED ANIMALS

Stimulation of the preganglionic nerve trunks produced relatively simple excitatory postsynaptic potentials (e.p.s.p.'s) in the ganglion cells, in agreement with previous investigations (6). Most often, stimulation evoked a large suprathreshold e.p.s.p. with the action potential superimposed on the peak of the synaptic depolarization (Fig. 3). The large e.p.s.p. generally outlasted the impulse and resulted in a residual depolarization, representing continued transmitter activation of the ganglion cells (6). In 58% of the neurons (215 of 373 cells), responses from two or more presynaptic axons could be evoked by increasing the stimulus intensity to one vagus nerve and/or by stimulating the opposite vagus nerve (Fig. 3). Usually each cell received one suprathreshold vagal synaptic input, and other responses, if present, were subthreshold. Subthreshold responses were often quite small; their size was similar to that of spontaneous e.p.s.p.'s (0.5–

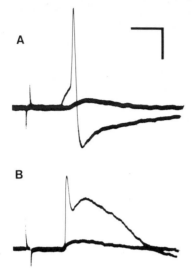

FIG. 3. Intracellular responses from a parasympathetic neuron in the frog cardiac ganglion. Synaptic potentials were evoked by stimulating the left **(A)** and right **(B)** cardiac branches of the vagus nerves. This recording was unusual in that four separate inputs (sub- and suprathreshold ones from both vagus nerves) to one cell were produced by increasing the stimulus strength to the vagus nerves. These records are shown to demonstrate how multiple innervation was detected in many of the ganglion cells. Note the large synaptic potential in **B** which outlasts and reduces the peak amplitude of the impulse (compare action potential with that in **A**) by the intense transmitter activation of the postsynaptic membrane (see Dennis, et al., ref. 6). Calibrations, 20 mV and 20 msec.

2mV), and their amplitude fluctuated in discrete steps during repeated activation even with supramaximal stimulation. These observations suggest that the subthreshold responses probably were composed of only a few quanta, although no special study was made of their quantal content.

The above proportion of neurons receiving multiple innervation by the vagus nerves is surely less than the true value since it was difficult to distinguish small subthreshold responses superimposed upon the powerful input; usually detecting subthreshold inputs depended upon the ability to stimulate their presynaptic axons separately from the suprathreshold input.

Presynaptic activation of the ganglion cells could also be achieved by drawing the distal (atrioventricular) ends of the interatrial branches into suction electrodes and stimulating the nerves antidromically (see Fig. 1). Because preganglionic axons synapsing *en passant* with ganglion cells extend the entire length of the interatrial branches, when the distal ends of the branches were stimulated, synaptic potentials and antidromic impulses were often produced in the neurons (cf. 6). Stimulating the distal branches had the disadvantage that it was not possible to tell whether the evoked responses were produced by left or right preganglionic axons, but it served as a useful check on possible dissection damage. Thus, if many cells could not be activated by preganglionic stimulation but synaptic responses were evoked by stimulating the distal ends of the ganglion, it suggested that the vagus nerves had been injured. (There are no intrinsic ganglionic synapses normally: cf., 6,27).

Innervation Pattern of the Cardiac Ganglion

The first objective of these experiments was to map electrophysiologically the innervation of the cardiac ganglion in normal frogs, and in particular, of

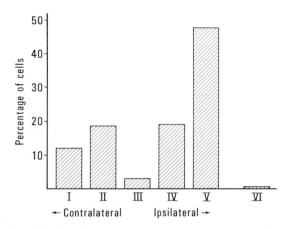

FIG. 4. Vagal dominance diagram for preganglionic innervation pattern of the left branch of the cardiac ganglion in the frog. This histogram shows the percentage of neurons in each of six categories as described in the text. Three hundred and seventy-three neurons from 15 unoperated frogs are included.

the left branch of the ganglion. As might be expected, ganglion cells tended to be innervated by the ipsilateral vagus nerve. Thus, of 373 cells recorded from the left branch in 15 control ganglia, 88% received synaptic input from the left vagus nerve and 52% from the right. Furthermore, the most powerful inputs were generated by stimulating the ipsilateral nerve; stimulating the contralateral nerve usually evoked subthreshold responses. In 0.5% of the cells no responses could be evoked by preganglionic stimulation.

Vagal dominance diagrams were constructed to map the innervation pattern in greater detail. A complete census was taken of the synaptic inputs to ganglion cells. Neurons were divided into six categories as follows: In category I are those which received synaptic input from the contralateral nerve only. Cells which received a suprathreshold response from the contralateral nerve and subthreshold one(s) from the ipsilateral nerve are listed in category II. Category III consists of the ganglion cells which had equal inputs from both vagus nerves, either both suprathreshold or both subthreshold responses. Category IV is the group of cells which received suprathreshold ipsilateral innervation and subthreshold contralateral input(s). Cells which were innervated only by the ipsilateral nerve were grouped into category V. Lastly, cells receiving no synaptic input were included in category VI.

The vagal dominance diagram of the left branch of ganglia from unoperated frogs is shown in Fig. 4. This figure clearly demonstrates that normally the ipsilateral vagus dominates the nerve supply to the cardiac ganglion cells.

Light Microscopy of Preganglionic Boutons

Synaptic boutons were stained with zinc iodide-osmium or methylene blue to establish the number, size, and position of vagal endings on ganglion cells.

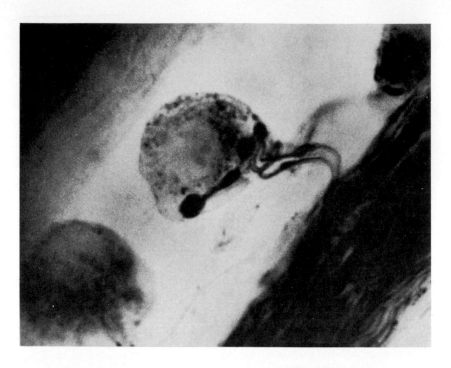

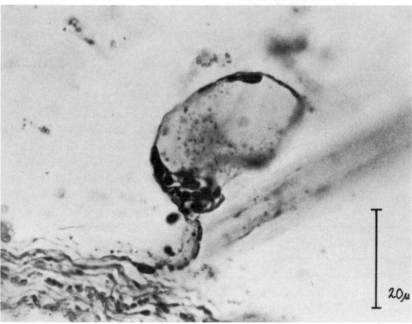

FIG. 5. Parasympathetic ganglion cells taken from a preparation stained with zinc iodide-osmium. On the *left* are photomicrographs of two different ganglion cells, and on the *right* are camera lucida drawings of the same cells. In the ganglion cell on *top*, the preganglionic

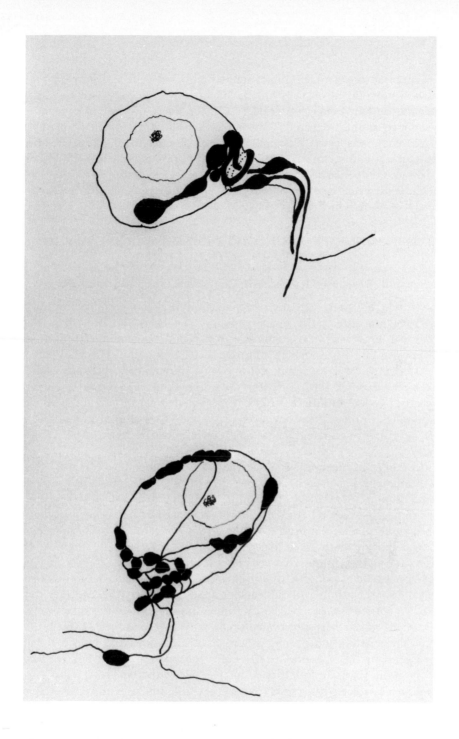

terminal can be seen to coil around the axon hillock before depositing boutons on the cell body (see Fig. 2). The neuron on the *bottom* has more synaptic boutons than average, whereas the neuron on top is more typical.

An example of zinc iodide-osmium-stained ganglion cells is shown in Fig. 5. Boutons were counted on cells on the left branch in normal ganglia. As had been found by McMahan and Kuffler (17), the mean number of boutons/cell body differed slightly depending upon whether the zinc iodide or methylene blue technique was used. Zinc iodide-stained ganglia from unoperated frogs yielded a mean number of boutons ($\pm$SD) = 8.9 ± 4.0 boutons/cell (99 neurons), and methylene blue yielded 7.1 ± 2.3 boutons/cell (195 neurons). Boutons were often clustered near the axon hillock or formed a loop encircling the ganglion cell body, as shown in Fig. 5.

PREGANGLIONIC SPROUTING AFTER PARTIAL DENERVATION OF THE CARDIAC GANGLION

Synaptic Responses Recorded in Ganglion Cells in Operated Frogs

To test whether there was any reorganization of synaptic connections in the cardiac ganglion after partial denervation of the heart, the left vagus nerve was crushed in a group of experimental frogs. Animals were anesthetized with 0.5% ethyl-m-aminobenzoate (Sigma) or in 10% ethanol. The skin was slit just posterior to the tympanum, the overlying musculature retracted, and the vagus nerves exposed near their exit from the skull. The large vagus nerve was gently freed from adjacent blood vessels and crushed two or three times with jewellers' forceps. The skin over the wound was sutured closed and the animal returned to running water tanks, maintained between 10 to 17°C for recovery.

When the vagal innervation of the ganglia was mapped several days (6–26) after the operation, a striking change in the preganglionic inputs had occurred; synaptic responses evoked by stimulating the intact right vagus nerve were recorded in nearly every cell and inputs from the crushed left vagus functionally degenerated (Fig. 6). Because there was no atrophy of ganglion cells, this suggests that vagal axons had sprouted to innervate the parasympathetic neurons. That is, had left vagal axons merely degenerated without any alteration in inputs from the opposite nerve, one would have expected to find a large proportion (nearly 50%) of neurons without synaptic input (category VI), contrary to the results. Synaptic responses evoked by stimulating the remaining intact preganglionic axons in partially denervated preparations were normal. Initially there were proportionately more subthreshold than suprathreshold e.p.s.p.'s, but 2 to 3 weeks after the operation nearly every cell had suprathreshold responses from the right vagus nerve. It was not possible with the present analysis to distinguish between e.p.s.p.'s produced at preexisting synapses and ones produced by sprouted nerve terminals.

In addition to the increase in the proportion of cells innervated by the opposite (intact) vagus nerve during the first days, there was a concomitant decline in neurons receiving inputs from the damaged left vagus nerve (Fig. 6). In some frogs it took up to 6 days for all signs of synaptic responses from the crushed nerve to disappear. At all stages after partial denervation, e.p.s.p.'s from the left vagus nerve, if present, were normal, and thus disappearance of functional transmission at degenerating vagal endings was apparently quite abrupt. Although not explored in depth, this finding is consistent with studies of synaptic transmission at degenerating nerve terminals in sympathetic ganglia of the frog (10).

These changes in the innervation pattern of the cardiac ganglion after partial denervation could be accounted for by collateral sprouting either of the preganglionic or of postganglionic axons. For example, had postganglionic axons established connections with adjacent ganglion cells, stimulation of the intact nerve would have produced responses directly in roughly half the neurons (from preexisting vagal connections), and the remaining neurons would have been activated secondarily by excitation of collateral synapses. Although we found no evidence for such multisynaptic activation of parasympathetic neurons, direct evidence that postganglionic axon collateral sprouting did not occur was shown by the following experiment. An initial operation was made as described above; in two frogs the left vagus nerve was crushed and the animals allowed to recover for 1 week, by which time the opposite nerve would have innervated the entire ganglion. The animals were then reanesthetized and the *right* vagus nerve was cut (in a second operation); the wound was closed, and the animals were allowed

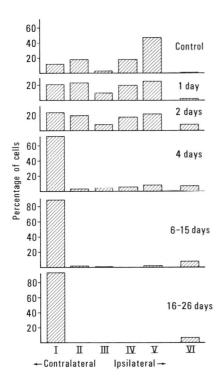

FIG. 6. Vagal dominance diagrams for the change in innervation of the left branch of the cardiac ganglion following partial denervation (see text and Fig. 4 for description of categories). Each histogram shows the data at different intervals after crushing the left vagus nerve (times shown to the *right* of each histogram). A detectable change in the innervation pattern is seen within 1 day after the operation, and the maximum change is seen after 6 days.

to recover for an additional 1 to 2 weeks to allow the right vagal axons to degenerate. The animals were killed before any regeneration of preganglionic axons had occurred, the ganglia dissected free, and the vagal innervation mapped. In 40 neurons from both frogs no synaptic responses were produced by stimulating vagal axons orthodromically (at the central end of the ganglion) or antidromically (at the atrioventricular end, see Fig. 1). If postganglionic axon sprouting had been the basis for the remodeling of ganglionic connections after partial denervation, in at least half the cells one would have expected stimulation of the atrioventricular stump to have produced e.p.s.p.'s by antidromic activation of collateral synapses (25,27), which is in clear contrast to our results.

Light Microscopy of Partially Denervated Ganglia

To determine whether sprouting after partial denervation resulted in morphologically abnormal innervation of the parasympathetic neurons, synaptic boutons were stained with zinc iodide or methylene blue at various times after crushing

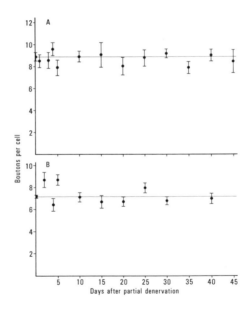

FIG. 7. The number of intact boutons per neuron on the *left* branch of the cardiac ganglion remains constant after partial denervation. **A:** Average number of boutons per cell as measured with zinc iodide-osmium staining. **B:** Average number of boutons per cell measured with methylene blue staining. Boutons were counted in whole-mounted preparations, observed with an oil immersion objective for zinc iodide stained preparations (overall magnification X1000) or a water immersion objective for methylene blue stained preparations (overall magnification X400). Abscissae, time after crushing the left vagus nerve (with data at time zero being from unoperated animals). Each point represents the averaged counts from 8–195 neurons, with standard error bars included. A line originating in the average number of boutons from unoperated animals has been drawn across the graphs.

the left vagus nerve. At all intervals, the number of intact boutons/cell was remarkably constant, even at times when electrophysiological and electron microscopical studies (Frenk and Roper, *in progress*) demonstrated that damaged vagal terminals had completely degenerated (Fig. 7). Furthermore, there was no apparent difference in either the size, the shape, or the position of the boutons in the operated ganglia. It was not possible to distinguish sprouted from preexisting vagal endings using these techniques. Nevertheless, collateral sprouting must have occurred to replace the synaptic boutons which degenerated, since otherwise an overall decrease in the number of boutons per cell would have been observed.

SPROUTING AND REGENERATION OF PREGANGLIONIC AXONS

Regeneration of Crushed Vagal Fibers

Several frogs were left to recover for long periods (up to 1 year and longer) after partial denervation to study the interrelationship between sprouting and regeneration. That is, would functional reinnervation of the cardiac ganglion by the crushed left vagus nerve occur when all the cells were innervated by the opposite (sprouted) nerve? If so, what is the fate of the sprouted synaptic connections?

Beginning about 6 weeks after crushing the left vagus nerve, synaptic responses in some ganglion cells were obtained by stimulating the operated nerve, signifying that functional reinervation had commenced. At this early stage of regeneration, the synaptic responses produced by the left vagus usually were subthreshold, and their latency was often 2 to 3 times that of synaptic responses produced by the opposite (sprouted) vagus nerve or synaptic responses in unoperated animals. At later times, increasing numbers of ganglion cells received input from the operated left vagus nerve, and supra- as well as subthreshold responses were obtained (Fig. 8).

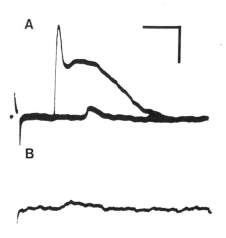

FIG. 8. Intracellular responses from a parasympathetic neuron on the left branch of the cardiac ganglion, 288 days after crushing the left vagus nerve. A: Responses evoked by stimulating the regenerating left vagus nerve. B: Response produced by stimulating the right vagus nerve. Two different inputs were evoked by stimulating the left vagus nerve, a sub- and a suprathreshold one. Although not as pronounced as in earlier stages of regeneration, the latency of the smaller left vagal response clearly differs from that of the other reponses. At earlier times (about 6 weeks) after partial denervation, most of the synaptic potentials produced by the left vagus nerve during reinnervation were subthreshold and few suprathreshold inputs were observed. Calibrations, 20 mV and 20 msec.

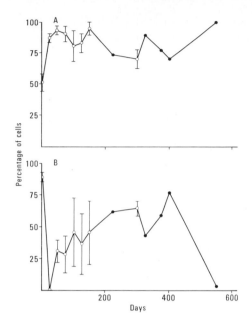

FIG. 9. Functional reinnervation of the left branch of the cardiac ganglion after crushing the left vagus nerve results in a slight loss of inputs from the (sprouted) right vagus nerve. **A:** Percentage of cells innervated by the right vagus nerve. **B:** Percentage innervated by the left vagus. Abscissae represent time after crushing the left vagus nerve. Innervation was tested by recording intracellular responses evoked by stimulating the right and left vagus nerves. *Open circles* are averages of data from 2–10 ganglia with standard error bars included. *Solid circles* are data from a single ganglion. Synaptic responses in 20–40 neurons were examined in each ganglion.

TABLE 1. *Loss of right vagal innervation at long intervals (101–546 days) after crushing the left vagus nerve (partial denervation), when reinnervation by the damaged axons is occurring[a]*

Experiment	No. of ganglia	No. of neurons	Percent innervation by right vagus ($\pm$ SEM)	Percent innervation by left vagus ($\pm$ SEM)
Control frogs	15	373	51.9 ± 6.2	87.6 ± 3.3
Days 14–100 after partial denervation	26	672	90.2 ± 2.3[b]	22.6 ± 5.5
Days 101–546 after partial denervation	14	429	82.6 ± 3.6[b]	48.9 ± 8.0

[a]At short intervals after partial denervation (14–100 days) the intact right vagal endings sprout; the proportion of parasympathetic neurons receiving right inputs increases from 52% to 90%. At longer intervals, the left vagal axons reinnervate the ganglia and the proportion of neurons innervated by the right nerve decreases to 83% (see Fig. 9).

[b]Values differ significantly from each other and from control value ($p < 0.05$).

On the other hand, after the initial increase following partial denervation of the ganglion, innervation from the right nerve declined somewhat as the left vagal fibers reestablished functional connections (Fig. 9). This decrease was significant at the 0.05 level (Table 1). Nevertheless, even up to 1½ years after partial denervation, the innervation of the cardiac ganglion did not return to normal, and many more neurons than usual were innervated by the right vagus nerve (Figs. 9,10). Because we were unable to distinguish between e.p.s.p.'s produced by sprouted endings and by normal endings from the same nerve (above), we could not determine from these experiments whether the sprouted terminals were preferentially lost during reinnervation by the original nerve.

The data in Fig. 9 suggest that the functional disappearance of right vagal innervation corresponds with the return of left vagal axons after partial denervation. This was tested further by preventing regeneration of the left vagus nerve altogether and examining the fate of right vagal innervation. In three frogs the left vagus nerve was repeatedly sectioned at about 1 month intervals for 19 to 34 weeks. In every instance there was no regeneration of left vagal axons and no decline in right vagal innervation. This suggests that sprouted nerve terminals form synaptic contacts with ganglion cells which remain stable at least until the original nerve supply regenerates.

When ganglia were stained with zinc iodide-osmium at long intervals after partial denervation, the number of intact boutons/cell we observed was not significantly different from that in normal ganglia or partially denervated ganglia at earlier times (Table 2). This suggests that when left vagal axons reestablish functional connections, some right vagal terminals regress morphologically.

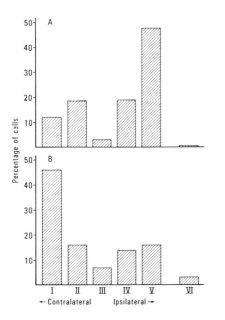

FIG. 10. Vagal dominance diagram for innervation pattern of partially denervated cardiac ganglia after reinnervation (see text and Fig. 4 for description of categories). **A:** Data from unoperated frogs (as in Fig. 4). **B:** Data from frogs 302–546 days after crushing the left vagus nerve. Even at this long interval, functional reinnervation by the damaged left vagus is incomplete. In **A** 373 neurons are included, and 147 neurons from 4 ganglia are included in **B**.

TABLE 2. *Average number of boutons per cell body in tne cardiac ganglion after partial denervation (crushing the left vagus nerve) remains constant* [a]

Experiment	No. of ganglia	No. of neurons	Average no. of boutons/cell (± SEM)
Control frogs	12	99	8.9 ± 0.4 [b]
Days 14–100 after partial denervation	27	241	8.8 ± 0.2 [b]
Days 101–546 after partial denervation	4	29	9.2 ± 0.6 [b]

[a] Ganglia were stained with zinc iodide-osmium and boutons counted on parasympathetic neurons on the left branch of the cardiac ganglia.
[b] None of the values in this column differ significantly from each other.

Experiments currently in progress are yielding information regarding another interesting aspect of regenerating vagal axons. We are finding that although functional reinnervation of partially denervated ganglia is successful, it occurs at a surprisingly slow rate. Even 1 to 1½ years after crushing the left vagus nerve, functional reinnervation is incomplete; damaged left vagal axons reestablish connections with only 49% of the neurons, compared with a normal value of 88% (see Table 1). In their studies in the brain of rats, Raisman and Field (22) suggested that the presence of sprouted nerve terminals impedes the reestab-

TABLE 3. *Functional reinnervation of the cardiac ganglion is impeded by the presence of sprouted synapses after partial denervation* [a]

Experiment	No. of ganglia	Percent innervation, left vagus (± SEM)	Percent innervation, right vagus (± SEM)
Unoperated frogs	15	87.6 ± 3.3	51.9 ± 6.2
Reinnervation 29–59 days after total vagotomy	12	83.8 ± 3.6 [b]	82.4 ± 4.4
Innervation 30–60 days after partial denervation	12	48.3 ± 6.6 [b]	93.2 ± 2.8

[a] Two experiments are compared—reinnervation after complete denervation (both vagus nerves crushed) and reinnervation when only the left vagus nerve is crushed and the right vagus has sprouted to innervate the ganglion. Significantly fewer functional connections are reestablished by the left vagus nerve when axons compete with established right vagal inputs (partial denervation experiments) as compared with regeneration after total vagotomy.
[b] Values are significantly different at $p < .01$.

lishment of the original synaptic contacts, and our experiments are providing direct evidence for this.

Using physiological recording techniques, we have compared reinnervation of the cardiac ganglion in two situations: (a) after complete denervation (crushing both vagus nerves), and (b) after the left vagus nerve only is crushed, allowing the right vagus to sprout and innervate all the cells. Although the findings are as yet incomplete, there was a striking difference between the two operations in the ability of damaged vagal axons to reestablish functional connections with ganglion cells. Reinnervation of cardiac ganglia by both left and right vagal inputs was rapid and complete after both nerves were crushed, demonstrating that both right and left vagal axons are quite capable of axonal regrowth and synapse formation after injury. In contrast, at comparable times after *partial* denervation, significantly fewer cells were functionally reinnervated by the operated left nerve, and most of the neurons received inputs from the (sprouted) right vagus (Table 3). The presence of sprouted vagal endings from the right vagus nerve after partial denervation clearly has an adverse effect on the ability of regenerating preganglionic axons to reestablish functional synapses.

DOES CHRONIC IMPULSE BLOCKADE IN VAGUS NERVES MIMIC PARTIAL DENERVATION?

The above experiments indicate that a profound remodeling of synaptic connections occurs after partial denervation of the cardiac ganglion. Many factors could be responsible for sprouting. For example, the cessation of propagated impulses in one nerve could stimulate sprouting in the other vagus nerve. Alternatively, interruption of axoplasmic transport could initiate sprouting in adjacent terminals. Products of nerve degeneration may themselves produce collateral sprouting.

It was possible to test and rule out the first of these possibilities by applying small tetrodotoxin (TTX)-impregnated implants (cuffs) around one vagus nerve in the frog, thereby blocking nerve impulses without interfering with axoplasmic transport (11,20). These cuffs were constructed similar to the technique described by Robert and Oester (24) and Lømo and Rosenthal (14). About 1.5% (by weight) TTX was mixed into a small amount of Dow Corning Silastic RTV A and then Dow Corning catalyst no. 4 was added. While the material was still fluid, small cylindrical cuffs were formed on a rotating spindle and the silastic allowed to polymerize. Subsequently, a thin layer of drug-free silastic was applied to the outside of the TTX cuff to encapsulate the toxin. Each cuff contained approximately 3 to 5 micrograms TTX. When the cuff was implanted on the vagus nerves in the frog, it blocked nerve conduction for periods of up to at least 10 days, although there was a great variability in the effectiveness of individual cuffs.

Cuffs were implanted on the vagus nerves in anesthetized frogs by carefully freeing the vagus from surrounding tissue with fire-polished glass probes and slipping the cuff around the exposed section of nerve. After implantation, the vagus nerves were visually inspected at X50 with the dissecting microscope to assure that small vessels within the nerve were still circulating blood, thereby indicating that the cuff had not compressed the nerve.

The effectiveness of the TTX cuffs in blocking conduction in the axons was tested by their ability to prevent cardioinhibition produced by electrically stimulating the vagus nerve trunk central to the cuff (see below).

Considerable difficulties were met in using TTX-impregnated cuffs, however. First, frogs took a long time to recover from the TTX implantation (about 1–3 days, in contrast with about 1 hr when frogs were submitted to other surgical procedures or when untreated cuffs were implanted), and many animals died. Even with precautions to reduce the diffusion of TTX from the cuff (coating the outside of the cuff with untreated silastic), TTX escaped in sufficient quantities to produce generalized toxic effects during the first days of implantation. However, control experiments showed that this generalized effect did not affect the analysis (see below). Second, the lumen of the cuff had to be significantly larger than the nerves to avoid compression damage (see ref. 4). Third, not every cuff was equally effective, presumably due to variability in the release of the toxin from different cuffs (see ref. 3). Nevertheless, in a sufficient number of experiments conduction was blocked with negligible damage to the nerves and yielded unequivocal evidence that chronic impulse blockade did not induce functional changes in the opposite, actively conducting nerve. This was shown by the following results.

TTX-impregnated cuffs were implanted on the left vagus nerves in several frogs for periods of 5 to 10 days (the interval after which sprouting is nearly complete following partial denervation). The frogs were then killed and the vagal innervation of the cardiac ganglion was mapped. To determine whether the TTX was effective and that only the left vagus nerve was blocked, a test was run on each animal before the ganglion was dissected free. This consisted of stimulating the vagus nerves and recording the electrocardiogram (EKG), testing for vagally mediated cardioinhibition. The frog was pithed, and both vagus nerves were severed close to the skull (central to the cuff on the left side). Stimulating the distal end of the right vagus nerve with a suction electrode with low intensity stimulation abruptly stopped the heart beat as shown in Fig. 11A. Similar results were obtained when the left vagus was stimulated *distal* to the TTX cuffs (Fig. 11C). On the other hand even prolonged intense stimulation had much less of an effect on the EKG when applied *central* to the TTX cuff (Fig. 11B). This test was repeated on every frog before the innervation pattern of the cardiac ganglion was mapped, and if the stimulus intensity which just blocked the heartbeat when applied central to the cuff did not exceed the threshold intensity distal to the cuff (or on the opposite nerve) by at least a factor of 10, the data were discarded from further analysis. Approximately 10% of the animals succeeded in meeting this stringent criterion, especially at

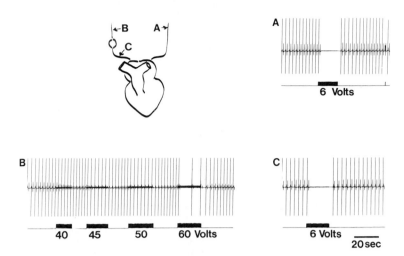

FIG. 11. Electrocardiogram (EKG) of frog in which a TTX cuff was implanted on the left vagus nerve for 6 days. The experiment was conducted on the intact, but pithed, frog prior to removing the heart and cardiac ganglion. Drawing in *upper left* is a schematic diagram of the experimental protocol showing where vagal stimuli were applied. The vagus nerves were severed from the brain before the experiment. **A:** A train of pulses (1 msec pulses at 10 Hz) applied to the untreated vagus nerves with a suction electrode inhibits the heart beat with a stimulation intensity of 6 volts. **B:** A train of pulses (1 msec, 10 Hz) applied central to the TTX cuff did not affect EKG to any extent until at least 60 volts were applied. **C:** Stimulating the vagus nerve distal to the cuff once again was effective at low stimulus intensities. The strong stimulation central to the cuff **(B)** presumably spread to unblocked regions of the vagus nerve distal to the cuff to effect cardio-inhibition. This test was used in every TTX experiment before mapping the innervation pattern of the cardiac ganglion to establish that the toxin-impregnated cuff had blocked propagated activity in the vagus nerve.

the longer recovery times when the effectiveness of the cuffs was wearing off (e.g., 8–10 days).

When the vagal innervation of these ganglia was mapped after propagated impulses in the left preganglionic nerve had been effectively blocked with a TTX cuff, there were no clear signs of synaptic remodeling (Table 4) in contrast to the results at comparable times after crushing the left vagus nerve. Although there appeared to be a slight increase in the proportion of cells innervated by the actively conducting (right) vagus nerve, this was not related to cessation of impulse traffic in the left vagus; control cuffs containing equivalent or greater amounts of citrate buffer or NaCl (neither substance affected impulse conduction) produced quantitatively identical results. The small change in innervation pattern, instead, is consistent with slight damage to the vagus nerves caused by the cuff technique (e.g., unavoidable compression or changes in tonicity). In fact, electron micrographs of cross sections taken from control and experimental material showed 1 to 10% of the vagal axons were degenerating in the cuff-implanted nerves (Roper, Ko, Frenk, and Frank, *in progress*).

TABLE 4. *Effect of TTX-impregnated cuffs on vagal innervation of the cardiac ganglion*[a]

Experiment	No. of ganglia	No. of neurons	Percent left innervation (± SEM)	Percent right innervation (± SEM)
Unoperated frogs	15	373	87.6 ± 3.3	52.0 ± 6.2
NaCl control cuffs	10	290	85.2 ± 3.3	61.0 ± 7.4
Citrate buffer control cuffs	11	336	77.4 ± 6.3	67.0 ± 6.9
TTX cuffs	13	382	77.3 ± 5.1	66.2 ± 7.8

[a] 1½% TTX cuffs were implanted on the left vagus nerve and left in place for 5–10 days before vagal innervation was mapped. Each frog was tested before mapping the innervation of the ganglion to ascertain that the left vagus nerve activity had been blocked by the TTX. For comparison, control cuffs containing 20% NaCl or 7.5% citrate buffer (pH 4.8) were implanted on the left nerves in other frogs. Citrate buffer was chosen because commercially available TTX is provided in a mixture of citrate buffer to TTX = 5 : 1. Neither NaCl nor citrate buffer blocked impulse conduction in the vagus nerves.

Although the above experiments showed that conduction block of one vagus nerve did not alter the functional innervation from the opposite actively conducting nerve, we cannot rule out some degree of morphological sprouting (see ref. 3). Zinc iodide-osmium staining of ganglia in which one nerve had been blocked did not show increased numbers of boutons on ganglion cells or any indications of synaptic remodeling, but small nerve terminal sprouts would have been beyond the resolution of this histological method as applied to the cardiac ganglion.

A corollary to these experiments was to crush the left vagus nerve and at the same time block conduction in the remaining intact nerve by applying a TTX cuff to the right vagus. This tested whether a TTX-treated nerve was capable of sprouting (as shown in ref. 3 at the neuromuscular junction), and also controlled whether the above lack of sprouting in TTX-implanted animals could be attributed to a generalized effect of the toxin. In a series of frogs, the left vagus was crushed, a TTX cuff placed on the intact right vagus, and the animals allowed to recover for 6 to 8 days. The TTX cuff was found to have blocked impulses in three of these animals. In every case, the TTX-treated nerve sprouted and innervated the ganglion (right innervation increased to 94 ± 7%, mean ± SD) at least as much, if not more, than in animals where the left nerve was crushed for the same period but no TTX cuff was present on the opposite nerve (right innervation increased to 81 ± 7%).

These data indicate that the mere cessation of propagated impulses has little effect on inducing functional sprouting in adjacent axons and does not prevent collateral sprouting by blocked nerves. In short, TTX application to one vagus nerve did not mimic partial denervation of the ganglion. Some other factor(s), as discussed below, must be important in causing the functional reorganization of nerve terminals after partial denervation.

DISCUSSION

Functional synaptic transmission at sprouting terminals has been investigated only indirectly in the central and autonomic nervous systems due to the difficulties in impaling cells, recording near the site of synapses, observing individual neurons, and selectively stimulating well-defined inputs. The parasympathetic ganglion in the heart of the frog is well suited for studying both structural and functional aspects of nerve terminal sprouting because of its simple organization and because of the clarity with which single cells can be seen. These studies have shown that after partial denervation of the ganglion, a striking remodeling of synaptic connections occurs; remaining intact preganglionic fibers sprout to form new synapses. Furthermore, synaptic transmission at the sprouted synaptic terminals appears normal, within the resolution of the present analyses. Although not yet investigated in detail, we were unable to distinguish between e.p.s.p.'s produced by a sprouted nerve terminal and by a normal ending, and it was not possible to identify selectively sprouted synaptic terminals with the light microscope. Experiments are being conducted to resolve collateral sprouting with quantitative electrophysiological analyses and with electron microscopic studies (Proctor, Frenk, and Roper, *in progress*).

An important advantage of recording from individual neurons during sprouting is that a very accurate census can be taken of the change in inputs, both sub- and suprathreshold. Because of this, it was possible to detect functional signs of collateral sprouting in the cardiac ganglion within 1 day after the operation. The rapidity with which changes in the innervation begins gave rise to concern that preexisting, nonfunctional synapses might have become active after partial denervation and that collateral sprouting did not occur. Histological studies made this highly unlikely, however. That is, the number of intact boutons on each cell, measured with two different histological techniques (each of which stained synaptic boutons and vagal preterminals), remained constant at all times after partial denervation. Because both zinc iodide-osmium and methylene blue stained the entire vagal terminal, bouton counts made with either method would have included putative nonfunctional synaptic boutons, had they been present in any significant number. Thus, if there had been no collateral sprouting to replace the degenerating vagal inputs, one would have expected a decrease in the average number of boutons per cell body, contrary to the findings. Instead, these data indicate that as boutons degenerate, intact nerve terminals rapidly sprout, confirming our electrophysiological findings. The rapidity with which collateral sprouting occurs is plausible; Speidel (29) observed growing nerve terminals in the tadpole advancing at rates up to 40 μm per hr. This distance is about one cell diameter in the cardiac ganglion.

We still do not know what controls collateral sprouting and why the same number of synaptic endings is preserved after partial denervation. If the presence of a vacant postsynaptic site is one of the factors responsible for collateral sprouting, this might explain why the number of vagal boutons remains constant after partial denervation; when all the vacated sites are filled by sprouting terminals, the impetus to sprout disappears. Hence, the ganglion cell itself would in part control the proliferation of presynaptic endings. However, it is not known whether the number of postsynaptic sites remains fixed after denervation in the cardiac ganglion (although there is evidence for this in the rat superior cervical ganglion; 23) or how a vacant postsynaptic site could attract sprouting nerve terminals.

Barker and Ip (1) and Tuffery (31) have suggested that a continued renewal of synaptic connections occurs at the neuromuscular junction; Speidel (29) and Sotelo and Palay (28) have suggested a similar process in the central nervous system. In his classic studies, Speidel (29) had actually observed spontaneous withdrawal and advance of free nerve endings in the living tadpole. As we have suggested elsewhere (26), a continual turnover of synaptic endings could explain some of the results at the frog cardiac ganglion. Namely, the rate of reinnervation of ganglia by regenerating fibers after partial denervation would be determined by the rate of spontaneous degeneration or withdrawal of existing synapses. Until an existing terminal withdrew from its postsynaptic site(s), regenerating vagal axons could not form functional synapses, even though they may be in the vicinity of the cell body. When the existing bouton withdrew, right and left preganglionic endings could compete for the vacant site. Thus, reinnervation would be delayed by the slow rate of spontaneous turnover. If this hypothesis is correct, one should be able to calculate an approximate rate of synaptic ending turnover based upon the rate of reinnervation after partial denervation and to examine normal ganglia with the electron microscope with some idea of how many spontaneously degenerating or withdrawing terminals might be expected.

If it is true that there is a continual turnover of synapses, we should not be looking for a specific factor which initiates sprouting, but rather, we should be searching for factors which inhibit the formation of collateral extensions under normal conditions. Diamond and his colleagues have elaborated on Cajal's suggestions that axonal sprouting is normally prevented by the release of substances from the axon terminals themselves and which neutralize a sprouting factor, produced by the target cells (reviewed in ref. 7). Additionally, contact of a growing terminal with a vacant postsynaptic site might establish some form of "contact inhibition," thereby retarding further growth. This might be mediated by molecular interactions on the pre- and postsynaptic surfaces (e.g., "chemoaffinity," see refs. 12,30). Surface interactions at the postsynaptic membrane, surrounding glial cells or basement membrane, might stabilize the presynaptic growth cone.

Wiesel and Hubel (32) demonstrated that blinding one eye of a kitten at birth but not of adult cats led to substantial remodeling of synaptic connections in the visual cortex. One possible explanation is that cessation of patterned activity in maturing nerve connections from the blinded eye allowed inputs from the functional eye to sprout and take over all the postsynaptic sites of cortical cells. More recent investigations have shown the importance of patterned activity in the development and maintenance of functional synaptic contacts in the immature visual cortex (reviewed in ref. 2, see also Pettigrew, *this volume*). The results of the present studies may bear upon this problem insofar as it was shown that rather large changes in the activity in one vagus nerve (i.e., the cessation of propagated impulses) did not lead to sprouting of functional ganglionic synapses in the adult frog. It would be interesting to know if a similar result would be obtained upon immature vagal connections in the amphibian cardiac ganglion, and thus whether this preparation will be useful as a model for investigating the cellular basis of developing neuronal connections in the mammalian central nervous system. Certainly, with regard to the phenomenon of collateral sprouting, this appears to be the case.

Many important questions regarding collateral sprouting remain unsolved. Perhaps the most salient question is what is the significance of sprouting? Are the newly formed synapses useful, and do they restore function to the damaged tissue? The results from intracellular recording in the cardiac ganglion indicate that ganglionic transmission is restored, and experiments utilizing vagally mediated cardiac reflexes are underway to test this at a behavioral level. Furthermore, what factors regulate sprouting? The present study indicates that cessation of propagated impulses does not lead to a reorganization of functional synapses and does not mimic partial denervation. An intriguing possibility is that factors acting upon the central autonomic neurons, in addition to interactions between the peripheral fields of the preganglionic axons, are important, and currently our attention is being directed to the fate of the cell bodies of the vagal axons during partial denervation of the cardiac ganglion.

ACKNOWLEDGMENTS

We would like to acknowledge Dr. Ken Courtney's participation in many of the early experiments reported here. Also, we are deeply grateful for the criticisms and comments by our colleagues, Drs. Samy Frenk, William Proctor, and William Betz. We would also like to thank Ms. Betty Aguilar and Denise Ryan for their assistance in preparing this manuscript. The work has been supported over the past few years by grants from the Mallinckrodt Foundation, the Colorado Heart Association, NIH (No. RO1 NS11505) and BRSG Grant RR-05357 awarded by the Biomedical Research Support Grant Program, Division of Research Resources, NIH.

REFERENCES

1. Barker, D., and Ip, M. C. (1966): Sprouting and degeneration of mammalian motor axons in normal and de-afferented skeletal muscle. *Proc. Roy. Soc. B,* 163:538–554.

2. Blakemore, C. (1974): Development of functional connexions in the mammalian visual system. *Brit. Med. Bull.,* 30:152–157.
3. Brown, M. C., and Ironton, R. (1977): Motor neurone sprouting induced by prolonged tetrodotoxin block of nerve action potentials. *Nature,* 265:459–461.
4. Cangiano, A., and Fried, J. A. (1977): The production of denervation-like changes in rat muscle by colchicine, without interference with axonal transport or muscle activity. *J. Physiol.,* 265:63–84.
5. Courtney, K., and Roper, S. (1976): Sprouting of synapses after partial denervation of frog cardiac ganglion. *Nature,* 259:317–319.
6. Dennis, M. J., Harris, A. J., and Kuffler, S. W. (1971): Synaptic transmission and its duplication by focally applied acetylcholine in parasympathetic neurons in the heart of the frog. *Proc. Roy. Soc. Lond. B,* 177:509–539.
7. Diamond, J., Cooper, E., Turner, C., and Macintyre, L. (1976): Trophic regulation of nerve sprouting. *Science,* 193:371–377.
8. Edds, M. V., Jr. (1953): Collateral nerve regeneration. *Q. Rev. Biol.,* 28:260–276.
9. Guth, L., and Bernstein, J. J. (1961): Selectivity in the reestablishment of synapses in the superior cervical ganglion of the cat. *Exp. Neurol.,* 4:59–69.
10. Hunt, C. C., and Nelson, P. G. (1965): Structural and functional changes in the frog sympathetic ganglion following cutting of the presynaptic nerve fibres. *J. Physiol.,* 177:1–20.
11. Lavoie, P.-A., Collier, B., and Tenenhouse, A. (1976): Comparison of α-bungarotoxin binding to skeletal muscles after inactivity or denervation. *Nature,* 260:349–350.
12. Letourneau, P. C. (1975): Possible roles for cell-to-substratum adhesion in neuronal morphogenesis. *Develop. Biol.,* 44:77–91.
13. Liu, C.-N., and Chambers, W. W. (1958): Intraspinal sprouting of dorsal root axons. *Arch. Neurol. Psychiatr.,* 79:46–61.
14. Lømo, T., and Rosenthal, J. (1972): Control of ACh sensitivity by muscle activity in the rat. *J. Physiol.,* 221:493–513.
15. Lynch, G., Deadwyler, S., and Cotman, C. (1973): Post lesion axonal growth produces permanent functional connections. *Science,* 180:1364–1366.
16. Lynch, G., Matthews, D. A., Mosko, S., Parks, T., and Cotman, C. (1972): Induced acetylcholinesterase-rich layer in rat dentate gyrus following entorhinal lesions. *Brain Res.,* 42:311–318.
17. McMahan, U. J., and Kuffler, S. W. (1971): Visual identification of synaptic boutons on living ganglion cells and of varicosities in postganglionic axons in the heart of the frog. *Proc. Roy. Soc. B,* 177:485–508.
18. Murray, J. G., and Thompson, J. W. (1957): The occurrence and function of collateral sprouting in the sympathetic nervous system of the cat. *J. Physiol.,* 135:133–162.
19. Nakamura, Y., Mizuno, N., Konishi, A., and Sato, M. (1974): Synaptic reorganization of the red nucleus after chronic deafferentation from cerebellorubral fibers: an electron microscope study in the cat. *Brain Res.,* 82:298–301.
20. Pestronk, A., Drachman, D. B., and Griffin, J. W. (1976): Effect of muscle disuse on acetylcholine receptors. *Nature,* 260:352–353.
21. Raisman, G. (1969): Neuronal plasticity in the septal nuclei of the adult rat. *Brain Res.,* 14:25–48.
22. Raisman, G., and Field, P. M. (1973): A quantitative investigation of the development of collateral reinnervation after partial deafferentation of the septal nuclei. *Brain Res.,* 50:241–264.
23. Raisman, G., Field, P. M., Ostberg, A. J. C., Iversen, L. L., and Zigmond, R. E. (1974): A quantitative ultrastructural and biochemical analysis of the process of reinnervation of the superior cervical ganglion in the adult rat. *Brain Res.,* 71:1–16.
24. Robert, E. D., and Oester, Y. T. (1970): Absence of supersensitivity to acetylcholine in innervated muscle subjected to a prolonged pharmacologic nerve block. *J. Pharmacol. Exp. Ther.,* 174:133–140.
25. Roper, S. (1976*a*): An electrophysiological study of chemical and electrical synapses on neurones in the parasympathetic cardiac ganglion of the mudpuppy, *Necturus maculosus:* evidence for intrinsic ganglionic innervation. *J. Physiol.,* 254:427–454.
26. Roper, S. (1976*b*): Sprouting and regeneration of synaptic terminals in the frog cardiac ganglion. *Nature,* 261:148–149.
27. Sargent, P. B., and Dennis, M. J. (1977): Formation of synapses between parasympathetic neurones deprived of preganglionic innervation. *Nature,* 268:456–458.

28. Sotelo, C., and Palay, S. L. (1971): Altered axons and axon terminals in the lateral vestibular nucleus of the rat. *Lab. Invest.,* 25:653–671.
29. Speidel, C. C. (1941): Adjustments of nerve endings. *Harvey Lectures,* 36:126–158.
30. Sperry, R. W. (1963): Chemoaffinity in the orderly growth of nerve fiber patterns and connections. *Proc. Natl. Acad. Sci. U.S.A.,* 50:703–710.
31. Tuffery, A. R. (1971): Growth and degeneration of motor end-plates in normal cat hind limb muscles. *J. Anat.,* 110:221–247.
32. Wiesel, T. N., and Hubel, D. H. (1963): Single-cell responses in striate cortex of kittens deprived of vision in one eye. *J. Neurophysiol.,* 26:1003–1017.

Neuronal Plasticity, edited by
Carl W. Cotman.
Raven Press, New York © 1978.

Trophic Maintenance of Synaptic Connections in Autonomic Ganglia

Dale Purves and Arild Njå

Department of Physiology and Biophysics, Washington University School of Medicine, St. Louis, Missouri 63110

INTRODUCTION

The orderly arrangement of the adult nervous system raises important questions about the mechanisms responsible for the development and maintenance of precise synaptic connections. Apart from the problem of how neurons recognize each other, it is necessary to account for the formation of an appropriate *number* of contacts between pre- and postsynaptic cells. That quantitative regulation of synapses occurs is evident in the mature nervous system: individual neurons innervate a functionally correct number of target cells, each of which receives an adequate number of synaptic contacts. The way in which this numerical balance is established in development, and maintained throughout life, is a central issue in neurobiology. Our purpose in this Chapter is to review some experiments which bear on this question. Most of the work that we will discuss concerns changes of synaptic connections in mature sympathetic ganglia after interruption of the axonal connection between ganglion cells and their targets.

These experiments provide some evidence for trophic signals arising from peripheral targets that influence many properties of the innervating neurons, including the number of synapses contacting the neuronal surface. Before a detailed discussion of this work, we consider more briefly other experiments that suggest a similar trophic influence of targets on innervating neurons during normal development.

We have made no attempt to review the relevant literature in a comprehensive way; more complete accounts of some of these topics are found in reviews by Lieberman (62), Harris (37), Watson (100), Hamburger (34,35), Purves (75), Levi-Montalcini (52,53), and Hendry (40). Some topics we mention are also discussed more fully in other Chapters in this volume. We have confined ourselves to a consideration of higher vertebrates, since a number of findings suggest that the rules which regulate synaptic connections in invertebrates may be somewhat different.

THE FORMATION OF NEURAL CONNECTIONS DURING DEVELOPMENT

Although the rules which govern the establishment of synaptic connections in development are not understood, two phenomena which play an important role in this process are cell death and elimination of a portion of the synapses initially formed.

Neuronal Death in Embryonic Development

The occurrence of neuronal death in the course of normal development was first recognized in the early part of this century (31). Subsequent studies have shown that in many (perhaps most) regions of the developing vertebrate nervous system, more neurons are present in early embryonic life than in maturity. Thus a substantial portion (on the order of 25–75%) of the original neuronal population dies in early life (see refs. 20,21,34,35,44 and 72 for reviews). The experiments of Hamburger and others suggest that neuronal death is not predetermined for individual cells, but rather is the result of competition at the level of the target organ. If a limb bud of a chick embryo is amputated at 2½ days of incubation, the neurons in the lateral motor column of the corresponding segments of the spinal cord continue to proliferate, migrate, and differentiate in an apparently normal way. However, starting at about the time when innervation of the missing limb would normally occur (6–7 days), nearly the entire population of limb motor neurons degenerates within 3 days (33). In the usual course of development only about 40% of these cells degenerate (33–36). On the other hand, grafting a supernumerary limb onto the embryo, so that the target provided the thoracic motor neurons is abnormally large, results in a significant decrease in the number of neurons that die (43). A sharp increase in neuronal death when the normal target is missing has been confirmed in other motor systems (23), in the peripheral autonomic system (48,49; see also ref. 4), as well as for projections entirely within the central nervous system (22,24; see also refs. 20,21). In each case, degeneration occurs about the time of synapse formation with the target. These results suggest that developing neurons can live for a limited time on their own, but ultimately must make a sufficient number of synaptic contacts with an appropriate target to insure survival. This view is supported by recent electron microscopical studies of Landmesser and Pilar (50,71) which show that preganglionic autonomic neurons can degenerate in spite of having made at least some synapses. It is possible, however, that the survival of presynaptic neurons depends on an interaction with their target other than the formation of synapses.

An attractive explanation of these findings is that neurons compete for some property of the target cells, presumably a trophic agent, which is required for neuronal survival and which is available in limited supply (35). The acquisition of this agent might depend on the formation of a sufficient number of synapses by each innervating neuron. Whatever its mechanism, the occurrence of neuronal death in development appears to be a major way in which an initial balance between pre- and postsynaptic elements is achieved.

Synapse Elimination in Early Life

A second phenomenon which determines the organization of the synaptic connections found in maturity is the elimination of a portion of the synaptic contacts initially formed. This process has been most thoroughly studied in mammalian muscle in which each mature fast-twitch skeletal muscle fiber receives a single motor terminal. Redfern (78) first observed that stimulation of nerves to neonatal skeletal muscle fibers elicits complex synaptic potentials characteristic of multiple innervation. Multiple innervation of neonatal fibers has been confirmed by Bennett and Pettigrew (9,10) and Brown et al. (17). Using both anatomical and electrophysiological techniques, these workers demonstrated that several motor axons initially contact each endplate, but that during the first several weeks of postnatal life, the endings from all but one motor axon are withdrawn. It is unlikely that this involves cell death, since Brown et al. (17) have shown that synapse elimination occurs without a substantial reduction in the number of motor units or a decrease in the number of axons supplying the muscle studied. Moreover, normal cell death generally occurs early in embryonic life, coincident with the initial formation of synaptic contacts with the target (see however ref. 79).

A similar reorganization of initial synaptic connections has recently been shown to occur in developing mammalian autonomic ganglia (61). The neurons of the rat submandibular ganglion are dominated in maturity by innervation from a single preganglionic fiber. At birth, however, each cell is contacted by five fibers, on average, several of which may elicit an approximately equal synaptic response. As at the neuromuscular junction, the transition from multiple to generally single innervation occurs during the first month of postnatal life. A reduction in the number of presynaptic neurons innervating each postsynaptic cell is also suggested by anatomical and physiological observations of developing cerebellar Purkinje cells and spinal motor neurons (25,80). Thus it may be that synapse elimination, like cell death, is a general feature of neural ontogeny. If the purpose of normally occurring cell death is to reduce the population of innervating neurons to a number appropriate to the size of the target as a whole, the purpose of synapse elimination may be to extend the balance to the level of the individual cells involved.

The mechanism of synapse elimination in skeletal muscle and parasympathetic ganglia is not known. It is hard to imagine how the final result (one endplate, one motor axon; or, one ganglion cell, one dominant preganglionic axon) could be achieved other than through some form of competition. However, when Brown et al. (17) partially denervated neonatal muscles, they found that synapse elimination still occurred, albeit with a somewhat prolonged time course. This suggests that an intrinsic motor neuron mechanism also plays a role. Thus it may be that the final synaptic balance is, on the one hand, dictated by the number of terminals each innervating neuron can support, and on the other hand by a local competition that reduces the number of axons which contact individual target cells.

MAINTENANCE OF SYNAPTIC CONNECTIONS IN MATURITY

The sequence of events in synaptogenesis raises the question of whether the underlying mechanisms are lost in maturity or whether the initial balance of connections is actively maintained throughout life. Several observations suggest that the mechanisms are, at least in part, retained: (a) the organization of connections to nerve and muscle cells formed during reinnervation has many normal features; (b) compensatory sprouting of intact nerve terminals occurs after partial denervation of tissues; and (c) synapses are lost from neurons separated from their target by axotomy, but are recovered coincidentally with target reinnervation. Since reinnervation and sprouting are treated elsewhere in this volume (see Chapter 1, for example, we have focused on the effects of interrupting the connection between neurons and their target)

General Features of the Reaction to Axotomy

As a rule, nerve cell bodies in the higher vertebrate nervous system undergo complex anatomical and metabolic changes after axotomy. The major morphological features of the reaction are a breaking up of Nissl bodies with a consequent loss of cytoplasmic basophilia (chromatolysis), movement of the nucleus to an eccentric position within the cell body, and an increase in the irregularity of the cellular and nuclear outline. Ultrastructural changes following axotomy in rat sympathetic neurons have been described in detail by Matthews (63) and

Matthews and Raisman (65). Corresponding to the break-up of Nissl bodies is a disaggregation of rough endoplasmic reticulum; in addition, there is an increase in the cytoplasmic content of dense bodies and autophagic vacuoles, while the number of cytoplasmic dense-core vesicles decreases. Evidence of neuronal sprouting is also described.

In parallel with these morphological changes are profound alterations in neuronal metabolism. These have been most extensively studied by Watson in the hypoglossal nucleus of the rat (96–99). Shortly after axotomy, both the total and nucleolar RNA content of brainstem motor neurons increases, and there is a net shift of RNA from the nucleus to the cytoplasm. These changes appear to be in part a result of the injury itself, since if the transected hypoglossal nerve is implanted into the innervated sternomastoid muscle where it is unlikely to form any functional synaptic connections, similar fluctuations in RNA metabolism occur after a second nerve section (97). Watson, however, has also presented evidence that some of these changes may depend on the functional connection between neurons and their targets (98,99).

In neurons surviving axotomy, these anatomical and metabolic features are reversed over a period of several weeks. On the other hand, cell death often follows axon interruption. In the hypoglossal nucleus after section of the 12th cranial nerve, estimates of cell death range from 10 to 75%, although less degeneration may occur after nerve crush (84,94–96). In the superior cervical ganglion, about half the neurons are lost after crushing the major postganglionic nerves; after nerve ligation, most (perhaps all) neurons whose axons are effectively enclosed in the ligature die within several months (73; see also ref. 3). Neurons in immature animals are generally thought to be even more sensitive to the effects of axon interruption. For example, axotomy of superior cervical ganglion cells in newborn rats causes degeneration of most neurons (90%) after nerve section alone (41). Neurons ramifying entirely within the central nervous system may also degenerate after axotomy (see ref. 62).

Changes in Synaptic Transmission to Neurons Whose Axons Have Been Interrupted

Depression of synaptic transmission after axotomy was first observed by Acheson et al. (1) in recordings of the discharge of respiratory motor neurons whose axons had been cut (Fig. 1). The time course of this phenomenon was generally similar to the course of chromatolytic changes in motor neurons after axotomy, and appeared to be due to impaired synaptic function, as there was little change in the ability of the phrenic nerve to conduct action potentials. Since these initial experiments, impairment of transmission to injured neurons has emerged as a general feature of the reaction to axotomy. Depressed synaptic function follows axotomy of spinal motor neurons (28,29,47,66), parasympathetic neurons (14,15,70), and sympathetic neurons (2,3,16,64,73). It is unclear whether synaptic depression occurs after axotomy of neurons projecting entirely within the central

FIG. 1. Depression of respiratory discharge recorded from the proximal portion of the phrenic nerve after section close to the diaphragm 15 days previously. **A:** Discharge recorded from the normal phrenic nerve. **B:** Discharge from cut phrenic nerve. Calibration bars are 50μV, 1 sec. (From ref. 1.)

nervous system, primarily because of difficulties in performing and interpreting analogous experiments.

The accessibility of peripheral autonomic ganglia, and the relative ease of carrying out electrophysiological and anatomical studies on these preparations, has led to a detailed picture of the synaptic changes that follow axotomy. In the superior cervical ganglion, a marked decrease in the synaptic response to preganglionic stimulation occurs within 3 to 4 days of interrupting the postganglionic axons (73) (Fig. 2). The amplitude of the intracellularly recorded synaptic potential is maximally depressed 4 to 7 days after axotomy, and gradually recovers thereafter if prompt regeneration of the postganglionic axons is allowed (73; see also ref. 91). Similar decreases in the amplitude of intracellularly recorded synaptic potentials after axotomy have been observed in parasympathetic neurons (14,15) and spinal motoneurons (28,29,47,66).

Synaptic depression after axotomy might be due to a defect in any of the steps in chemical synaptic transmission. In mammals, several studies are in general agreement that axotomy is followed by a loss of synapses from the surface of the affected cells (12,26,32,64,73,89,92,94,95). This effect has been studied quantitatively in sympathetic ganglia, and in the hypoglossal nucleus, where, because of the relative uniformity of the neuronal population, counts of synapses per unit area can be taken as representative. In the superior cervical ganglion of both the rat and the guinea pig, the number of ganglionic synapses is reduced to about 30% of normal within several days of axotomy (64,73). Synapse counts in the hypoglossal nucleus after section of the 12th cranial nerve show a similar reduction (89,92). The number of vesicle-filled profiles per unit area of electron microscopical section from sympathetic ganglia after axotomy declines by nearly the same amount as the number of synapses (64,73), although the volume of sympathetic ganglia and the distribution of neurons remains normal during this time (up to 7 days after the initial injury) (69,73). Thus it appears that, in addition to the disjunction of most endings, the pregan-

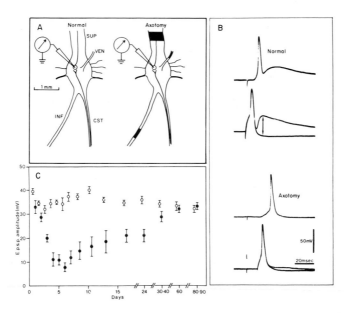

FIG. 2. Depression of synaptic transmission recorded intracellularly in guinea pig superior cervical ganglion cells after postganglionic axotomy. **A:** Diagram of control and experimental ganglia. The three major postganglionic nerves were crushed, thus allowing prompt regeneration. CST, cervical sympathetic trunk. SUP, superior postganglionic branch. VEN, ventral postganglionic branch. INF, inferior postganglionic branch. **B:** Intracellular recording from a normal neuron, and a neuron 6 days after axotomy. The response to supramaximal stimulation of the preganglionic nerve is shown in the *uppermost record* of each pair. After axotomy, the threshold is reached more slowly, and the depolarization that arises from maintained transmitter action following the action potential is reduced. A relative measure of the postsynaptic potential amplitude was obtained by causing transmitter release to occur during the refractory period of a preceding action potential (*lower traces* of each pair). The excitatory postsynaptic potential (e.p.s.p.) after axotomy is markedly reduced. **C:** Time course of the development of, and recovery from, synaptic depression after axotomy. *Filled circles* represent the mean ±SE of synaptic responses from 5 to 28 neurons in ganglia after postganglionic axotomy; *open circles* are responses measured in neurons from contralateral control ganglia. (After ref. 73.)

glionic terminals undergo some degree of involution. Whether this involves frank degeneration, or simply terminal retraction, is not known.

Considerable evidence suggests that abnormalities of transmission precede disjunction. In the superior cervical ganglion, each ganglion cell retains some degree of innervation, even in the period of maximal synaptic depression which follows axotomy. During this time, spontaneously occurring potentials (presumably corresponding to quantal release of acetylcholine at the remaining synapses) are reduced in amplitude (73; see also ref. 16). Transmission at residual synapses on spinal motor neurons after axotomy is also abnormal; based on the time course of evoked responses, Kuno and Llinás (47) have suggested that proximal contacts are lost preferentially during the axotomy reaction (see also ref. 92). In the hypoglossal nucleus, morphological evidence suggests that excitatory synapses are lost more readily than inhibitory ones (90). A more detailed study of transmission at intact synapses after axotomy has been made in the ciliary ganglion of the chick (14,15). In this ganglion, synapse loss is less apparent, perhaps because of the anatomy of the presynaptic terminals which make calici-form endings on the ganglion cells. The basis of postaxotomy synaptic depression in this preparation involves both hyposensitivity of the postsynaptic cell to acetyl-choline and a decrease in the ability of the presynaptic terminal to release the normal number of transmitter packets.

In addition to chromatolysis and synapse loss, electrophysiological and mor-phological changes are apparent in neurons after axotomy. In both spinal motor neurons and sympathetic ganglion cells, fast-rising depolarizations superimposed on subthreshold synaptic potentials are often observed within several days of axotomy; these are thought to represent action potentials in dendrites (29,46,73). In sympathetic neurons, injection of horseradish peroxidase shows numerous swellings along the course of dendrites; these may correspond to abnormal pro-files filled with tubular and vesicular organelles (including dense-core vesicles) which are seen in electron microscopical sections (69,73,74). Sprouting within sympathetic ganglia probably occurs after axotomy (65), and this process may take place in both axons and ganglion cell dendrites; the dendritic arborization of hypoglossal motor neurons has also been reported to contract (and eventually reexpand) after axotomy (93). The changes in the pattern of neuronal processes that occur after axotomy will probably remain uncertain until quantitative studies are undertaken with intracellular marking techniques.

Causes of Synapse Loss After Axotomy

The mechanism of synapse loss after axotomy is not fully known. In sympa-thetic ganglia, intact preganglionic terminals are sometimes seen separated from the postsynaptic element by a finger of satellite cell cytoplasm (64) (Fig. 3), a finding which has also been noted in brainstem nuclei after axotomy (12,94,95). This has led to the suggestion that glial cells play an active role in the process of synaptic detachment (64,94,95). Although some vacated postsynaptic thicken-

FIG. 3. Electron micrographs of the superior cervical ganglion of the adult rat, suggesting that detachment of synapses after axotomy is preceded by loss of membrane specializations for attachment in the postsynaptic element and that the final separation may be effected by the insinuation of a satellite cell process. Calibration bars are 0.5 µm. **A:** Synapse at which the presynaptic profile shows a band of dense material (*arrow*) applied to its membrane. No corresponding band is seen in the postsynaptic element. This is interpreted as representing a desmosome of which the postsynaptic half has disappeared, allowing the satellite cell to separate the pre- and postsynaptic profiles. Twenty-seven days after axotomy. **B:** Synapse partly attached (single arrow, left-hand side), partly detached *(two arrows, right-hand side);* a slender tongue of satellite cytoplasm intervenes. In the detached portion of the synapse there is a well defined presynaptic thickening, but there is no evidence of any vacated postsynaptic thickening in the corresponding zone of the postsynaptic dendrite (d). The attached region, however, still shows some dense material apposed to the postsynaptic membrane. Four days after axotomy. (From ref. 64.)

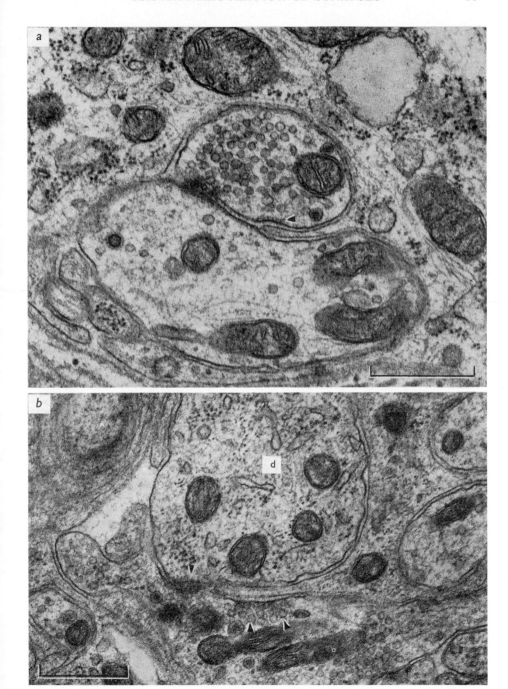

ings in dendrites of denervated superior cervical ganglion cells can be observed for at least several months after degeneration of the preganglionic fibers (77), thickenings unopposed by presynaptic elements are not seen after axotomy (64,73). The apparent lability of postsynaptic specializations after axotomy is consistent with physiological evidence showing that the postsynaptic cells become hyposensitive to neurotransmitter (15). Some morphological evidence using a labeled binding agent also suggests a decrease in postsynaptic receptors in the hypoglossal nucleus after cutting the 12th cranial nerve (81). Whether these receptor changes (or, more broadly, changes in the postsynaptic specialization) bear a causal relation to synapse loss is uncertain.

Although the immediate cause of synaptic disjunction is unclear, in a more general sense the loss of synaptic contacts probably stems from interrupting the injured neuron's connection with its target. This is most strongly suggested by the recovery of synaptic contacts on neurons coincident with the regeneration of postsynaptic axons and the reestablishment of functional peripheral connections (26,73,89,91,92). If postganglionic axons are delayed or prevented from reaching the periphery by ligation, synaptic contacts are not regained for at least 3 months, and most (perhaps all) of the neurons whose axons are ligated eventually die (73). A similar inhibition of synaptic recovery has been described in the hypoglossal nucleus after implantation of the cut nerve into an innervated muscle; in this case, however, cell death was not observed (91).

Because crushing or ligating axons disconnects the cell body from the bulk of the neuronal cytoplasm, amputation per se might be a major cause of synapse loss (and perhaps other postaxotomy effects). As noted, changes in RNA metabolism appear to derive in part from the nerve injury itself (97). Most of the functional and morphological effects of axotomy in autonomic ganglia, however, can be elicited in the absence of nerve injury by agents which block the fast component of axoplasmic transport. This was first demonstrated by Pilar and Landmesser (70); within a few days of local colchicine application to the postganglionic nerves, chromatolysis and depression of transmission through the avian ciliary ganglion occurred. In the mammalian superior cervical ganglion, local colchicine treatment of postganglionic nerves leads to most of the electrophysiological and ultrastructural changes associated with axotomy (74). Four to 7 days after briefly exposing one of the postganglionic nerves to a colchicine solution, intracellular recordings from neurons whose axons ran to the periphery in the treated nerve (but not nearby neurons whose axons ran in an untreated nerve) showed a marked reduction in the amplitude of evoked synaptic potentials (Fig. 4). Moreover, many affected neurons showed regenerative dendritic responses superimposed on subthreshold synaptic potentials. By antidromic stimulation distal to the region exposed to colchicine, the axons of affected cells were shown to be intact across the segment of nerve where the drug had been applied. Counts of synapses per unit area from the region of the ganglion containing the treated cells showed a reduction in the number of contacts, suggesting that loss of synapses is a major cause of synaptic depression following drug treatment (see Fig. 4). Light microscopy using the zinc iodide-osmium method

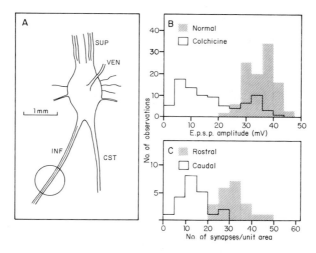

FIG. 4. Ability of local colchicine application to mimic the effects of postganglionic axotomy in the superior cervical ganglion of the guinea pig. **A:** A drop of saturated colchicine solution *(circle)* was applied to the inferior postganglionic nerve for 30 min; the drug was then washed away and the animal allowed to recover. **B:** Four to 7 days after this procedure postsynaptic potential amplitudes (measured as in Fig. 2B) in neurons whose axons ran in the treated nerve were reduced when compared with synaptic responses in neurons from the same ganglion whose axons ran in the untreated superior nerve. **C:** The neurons whose axons run in the inferior nerve are located in the lower half of the ganglion. Thus the number of synapses made on treated and untreated cells in the same ganglion could be examined by counting synapses per unit area in blocks from the rostral and caudal regions. Counts from the caudal region of treated ganglia were reduced when compared with the rostral region, indicating that synaptic depression is accompanied by a loss of synaptic contacts from the cells whose axons were exposed to colchicine. The area surveyed for each determination was 10 400-mesh grid squares. (After ref. 74.)

also suggests a decrease in synapses on hypoglossal motor neurons after chronic application of a colchicine- or vinblastine-impregnated cuff to the 12th cranial nerve (27).

The apparent dependence of synapses on the integrity of the recipient neuron's axoplasmic transport system suggests that maintenance of synaptic contacts depends on the removal of some material from the neuron by anterograde transport or the supply of something brought to the cell by retrograde transport. In the peripheral sympathetic system, recent evidence suggests that the retrograde transport of nerve growth factor (NGF) plays a part in the development and maintenance of synaptic contacts on ganglion cells.

INFLUENCE OF NERVE GROWTH FACTOR AND ITS ANTISERUM ON SYNAPTIC CONNECTIONS IN SYMPATHETIC GANGLIA

Nerve Growth Factor

Trophic interactions between neurons and their targets have been described in several regions of the nervous system, although the agents which mediate these effects are, for the most part, unknown (see refs. 34,35,37,75 for reviews). An exception is the protein NGF which appears to play a trophic role in the peripheral sympathetic system.

NGF was discovered in the course of investigating the growth-promoting effects of certain mouse sarcomas on sensory and sympathetic ganglia (19,51, 59,60). The persistance of this effect when the tumors were implanted on the chorioallantoic membrane of chick embryos showed that the agent was a humoral one. The subsequent (and fortuitous) discovery of large amounts of the protein in snake venom (18) led to an investigation of the submaxillary glands of adult male mice, currently the major source of NGF (58). The protein extracted from the mouse salivary gland has three different subunits, of which the β-subunit (equivalent to 2.5S NGF) is the biologically significant part. The β-subunit has two identical polypeptide chains each with a molecular weight of about 13,000 (see refs. 13,55 for reviews).

Although the potency of its effect on sympathetic (and dorsal root) ganglion cells has never been in doubt, the normal biological role of NGF has been controversial. Over the years, however, considerable evidence has accumulated to support the view that NGF mediates a retrograde trophic influence between sympathetic targets and the ganglion cells which innervate them: (a) neurite outgrowth from embryonic ganglion cells is promoted by NGF *in vitro* (55,60); (b) growth and survival of sympathetic ganglion cells are enhanced in newborn mice injected with NGF (41,56); (c) the majority of developing sympathetic neurons are destroyed by administration of NGF-antiserum (55,57); (d) exogenous NGF is specifically taken up by sympathetic nerves and retrogradely transported to ganglion cell bodies (86,88); (e) exogenous NGF counteracts some of the biochemical and morphological changes which follow axotomy in developing sympathetic ganglion cells (38,40); (f) sympathetic ganglion cells (but not dorsal root ganglion cells) continue to respond to NGF throughout life (6,7).

In spite of this evidence, lack of information about the source of endogenous NGF and the site of its interaction with sensitive neurons has argued for continued caution in accepting the proposition that NGF normally acts after peripheral uptake and retrograde transport. Although NGF (or a very similar molecule) can be synthesized by cultured mesenchymal cells (see, for example, ref. 101), it has not been shown unequivocally that it is produced by normal sympathetic targets. Moreover, the purpose of the demonstrable synthesis of NGF by the salivary gland in the mouse remains uncertain and may be related to endocrine functions which have little or nothing to do with nerve cells. The site of NGF's interaction with sensitive neurons is not completely understood. It appears that NGF affects sympathetic ganglion cells in two ways: by binding to receptors on the cell body surface (8,13,30,85) and by uptake into peripheral nerve terminals and retrograde axonal transport to the cell soma (42,85,86,88). The relative importance of these two routes of access is not clear. While accumulation of ^{125}I-NGF in ganglion cell bodies after intraocular or intravenous injection occurs largely by means of retrograde axonal transport (85,87) (Fig. 5), neurons also

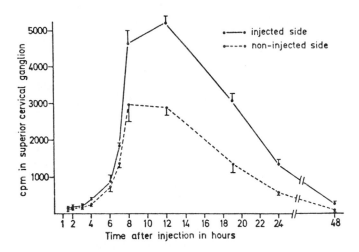

FIG. 5. Evidence for the retrograde transport of NGF. Time course of the accumulation of radioactivity in the superior cervical ganglion after unilateral injection of labeled NGF into the anterior eye chamber of rats weighing 150 to 200 g (9 µCi of ^{125}I-NGF were injected). Ganglia from the injected and noninjected sides were removed after 1.5 to 48 hr and counted in a γ-counter at an efficiency of 50%. Each point represents the mean ± SE of five to seven animals. The difference in counts between the two sides is interpreted to represent retrograde transport of labeled NGF to cell bodies in the superior cervical ganglion. (From ref. 87.)

respond to NGF after axotomy or destruction of adrenergic nerve terminals with 6-hydroxydopamine (5,38,54). Some aspects of the response to exogenous NGF are more pronounced after axotomy or 6-hydroxydopamine treatment, for instance the increase in ganglion volume, the proliferation of ganglion cell processes, and the increase in tyrosine hydroxylase activity (5,54). Thus it is possible that binding of NGF to cell bodies is enhanced after elimination of peripheral mechanisms (see ref. 53).

These uncertainties notwithstanding, the importance of NGF in the normal development of sympathetic and dorsal root ganglion cells is well supported. The finding that postganglionic axotomy, or antiserum treatment, causes degeneration of the vast majority of ganglion cells, as well as evidence for the specific uptake and retrograde transport of exogenous NGF, makes it attractive to suppose that normally occurring cell death in this system may result when sympathetic ganglion cells fail to compete successfully for endogenous NGF at the level of the target organ. Similarly, the effects of axotomy in adult sympathetic ganglion cells might reflect a continued dependence of mature neurons on NGF.

Effects of NGF on Synapses After Axotomy

Results suggesting that the maintenance of synaptic connections in mature sympathetic ganglia require the transport of some material to or from the neuronal periphery lead naturally to the question of whether impaired retrograde transport of NGF might be the basis of the synapse loss which follows axotomy. It is known that mature ganglion cells are responsive to NGF (6,7). Moreover, when the number of developing ganglion cells is reduced, the ganglionic content of choline acetyltransferase (an enzyme which reflects the development of preganglionic nerve terminals) fails to reach normal levels (11,39), and some preganglionic neurons undergo degeneration (4,45). The enzyme activity increases, however, if ganglia are supplied with exogeneous NGF after axotomy (39).

In order to test whether NGF plays a role in the maintenance of synaptic connections in mature sympathetic ganglia, we asked whether exogenous NGF could prevent the loss of ganglionic synapses which follows postganglionic axotomy (69,76). At the time of a crush injury to one of the major postganglionic nerves of the guinea pig superior cervical ganglion, we implanted a silicone rubber pellet impregnated with purified NGF (Fig. 6A). Since the pellets released NGF for at least a week, we could study whether the development of synaptic depression followed its usual course under these conditions. The outcome of this experiment is shown in Fig. 6B. Although some depression of transmission was observed, the synaptic responses recorded in most ganglion cells were of normal amplitude at a time (4–7 days after crush) when ganglionic transmission

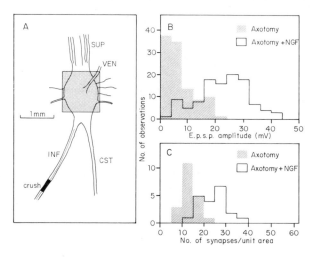

FIG. 6. Ability of exogenous nerve growth factor to prevent synapse loss when applied locally to guinea pig superior cervical ganglia after axotomy. **A:** NGF-containing pellets (100–500 μg of purified 2.5S mouse salivary gland NGF in silastic) were implanted near the ventral surface of ganglia at the time of inferior branch crush. The approximate size and location of the pellet is shown by the *stippled area*. **B:** Four to 7 days later, synaptic responses were measured in neurons antidromically driven from the crushed inferior branch (in NGF-treated and contralateral control ganglia which had undergone inferior branch) axotomy. The synaptic responses were generally larger in the NGF-treated ganglia. **C:** Synapse counts per unit area of electron microscopical sections from NGF-treated ganglia after axotomy compared with untreated ganglia after axotomy. All three major postganglionic branches were crushed; the unit area was 10 400-mesh grid squares. Fewer synapses were observed in the untreated ganglia, suggesting that exogenous NGF acts by preventing synapse loss. (After ref. 69.)

is markedly depressed after axotomy alone (see Fig. 2). In other animals, we determined morphologically whether the sparing effect of exogenous NGF was due to retention of ganglion cell synapses. Counts of synapses in NGF-treated ganglia after axotomy showed that more synaptic profiles were present than in similarly operated ganglia treated with a silicone rubber pellet which did not contain NGF (Fig. 6C). Thus, a major cause of NGF's remedial effect is the maintenance of synapses usually lost after axotomy. NGF also prevented (fully or in part) other effects of axotomy such as the dispersion of rough endoplasmic reticulum (chromatolysis), the appearance of abnormal neuronal processes filled with tubular and vesicular organelles, and the occurrence of regenerative dendritic responses.

The ability of NGF to prevent most of the synaptic changes which normally follow axotomy in adult animals might be due to a direct effect of the protein on preganglionic endings. While a primary preganglionic effect is difficult to rule out, the recent experiments of Schwab and Thoenen (82,83) argue against this possibility. They found that retrogradely transported tetanus toxin labeled with ^{125}I appeared in presynaptic terminals contacting both motor neurons and sympathetic ganglion cells. When the experiment was repeated with NGF, however, label was evident in ganglion cell bodies, but not in the preganglionic endings. Consistent with these results is our finding that NGF pellets applied to *normal* superior cervical ganglia had little or no effect on synaptic transmission measured intracellularly or on the prevalence of ganglionic synapses (69).

Effects of NGF-Antiserum on Synapses in Normal Sympathetic Ganglia

If the reaction to axotomy in sympathetic ganglia is due to a relative deficiency of NGF reaching affected cell bodies by retrograde transport, then one might expect treatment of adult animals with NGF-antiserum to cause depression of transmission and loss of synapses. To examine this possibility, we injected a series of guinea pigs ranging in age from a few days to sexual maturity with antiserum to purified mouse salivary gland NGF raised in rabbits (69). One week after the end of a 5-day course of antiserum, the superior cervical ganglia were removed and studied electrophysiologically and with the electron microscope. A series of control animals received injections of normal rabbit serum. The synaptic responses recorded in ganglion cells from animals treated with antiserum were smaller than those in control animals (Fig. 7A), although the average input resistance and resting potential were similar for the two groups. Counts of synapses in thin sections from antiserum-treated ganglia confirmed that many synapses had been lost: the mean number of synaptic contacts in treated ganglia was only about half that in the control ganglia (Fig. 7B). Counts of neurons per unit area showed that synapse loss occurred in the absence of significant neuronal degeneration. Although other interpretations are possible (69), the results of these experiments suggest that the synaptic contacts made on adult sympathetic neurons depend, in some say, on NGF. It seems likely

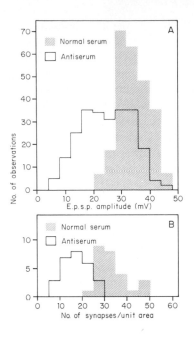

FIG. 7. Effect of NGF antiserum on synapses in the superior cervical ganglion of the guinea pig. **A:** Five to 8 days after the end of a 5-day course of rabbit antiserum (0.3–0.5 ml/g body wt/day; titre 1,000–3,000), synaptic responses were reduced compared to postsynaptic potentials elicited in neurons from control animals which received a similar course of normal rabbit serum. **B:** Synapse counts per unit area of electron microscopical sections were also reduced in ganglia from antiserum-treated animals, suggesting that endogenous NGF is required for the maintenance of ganglionic synapses. (After ref. 69.)

that this dependency is similar in its mechanism to the NGF dependence of preganglionic endings in development (11,39).

An attractive explanation of these results, as well as the experiments on cell death and synapse elimination described earlier, is that target cells, whether neuronal or not, provide specific trophic factors to the nerve cells which innervate them. Such factors would serve to maintain presynaptic contacts, and would ultimately be required for the survival of the presynaptic cells. In this view, NGF might produce its effects on ganglionic synapses by controlling the production or secretion of the analogous agent on which preganglionic fibers depend.

CONCLUSION

The establishment and maintenance of precise neural connections requires highly efficient regulatory mechanisms. Although the way in which neurons locate and recognize one another remains obscure, some aspects of the way a numerical balance between pre- and postsynaptic elements is achieved are understood. Initially, overproduction of neurons followed by cell death appears to provide a rough matching between the size of a target and the size of the neuronal population which is to innervate it. Cell death probably occurs because the original population of neurons competes for some property of the target which is in limited supply. In the peripheral sympathetic nervous system, nerve growth factor is essential for ganglion cell survival, and could be the object of competition. In addition to cell death, elimination of a portion of the synapses initially formed may be a more subtle means of achieving an appropriate numerical balance. The underlying mechanism is not known, but some form of local competition is probably required to explain the mature synaptic pattern in skeletal muscle and parasympathetic ganglia where each cell is innervated exclusively, or predominantly, by a single axon. An economical view would be that the basis for this competition is similar to that during competition for survival. A related question, largely unexplored, is whether the ability of nerve cells to compete for trophic factors is influenced by neuronal activity.

Since reinnervation of autonomic neurones in mature mammals establishes the original connections in a rather precise way (see, for example, refs. 67,68), it seems likely that, at least to some extent, the mechanisms present in development persist throughout life. The phenomena of sprouting after partial denervation and the reversible loss of synapses which occurs after axotomy also suggest that the initial synaptic balance is actively maintained. If the target presented to a neuron is increased, then that cell is stimulated to make additional synaptic connections. Conversely, if a neuron is cut off from its target, the number of synapses made on that nerve cell is reduced. The role of NGF in the sympathetic nervous system provides some basis for thinking that synaptic balance throughout life depends on trophic factors associated with (perhaps secreted by) the target cells.

REFERENCES

1. Acheson, G. H., Lee, E. S., and Morison, R. S. (1942): A deficiency in the phrenic respiratory discharges parallel to retrograde degeneration. *J. Neurophysiol.*, 5:269–273.
2. Acheson, G. H., and Remolina, J. (1955): The temporal course of the effects of postganglionic axotomy on the inferior mesenteric ganglion of the cat. *J. Physiol. (Lond)*, 127:603–616.
3. Acheson, G. H., and Schwarzacher, H. G. (1956): Correlations between the physiological changes and the morphological changes resulting from axotomy in the inferior mesenteric ganglion of the cat. *J. Comp. Neurol.*, 106:247–265.
4. Aguayo, A. J., Peyronnard, J. M., Terry, L. C. Romine, J. S., and Bray, G. M. (1976): Neonatal neuronal loss in rat cervical ganglia: retrograde effects on developing preganglionic axons and Schwann cells. *J. Neurocytol.*, 5:137–155.
5. Aloe, L., Mugnaini, E., and Levi-Montalcini, R. (1975): Light and electron microscopic studies on the excessive growth of sympathetic ganglia in rats injected daily from birth with 6-OHDA and NGF. *Arch. Ital. Biol.*, 113:326–353.
6. Angeletti, P. U., Levi-Montalcini, R., and Caramia, F. (1971): Ultrastructural changes in sympathetic neurons of newborn and adult mice treated with nerve growth factor. *J. Ultrastruct. Res.*, 36:24–36.
7. Angeletti, P. U., Levi-Montalcini, R., and Caramia, F. (1971): Analysis of the effects of the antiserum to the nerve growth factor in adult mice. *Brain Res.*, 27:343–355.
8. Banerjee, S. P., Synder, S. H., Cuatrecasas, P., and Greene, L. A. (1973): Binding of nerve growth factor in sympathetic ganglia. *Proc. Natl. Acad. Sci. USA*, 70:2519–2523.
9. Bennett, M. R., and Pettigrew, A. J. (1974): The formation of synapses in striated muscle during development. *J. Physiol. (Lond)*, 241:515–545.
10. Bennett, M. R., and Pettigrew, A. G. (1976): The formation of neuromuscular synapses. *Cold Spring Harbor Symposia on Quantitative Biology*, 40:409–424.
11. Black, I. B., Hendry, I. A., and Iversen, L. (1972): The role of post-synaptic neurones in the biochemical maturation of presynaptic cholinergic nerve terminals in a mouse sympathetic ganglion. *J. Physiol. (Lond)*, 221:149–159.

12. Blinzinger, K., and Kreutzberg, G. (1968): Displacement of synaptic terminals from regenerating motoneurons by microglial cells. *Z. Zellforsch. Mikrosk. Anat.,* 85:145–157.
13. Boyd, L. F., Bradshaw, R. A., Frazier, W. A., Hogue-Angeletti, R. A., Jeng, I., Pulliam, M. W., and Szutowicz, A. (1974): Nerve growth factor. *Life Sci.,* 15:1381–1391.
14. Brenner, H. R., and Johnson, E. W. (1976): Physiological and morphological effects of postganglionic axotomy on presynaptic nerve terminals. *J. Physiol. (Lond),* 26:143–158.
15. Brenner, H. R., and Martin, A. R. (1976): Reduction in acetylcholine sensitivity of axotomized ciliary ganglion cells. *J. Physiol. (Lond),* 260:159–175.
16. Brown, G. L., and Pascoe, J. E. (1954): The effect of degenerative section of ganglionic axons on transmission through the ganglion. *J. Physiol. (Lond),* 123:565–573.
17. Brown, M. C., Jansen, J. K. S., and Van Essen, D. (1976): Polyneuronal innervation of skeletal muscle in newborn rats and its elimination during maturation. *J. Physiol. (Lond),* 216:387–422.
18. Cohen, S., and Levi-Montalcini, R. (1956): A nerve growth stimulating factor isolated from snake venom. *Proc. Natl. Acad. Sci. USA,* 42:571–574.
19. Cohen, S., Levi-Montalcini, R., and Hamburger, V. (1954): A nerve growth stimulating factor isolated from sarcomas 37 and 180. *Proc. Natl. Acad. Sci. USA,* 40:1014–1018.
20. Cowan, W. M. (1970): Anterograde and retrograde transneuronal degeneration in the central and peripheral nervous system. In: *Contemporary Research Methods in Neuroanatomy,* edited by S. O. E. Ebbesson and W. J. H. Nauta, pp. 217–251. Springer-Verlag, New York.
21. Cowan, W. M. (1973): Neuronal death as a regulative mechanism in the control of cell number in the nervous system. In: *Development and Aging in the Nervous System,* edited by M. Rockstein and M. L. Sussman, pp. 19–41. Academic Press, New York.
22. Cowan, W. M., and Clarke, P. G. H. (1976): The development of the isthmo-optic nucleus. *Brain Behav. Evol.,* 13:345–375.
23. Cowan, W. M., and Wenger, E. (1967): Cell loss in the trochlear nucleus of the chick during normal development and after radical extirpation of the optic vesicle. *J. Exp. Zool.,* 164:267–278.
24. Cowan, W. M., and Wenger, E. (1968): The development of the nucleus of origin of centrifugal fibers to the retina in the chick. *J. Comp. Neurol.,* 133:207–239.
25. Crepel, F., Mariani, J., and Delhaye-Bouchaud, N. (1976): Evidence for a multiple innervation of Purkinje-cells by climbing fibers in the immature rat cerebellum. *J. Neurobiol.,* 7:567–578.
26. Cull, R. E. (1974): Role of nerve-muscle contact in maintaining synaptic connections. *Exp. Brain. Res.,* 20:307–316.
27. Cull, R. E. (1975): Role of axonal transport in maintaining central synaptic connections. *Exp. Brain Res.,* 24:97–101.
28. Dowman, C. B. B., Eccles, J. C., and McIntyre, A. K. (1953): Functional changes in chromatolysed motoneurones. *J. Comp. Neurol.,* 98:9–36.
29. Eccles, J. C., Libet, B., and Young, R. R. (1958): The behaviour of chromatolysed motoneurones studied by intracellular recording. *J. Physiol. (Lond),* 143:11–40.
30. Frazier, W. A., Boyd, L. F., and Bradshaw, R. A. (1973): Interaction of nerve growth factor with surface membranes: biological competence of insolubilized nerve growth factor. *Proc. Natl. Acad. Sci. USA,* 70:2931–2935.
31. Glücksman, A. (1951): Cell deaths in vertebrate ontogeny. *Biol. Rev.,* 26:59–86.
32. Hamberger, A., Hansson, H-A., and Sjöstrand, J. (1970): Surface structure of isolated neurons. Detachment of nerve terminals during axon regeneration. *J. Cell Biol.,* 47:319–331.
33. Hamburger, V. (1958): Regression versus peripheral control of differentiation in motor hypoplasia. *Am. J. Anat.,* 102:365–410.
34. Hamburger, V. (1975): Changing concepts in developmental neurobiology. *Perspectives in Biol. and Med.,* 18:162–178.
35. Hamburger, V. (1977): The developmental history of the motor neuron. The F. O. Schmitt lecture in neuroscience 1976. *Neurosci. Res. Prog. Bull.,* 15:Suppl. 1–37.
36. Hamburger, V., and Levi-Montalcini, R. (1949): Proliferation, differentiation and degeneration in the spinal ganglia of the chick embryo under normal and experimental conditions. *J. Exp. Zool.,* 111:457–501.
37. Harris, A. J. (1974): Inductive functions of the nervous system. *Ann. Rev. Physiol.,* 36:251–305.

38. Hendry, I. A. (1975*a*): The response of adrenergic neurones to axotomy and nerve growth factor. *Brain Res.,* 94:87–97.
39. Hendry, I. A. (1975*b*): The retrograde trans-synaptic control of the development of cholinergic terminals in sympathetic ganglia. *Brain Res.,* 86:483–487.
40. Hendry, I. A. (1976): Control in the development of the vertebrate sympathetic nervous system. In: *Reviews of Neuroscience, Vol. 2,* edited by S. Ehrenpreis and I. J. Kopin, pp. 149–194. Raven Press, New York.
41. Hendry, I. A., and Campbell, J. (1976): Morphometric analysis of the rat superior cervical ganglion after axotomy and nerve growth factor treatment. *J. Neurocytol.,* 5:351–360.
42. Hendry, I. A., Stöckel, K., Thoenen, H., and Iversen, L. L. (1974): The retrograde axonal transport of nerve growth factor. *Brain Res.,* 68:103–121.
43. Hollyday, M., and Hamburger, V. (1976): Reduction of the naturally occurring motor neuron loss by enlargement of the periphery. *J. Comp. Neurol.,* 170:311–320.
44. Hughes, A. F. W. (1968): *Aspects of Neural Ontogeny.* Academic Press, London.
45. Johnson, E., Caserta, M. T., and Ross, L. L. (1977): Effect of destruction of the post-ganglionic sympathetic neurons in neonatal rats on development of choline-acetyltransferase and survival of preganglionic cholinergic neurons. *Brain Res.,* 136:455–464.
46. Kuno, M., and Llinás, R. (1970): Enhancement of synaptic transmission by dendritic potentials in chromatolysed motoneurones of the cat. *J. Physiol.(Lond),* 210:807–821.
47. Kuno, M., and Llinás, R. (1970): Alterations of synaptic action in chromatolysed motoneurones of the cat. *J. Physiol. (Lond),* 210:823–838.
48. Landmesser, L., and Pilar, G. (1974): Synaptic transmission and cell death during normal ganglionic development. *J. Physiol. (Lond),* 241:737–749.
49. Landmesser, L., and Pilar, G. (1974): Synapse formation during embryogenesis on ganglion cells lacking a periphery. *J. Physiol. (Lond),* 241:715–736.
50. Landmesser, L., and Pilar, G. (1976): Fate of ganglionic synapses and ganglion cell axons during normal and induced cell death. *J. Cell. Biol.,* 68:357–374.
51. Levi-Montalcini, R. (1952): Effects of mouse tumor transplantation on the nervous system. *Ann. N.Y. Acad. Sci.,* 55:330–343.
52. Levi-Montalcini, R. (1975): Regulatory processes in the sympathetic adrenergic neuron. In: *Golgi Centennial Symposium Proceedings,* edited by M. Santini, pp. 437–448. Raven, New York.
53. Levi-Montalcini, R. (1976): The nerve growth factor: its widening role and place in neurobiology. *Adv. Biochem. Psychopharmacol,* 15:237–250.
54. Levi-Montalcini, R., Aloe, L., Mugnaini, E., Oesch, F., and Thoenen, H. (1975): Nerve growth factor induces volume increase and enhances tyrosine hydroxylase synthesis in chemically axotomized sympathetic ganglia of newborn rats. *Proc. Natl. Acad. Sci. USA,* 72:595–599.
55. Levi-Montalcini, R., and Angeletti, P. U. (1968): Nerve growth factor. *Physiol. Rev.,* 48:534–569.
56. Levi-Montalcini, R., and Booker, B. (1960): Excessive growth of the sympathetic ganglia evoked by a protein isolated from mouse salivary glands. *Proc. Natl. Acad. Sci. USA,* 46:373–384.
57. Levi-Montalcini, R., and Booker, B. (1960): Destruction of the sympathetic ganglia in mammals by an antiserum to a nerve-growth protein. *Proc. Natl. Acad. Sci. USA,* 46:384–391.
58. Levi-Montalcini, R., and Cohen, S. (1960): Effects of the extract of the mouse submaxillary glands on the sympathetic system of mammals. *Ann. N.Y. Acad. Sci.,* 85:324–341.
59. Levi-Montalcini, R., and Hamburger, V. (1951): Selective growth stimulating effects of mouse sarcoma on the sensory and sympathetic nervous system of the chick embryo. *J. Exp. Zool.,* 116:321–363.
60. Levi-Montalcini, M., Meyer, H., and Hamburger, V. (1954): In vitro experiments on the effects of mouse sarcomas 180 and 37 on the spinal and sympathetic ganglia of the chick embryo. *Cancer. Res.,* 14:49–57.
61. Lichtman, J. W. (1977): The reorganization of synaptic connexions in the rat submandibular ganglion during postnatal development. *J. Physiol (Lond),* 273:155–177.
62. Lieberman, A. R. (1971): The axon reaction: a review of the principal features of perikaryal responses to axon injury. *Int. Rev. Neurobiol.* 14:49–124.
63. Matthews, M. R. (1973): An ultrastructural study of axonal changes following constriction of postganglionic branches of the superior cervical ganglion in the rat. *Phil. Trans. Roy. Soc. B.,* 264:479–505.

64. Matthews, M. R., and Nelson, V. (1975): Detachment of structurally intact nerve endings from chromatolytic neurones of the rat superior cervical ganglion during depression of synaptic transmission induced by post-ganglionic axotomy. *J. Physiol. (Lond),* 245:91–135.
65. Matthews, M. R., and Raisman, G. (1972): A light and electron microscopic study of the cellular response to axonal injury in the superior cervical ganglion of the rat. *Proc. Roy. Soc. B.,* 181:43–79.
66. Mendell, L., Munson, J., and Scott, J. (1976): Alterations of synapses on axotomized motoneurones. *J. Physiol. (Lond),* 255:67–79.
67. Njå, A., and Purves (1977): Specific innervation of guinea-pig superior cervical ganglion cells by preganglionic fibres arising from different levels of the spinal cord. *J. Physiol. (Lond),* 264:565–583.
68. Njå, and Purves, D. (1977): Re-innervation of guinea-pig superior cervical ganglion cells by preganglionic fibres arising from different levels of the spinal cord. *J. Physiol. (Lond),* 272:633–651.
69. Njå, A., and Purves, D. (1978): The effects of nerve growth factor and its antiserum on synapses in the superior cervical ganglion of the guinea-pig. *J. Physiol. (Lond).* (in press).
70. Pilar, G., and Landmesser, L. (1972): Axotomy mimicked by localized colchicine application. *Science,* 177:1116–1118.
71. Pilar, G., and Landmesser, L. (1976): Ultrastructural differences during embryonic cell death in normal and peripherally deprived ganglia. *J. Cell Biol.,* 68:339–356.
72. Prestige, M. C. (1974): Axon and cell numbers in the developing nervous system. *Br. Med. Bull.,* 30:107–111.
73. Purves, D. (1975): Functional and structural changes of mammalian sympathetic neurones following interruption of their axons. *J. Physiol. (Lond),* 252:429–463.
74. Purves, D. (1976): Functional and structural changes in mammalian sympathetic neurones following colchicine application to post-ganglionic nerves. *J. Physiol. (Lond),* 259:159–175.
75. Purves, D. (1976): Long-term regulation in the vertebrate peripheral nervous system. In: *International Review of Physiology, Neurophysiology II, Vol. 10.,* edited by R. Porter, pp. 125–177. University Park Press, Baltimore.
76. Purves, D., and Njå, A. (1976): Effect of nerve growth factor on synaptic depression following axotomy. *Nature,* 260:535–536.
77. Raisman, G., Field, P. M., Ostberg, A. J. C., Iversen, L. L., and Zigmond, R. E. (1974): A quantitative and biochemical analysis of the process of re-innervation of the cervical ganglion in the rat. *Brain Res.,* 71:1–16.
78. Redfern, P. A. (1970): Neuromuscular transmission in new-born rats. *J. Physiol. (Lond),* 209:701–709.
79. Romanes, G. S. (1946): Motor localization and the effects of nerve injury on ventral horn cells in the spinal cord. *J. Anat.,* 80:177–181.
80. Ronnevi, L., and Conradi, S. (1974): Ultrastructural evidence for spontaneous elimination of synaptic terminals on spinal motor neurons in the kitten. *Brain Res.,* 80:335–339.
81. Rotter, A., Birdsall, N. J. M., Burgen, A. S. V., Field, P. M., and Raisman, G. (1977): Axotomy causes loss of muscarinic receptors and loss of synaptic contacts in the hypoglossal nucleus. *Nature,* 266:734–735.
82. Schwab, M. E., and Thoenen, H. (1976): Electron microscopic evidence for a transynaptic migration of tetanus toxin in spinal cord motoneurons: an autoradiographic and morphometric study. *Brain Res.,* 105:213–227.
83. Schwab, M., and Thoenen, H. (1977): Selective transynaptic migration of tetanus toxin after retrograde axonal transport in peripheral sympathetic nerves: A comparison with nerve growth factor. *Brain Res.,* 122:459–474.
84. Sjöstrand, J. (1971): Neuroglial proliferation in the hypoglossal nucleus after nerve injury. *Exp. Neurol.,* 30:178–189.
85. Stöeckel, K., Guroff, G., Schwab, M., and Thoenen, H. (1976): The significance of retrograde axonal transport for the accumulation of systemically administered nerve growth factor (NGF) in the rat superior cervical ganglion. *Brain Res.,* 109:271–284.
86. Stöeckel, K., Paravicini, U., and Thoenen, H. (1974): Specificity of the retrograde axonal transport of nerve growth factor. *Brain Res.,* 76:413–421.
87. Stöeckel, K., Schwab, M., and Thoenen, H. (1975): Comparison between the retrograde axonal transport of nerve growth factor and tetanus toxin in motor, sensory, and adrenergic neurons. *Brain Res.,* 99:1–16.

88. Stöeckel, K., and Thoenen, H. (1975): Retrograde axonal transport of nerve growth factor: specificity and biological importance. *Brain Res.,* 85:337–341.
89. Sumner, B. E. H. (1975): A quantitative analysis of the response of presynaptic boutons to postsynaptic motor neuron axotomy. *Exp. Neurol.,* 46:605–615.
90. Sumner, B. E. H. (1975): A quantitative analysis of boutons with different types of synapse in normal and injured hypoglossal nuclei. *Exp. Neurol.,* 49:406–417.
91. Sumner, B. E. H. (1976): Quantitative ultrastructural observations on the inhibited recovery of the hypoglossal nucleus from the axotomy response when regeneration of the hypoglossal nerve is prevented. *Exp. Brain Res.,* 26:141–150.
92. Sumner, B. E. H., and Sutherland, F. I. (1973): Quantitative electron microscopy on the injured hypoglossal nucleus in the rat. *J. Neurocytol.,* 2:315–328.
93. Sumner, B. E. H., and Watson, W. E. (1971): Retraction and expansion of the dendritic tree of motor neurones of adult rats induced *in vivo. Nature,* 233:273–275.
94. Torvik, A., and Skjörten, F. (1971): Electron microscopic observations on nerve cell regeneration and degeneration after axon lesions. I. Changes in the nerve cell cytoplasm. *Acta Neuropathol.,* 17:248–264.
95. Torvik, A., and Skjörten, F. (1971): Electron microscopic observations on nerve cell regeneration and degeneration after axon lesions. II. Changes in the glial cells. *Acta Neuropathol.,* 17:265–282.
96. Watson, W. E. (1965): An autoradiographic study of the incorporation of nucleic-acid precursors by neurones and glia during nerve regeneration. *J. Physiol. (Lond),* 18:741–753.
97. Watson, W. E. (1968): Observations on the nucleolar and total cell body nucleic acid of injured nerve cells. *J. Physiol. (Lond),* 196:655–676.
98. Watson, W. E. (1969): The response of motor neurones to intramuscular injection of botulinum toxin. *J. Physiol. (Lond),* 202:611–630.
99. Watson, W. E. (1970): Some metabolic responses of axotomized neurones to contact between their axons and denervated muscle. *J. Physiol. (Lond),* 210:321–343.
100. Watson, W. E. (1974): Cellular responses to axotomy and to related procedures *Br. Med. Bull.,* 30:112–115.
101. Young, M., Oger, J., Blanchard, M. H., Asdourian, H., Amos, H., and Arnason, B. G. W. (1975): Secretion of a nerve growth factor by primary chick fibroblast cultures. *Science,* 187:361–363.

Neuronal Plasticity, edited by
Carl W. Cotman.
Raven Press, New York © 1978.

Spinal Cord Regeneration: Synaptic Renewal and Neurochemistry

Jerald J. Bernstein, Michael R. Wells, and Mary E. Bernstein

Departments of Neuroscience and Opthalmology, University of Florida College of Medicine, Gainesville, Florida 32601

The regenerative capacity of the spinal cord of mammals is extremely limited (54). This phenomenon appears to be due, in part, to the problem of obtaining a central source of axons for growth across the site of lesion (49,50). At first sight there would appear to be two available sources of centrally derived axons: the long spinal tracts which have been severed or the intrinsic interneuronal pools within the spinal cord proper. However, recent experiments have shown that the partial denervation of a neuron can induce the remaining afferent axons to sprout (11,28,40,41,45,52,53). These nerve fibers may provide an additional source of central nervous system axons. Since long tracts in adult mammals do not tend to regenerate after central axotomy, a variety of studies have been carried out to chemically induce growth of the severed axons.

Besides the problem of a source of nerve fibers for regeneration, the factors most significant in regeneration and functional recovery of the injured spinal cord must be established. Is age a dependent factor in regenerative capacity? Do all the long tracts have to regenerate in order to restore function? Is the restoration of function dependent upon reestablishment of the original connectivity? Is the neuroglial scar a barrier to successful axonal regeneration as has been postulated in the mammalian spinal cord? Are there specific neurochemical events essential for the regenerative process? If centrally derived axons could be induced, would the microenvironment of the cicatrix or scar at the lesion site be compatable with sustained maintenance of the regenerated nerve fibers? These problems will be explored in the following chapter utilizing mammalian spinal cord and a lower vertebrate animal model in which the spinal cord does regenerate.

SPINAL CORD REGENERATION IN THE FISH

Following transection of the spinal cord of the fish, the severed axons of the long tracts regenerate, and function is returned with the fish appearing to swim normally. This is a model for successful regeneration of the spinal cord. The return of function (normal swimming) is age dependent. The younger the fish, the more rapid the return of swimming. One-year-old goldfish swam normally 20 to 25 days after spinal cord transection whereas 2- and 3-year-old fish had a return of swimming at 25 to 30 and 35 to 40 days after operation, respectively (2). Although goldfish of all ages swim normally at the time of spinal cord transection, the ability to regenerate axons across the site of lesion decreased dramatically with age. One-year-old fish regenerated 90% of the available nerve fibers across the site of lesion whereas 2- and 3-year-old animals regenerated only 50% of the available nerve fibers across the site of injury. Although 90% of the available nerve fibers from the rostral spinal cord stump crossed the site of lesion, many of these nerve fibers appeared to terminate in the first segment distal to the transection (5). This fact has been verified by studying the spinal cord 2 cm distal to a spinal cord transection in the same goldfish. Using 1-year-old goldfish, spinal cord transection resulted in the restitution of 35 to 49% of the expected number of nerve fibers in a segment 2 cm from the site of lesion in the descending tectospinal, cerebellospinal and ventral tracts (9). Interestingly, 94% of the regenerated nerve fibers were approximately 4 to 8 times the fiber diameter usually found in these tracts. Retransection of the spinal cord resulted in the degeneration of these large nerve fibers and paralysis. However, the remaining 6% of the nerve fibers were of small diameter and did not degenerate upon spinal cord retransection. This indicates that these small diameter nerve fibers did not cross the original site of transection and most probably represented axonal sprouts that had grown into the degenerating and then regenerating long tracts (9).

The neuroglial scar has been blamed for the lack of regeneration of spinal cord axons in the mammalian spinal cord. This hypothesis can be tested in the spinal cord of the goldfish where the neuroglial scar forms simultaneously with the arrival of the axons growing from higher centers and, thus, is not a problem in regeneration. Perhaps the most convincing argument about the efficacy of the scar as a mechanism for abortive growth comes from a series of experiments in which the goldfish spinal cord was transected and blocked with a sheet of teflon (4,5). The presence of the teflon at the site of transection resulted in a lack of regeneration (after 30 days of teflon insertion) with a neuroglial-ependymal scar at the spinal cord-teflon-interface). If the teflon was removed after 30 days and the spinal cord transected against one segment rostral to the initial transection, nerve fibers regenerated across the second transection and through the neuroglial-ependymal scar at the site of the original transection (4). These data show that in the goldfish the neuroglial scar was not a barrier to the regeneration of centrally derived nerve fibers.

In another series of experiments, an attempt was made to determine the mechanism by which the teflon block induces abortive regeneration of the goldfish spinal cord. What causes the goldfish spinal cord to change from a model for spinal cord regeneration into a model for a nonregenerating system? In these experiments, the spinal cord of the goldfish was transected and a teflon sheet placed between the transected spinal stumps as before. The teflon was left in place for 30 days or more rendering the goldfish spinal cord unable to regenerate after teflon removal. The spinal cord was then examined elecronmicroscopically from 1 to 3 months posttransection and teflon insertion. These studies revealed that the regenerated central axons of the spinal cord had been forced to grow out of their original tracts, presumably because of the presence of the teflon block. The fine tips of these axons had short bouton projections from their ends that made myriads of axo-axonic synapses on contiguous axons from displaced regenerated axons that had grown beneath the neuroglial-ependymal scar. Removal of the teflon block 30 days after the operation did not result in the resumption of growth of these nerve fibers (5). The goldfish neuroglial-ependymal scar is not a barrier to regeneration, but neurons appear, at least in part, to be inhibiting their own growth by the formation of synaptic junctional complexes. In this case, the complexes are inappropriate and form axo-axonic synapses subjacent to the neuroglial-ependymal scar. Perhaps neurons are genetically programed to possess a minimum-to-maximum number of presynaptic boutons which make functional synapses and will suspend growth (perhaps due to the cessation of arrival at the soma of specific chemical substances carried by retrograde axoplasmic flow) when a predetermined number of connecting terminals are established.

One of the most interesting factors in the successful regeneration of the lower vertebrate central nervous system (48) has been the postulate that the regenerated nerve fibers reconnect point-to-point to reduplicate the original pattern of synaptic innervation (3). Experiments have been carried out in the regenerated fish spinal cord to ascertain the return of the synaptic profile, in absolute numbers, on spinal neurons 2 cm caudal to the site of spinal cord transection in the goldfish in order to determine if, following regeneration, the synaptic complement of reinnervated spinal neurons returned to normal (10). Goldfish were subjected to spinal cord transection just anterior to the dorsal fin. From 5 to 60 days postregeneration, a segment of spinal cord 2 cm from the site of transection was impregnated by the Rasmussen technique (55) for the light microscopic demonstration of presynaptic boutons. Counts of boutons on motorneuron soma (carried out blind on coded material) revealed some interesting points (Fig. 1, A; 10). Initially approximately one-half of the innervation to the motorneuron soma was derived from the long descending tracts as seen from the drop in the number of bouton 5 days after transection (Fig. 1, A). There was then a significant rise in the numbers of boutons until 20 days after the operation. This increase in numbers could not be due to the long tracts since, with the delay caused by the scar, the severed nerve fibers could not have regenerated

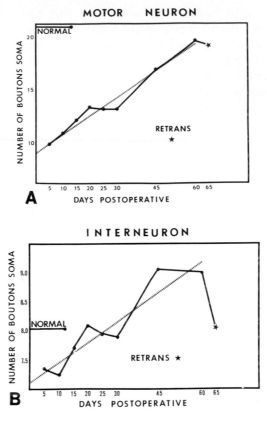

FIG. 1. A. Number of boutons on goldfish motorneuron soma over days after spinal cord transection. Counts were made from Rasmussen-impregnated material from neurons 2.0 cm from the site transection. The *dotted curve* indicates best fit data determined from a polynomial regression. The *star* at 65 days represents counts obtained 5 days after second transection. **B.:** Number of boutons on the soma of goldfish interneurons over days after spinal cord transection. Parameters as described above (7).

that distance in that period of time. The increases in presynaptic boutons then must be due to the spinal segmental afferents which could be derived from axonal sprouts as has previously been described in the descending tracts (10). There was a dramatic increase in the numbers of boutons from 30 to 60 days presumably indicating the arrival of the long tracts. At 60 days the numbers of boutons were statistically indistinguishable from normal. To properly control for the source of these boutons to the motorneuron soma the spinal cord of a group of regenerates was retransected at the initial site of transection. If the boutons were from regenerated axons, one would expect that the number of boutons would fall to the 5-day level. However, this was not the case. As shown in Fig. 1A (star, 65 days postoperative), the number of boutons after retransection was statistically indistinguishable from normal- and 60-day regenerates. These data show that the reinnervating boutons which form 30 to 60 days after the operation were not derived from the descending long tracts. All regenerates swam normally and were paralyzed following the second lesion as in former experiments, even though the motorneuron soma was hardly, if at all, reinnervated by the long tracts.

Where then did the long tracts terminate? When the synaptic profile on the soma of interneurons in the same segment was examined (Fig. 1, B), the same increases as on motorneurons were seen over the first 30 days (probably due to segmental axonal sprouting). However, with the arrival of the long tracts, the interneuron soma become hyperinnervated (30–60 days). When the spinal cord was retransected (star, 65 days postoperative, Fig. 1, B) the number of boutons returned to normal.

These data show that the ventral horn interneuron was a recipient of the regenerated long tracts which hyperinnervated the cell, whereas motorneurons did not receive boutons from the long tracts. A proposed mechanism of the revised circuitry of the spinal cord is shown in Fig. 2. Although the exact placement of all boutons is not known, there appears to be an establishment of new local circuits in the spinal cord of the fish following spinal cord regeneration. The motorneurons are innervated only by interneurons and lose their long-tract input even though the motorneuron synaptic profile returns to the normal number of presynaptic boutons. In essence, the fish spinal cord that normally has large numbers of direct projections to the motorneuron soma now appears to be rewired so as to resemble the rat or cat spinal cord in which motorneurons are only innervated by suprasegmental, infrasegmental, and segmental interneu-

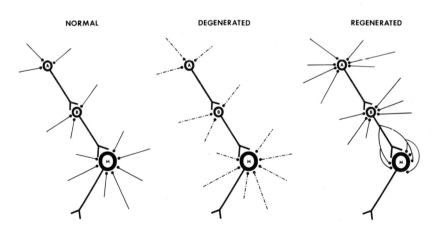

NORMAL   **DEGENERATED**   **REGENERATED**

FIG. 2. Schematic of proposed altered neuronal circuits in a regenerated goldfish spinal cord in a spinal cord segment 2.0 cm from the transection. In the normal cord there are long tract afferents and interneuronal afferents on interneurons (A,B) and motorneurons (M). Initially after transection the long-tract afferents degenerate (degenerated). Following regeneration (regenerated) the long tracts hyperinnervate the interneurons which have solely reinnervated the motorneuron by axonal sprouting to return the number of boutons to normal.

rons (16,63). The single or double synaptic relay in the new circuit may result in behavioral changes, but if so, these changes are not detectable by behavioral observations on swimming. A major source of boutons for the goldfish motorneuron could be axonal sprouts produced by hyperinnervated segmental interneurons with the presynaptic bouton hyperinnervation of interneurons involved in the production of axonal sprouts as shown in Fig. 2. This raises the interesting possibility that the number of presynaptic boutons, axonal collaterals, and/or telodendria of a given neuron could be influenced by the afferent innervation of that spinal neuron.

These data on the goldfish spinal cord have yielded extremely useful information which can be summarized as follows: (a) The neuroglial scar is not necessarily a barrier to the regenerative capacity of the spinal cord. (b) The regenerating nerve fibers from long tracts will form synaptic junctional complexes if forced to grow into a different area of the spinal cord. However, this process is deleterious and results in abortive regeneration. (c) Regenerated nerve fibers form synaptic complexes on partially deafferented neurons in the spinal cord distal to the transection. A sufficient number of these synapses are functional so as to restore the fish's ability to swim. (d) The regenerated nerve fibers and the reestablished presynaptic boutons are sustained for a long period of time. (e) The numbers of nerve fibers required to regenerate and restore function can be less than 50% of normal. (f) Axonal sprouting is a mechanism of increasing nerve fibers distal to the lesion but, in the goldfish, these sprouts cannot sustain function. (g) The specificity of the regenerated nerve fibers need not restore the original (point-to-point) synaptic profile on individual motorneurons. However, specificity for a particular segment or segmental neuronal circuit may be necessary to restore function.

DRUG-INDUCED SPINAL CORD REGENERATION

The actions of drugs which have shown some promise in the enhancement of CNS regeneration are important in determining the mechanisms of CNS metabolic reaction to injury and in the development of a rational therapy. The drugs reviewed here have been limited to those used to promote regeneration. Agents utilized in the acute aspects of spinal injury have been excluded since reviews are available elsewhere (47,51). Some of the more successful drugs which have been shown to enhance fiber growth after spinal cord lesions include: piromen (25,37,51), nerve growth factor (15,60), adrenocorticotropic hormone (ACTH) and corticosteroids (24,43), triiodothyronine or thyroxine (18,24,31,57), hydrolytic enzymes (26,42), and cyclophosphamide (15,23). Although there are many possible effects from any one of these drugs, their role has been primarily to alter the properties of the neuroglial cicatrix or surrounding tissue at the site of lesion (piromen, hydrolytic enzymes, and to some extent ACTH and thyroxine), or to facilitate some aspect of CNS metabolism (nerve growth factor, cyclophosphamide, ACTH, and thyroxine or triiodothyronine).

Piromen and other bacterial polysaccharides have been used in cats (25,37,51) to enhance regeneration. Some return of function and fiber growth across the site of lesion after spinal transection has been noted, but the success rate was low and there were some indications that the effects might be temporary. However, other investigators have not reported similar success. The bacterial pyrogens have many systemic effects which may be related to their enhancement of regeneration (51,62). Among these are their reactions with the pituitary adrenal axis, and direct or indirect actions on leukocytes, fibroblasts, and neuroglia. Other factors believed to be the source of regenerative enhancement of the pyrogens, particularily at the lesion site, include increased vascularity, reduction of edema, increased macrophage activity, and alterations of neuroglial scar formation. Presumably these effects produce a more suitable environment through which central nerve fibers may grow.

Adrenocorticotropic hormone (ACTH) has been utilized to enhance regeneration of central fibers both in rat somatomotor cortex (17,24) and spinal cord (43). After spinal cord transection (43), the regrowth of a small number of CNS fibers has been demonstrated in a few animals with some return of sensation in areas below the lesion. Similarly, some regrowth of central fibers into scar regions after cortical injury and ACTH treatment, has been demonstrated (24). ACTH and/or its induced release of corticosteroids seems to reduce inflammation, connective tissue scarring, and neuroglial scar formation (17). However, another possible effect may lie in a direct stimulation of CNS protein metabolism by ACTH (22).

The interrelationship of the bacterial pyrogens, ACTH and corticosteroid treatment with desoxycortisone acetate or cortisone (17,62), are interesting in their common relationship with the pituitary-adrenal axis. However, the morphological effects on scarring do differ somewhat, indicating multiple causes may produce the observed effects on scar formation.

Hydrolytic enzymes have been used to enhance regeneration of spinal cord with the primary objective being the reduction of scar tissue and removal of degenerating debris. Early studies (26) demonstrated that a modified trypsin treatment given to dogs after spinal lesions enhanced regeneration of spinal nerve fibers and reduced scarring. Further studies by Matinian and Andreasian (42) utilized treatments of hyaluronidase, trypsin, elastase, pyrogeneal, proserine, lidase, and combinations of these enzymes to enhance spinal cord regeneration. These authors claimed a high degree of functional, electrophysiological, and anatomical regeneration after hemisection and transection of the rat spinal cord. The results of other workers have not been as pronounced as these, suggesting that the results of Matinian and Andreasian should be considered with caution. However, hyaluronidase and other hydrolytic enzymes have been reported to reduce the density of the neuroglial scar and enhance phagocytic activity by leukocytes, as well as their action on the extracellular ground substance. The resulting reduction of scar tissue is perhaps more permeable to nerve fiber growth.

Another possible effect of hyaluronidase may be to reduce the accumulation of blood and serum proteins in spinal tissues after injury due to blood-brain barrier alterations. In order to examine this possibility, two groups of rats were hemisected at the T1-T2 vertebral interface. One group served as controls, and the other group of animals was treated by injection of 0.07 mg/kg of hyaluronidase (Sigma) into the cavity made by the surgery above the Gelfoam-covered post hemisection spinal cord, a procedure very similar to that of Matinian and Andresian (42). Injections were given daily with the first treatment 1 hr after hemisection. Following postoperative periods of 3, 7, and 14 days, animals were perfused with saline, and tissue segments (2.0 mm on either side of the spinal cord), including the lesion site and sites rostral and caudal, were processed. The protein profile was determined by SDS polyacrylamide gel electrophoresis and Coomassie blue (R-250) staining. Samples were run on 0.75-mm slab polyacrylamide gel with a linear exponential gradient (8.75–18.75%), according to published procedures (34). Equal amounts of protein were loaded for all samples. Compared with normal tissue, the protein spectrum in the lesioned area of the spinal cord from untreated hemisected animals (Fig. 3A) showed an increase in the staining intensity of bands in the 110K, 80K, 75K, and 10- 20K-molecular weight regions (calibrated by comparison with the mobility of proteins of known molecular weight). The increased staining in the 80K- and 75K-molecular weight regions was also found in tissue taken several millimeters rostral and caudal to the lesion. The molecular weight regions in which the increased staining intensity was observed correspond to those in which the major protein components of blood are found (Fig. 3, B). Specifically, albumin migrates in the 70 to 75K region, hemoglobin migrates in the 10 to 20K region, and the 110 K and 80 K bands are globulin fragments. The high concentration of hemoglobin at the site of hemisection probably was due to clotted blood, whereas the presence of serum proteins in the lesion site and in adjacent areas may be an indicator of a breakdown of the blood-brain barrier and edema (1,35,46).

Hyaluronidase treatment following hemisection appears to accelerate the loss of the presumed exogenous proteins from the site of lesion and adjacent areas compared with untreated hemisected animals (Fig. 3, A). The presence of relatively high concentrations of these exogenous proteins in spinal tissues may affect synaptic activity or perhaps regenerative growth. The mechanism by which hyaluronidase treatment aids in the removal of the exogenous proteins from

————————————————————▶

FIG. 3. A. Protein separation of spinal cord from a 2.0- mm area rostral and caudal to the site of spinal hemisection with and without hyalurondase treatment on a linear/exponential SDS polyacrylamide slab gel (7.5–18.75%). Labels (K) represent the approximate molecular weight in thousands calculated from known protein standards. Gel tracks: N, normal; 3D, 7D, 14D, untreated spinal hemisected animals over 3, 7, and 14 days postoperative; 3H, 7H, 14H, hyaluronidase-treated spinal hemisected animals over 3, 7, and 14 days postoperative. **B.** Protein separation of spinal cord and blood proteins from normal rats. S, normal spinal cord; P, blood plasma proteins; B, red blood cell proteins; 1 : 1 S + P, 1 : 1 S + B, a 1 : 1 mixture of normal spinal cord and plasma (P) or blood cell proteins (B); 3 : 1 S + P, 3 : 1 S + B, a 3:1 mixture of normal spinal cord protein to plasma or blood cell proteins. **A.** Mixtures of normal spinal cord and blood proteins can be made to approximate the appearance of experimentally injured spinal cord.

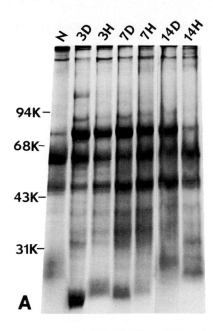

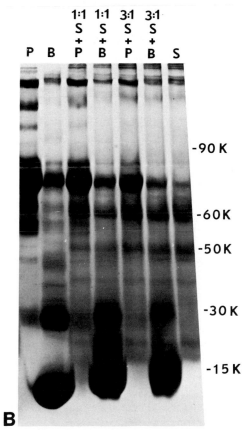

the spinal tissue is not known, but it may contribute to a general enhancement of functional recovery, such as bladder function (42), which has been reported following treatment with this and other hydrolytic enzymes.

The use of nerve growth factor (NGF; 38) is an attempt to induce CNS regeneration by altering metabolism. This protein can stimulate the growth of cell processes from sensory neurons *in vitro* and *in vivo,* and appears to be, for sympathetic neurons, a trophic factor involved in cell development, maintenance, and chromatolytic changes after injury (33,67). NGF is believed to produce its effects by stimulating RNA production in nerve cells. NGF has been utilized to promote regeneration of the spinal cord in kittens after dorsal column lesions (60). In more recent studies, NGF has been used to increase the degree and rate of regeneration of catecholaminergic pathways in rat brain (15). However, NGF does not seem to stimulate other types of nerve fiber growth.

The general metabolic stimulants, triiodothyronine and L-thyroxine have been utilized to enhance spinal cord regeneration in the hope that these drugs may stimulate protein synthesis in injured nerve cells directly to enhance regrowth (19,57). However, this hormone may also affect the pituitary adrenal system to produce corticosteroids and in part stimulate regeneration in this manner. In the spinal cord, Harvey and Srebnik (31) observed that L-thyroxine might enhance axon regrowth and functional recovery after spinal cord compression. More recent studies using a spinal transection model and L-thyroxine treatment (27) have failed to show any significant amount of regeneration. However, triiodothyronine has been reported to enhance fiber growth into lesioned areas of rat cortex (24,32) with slight effects on scarring. In the peripheral nervous system, triiodothyronine treatment has been reported to enhance nerve regeneration after lesions (18,19).

The use of immunosuppressive agents such as azathioprine and cyclophosphamide to induce regeneration after spinal cord injury (23) was proposed from experiments in demyellinating diseases which indicated that some components of degenerating CNS tissues may act as antigens for peripheral immune mechanisms. In a spinal transection model in the rat, cyclophosphamide in particular seemed to enhance the regeneration of spinal cord fibers as determined by both histological and electrophysiological analyses (23). However, the incidence of regrowth was slight, and functional regeneration was not obtained. Recent studies (68) have cast some doubt upon the formation of autoantibodies to CNS tissues after injury.

These data show that small numbers of axons can be induced to regenerate across the site of spinal cord injury in mammals. However, there are problems in the interpretation of these results. The actions of the drugs on the injured spinal cord remain unknown. Most of the drugs used are thought to have some effect on "loosening" the neuroglial scar, and in some manner affect the neuronal and neuroglial cells. Some drugs resulted in at least transient axonal growth through the scar into the cicatrix. The source of the nerve fibers in the cicatrix remains unknown although there are indications of a central derivation of these nerve fibers. The fact that these regenerated nerve fibers can establish synaptic contact with partially denervated neurons in the distal spinal cord can be inferred from limited electrophysiological studies. However, the regenerated nerve fibers in the mammalian spinal cord do not appear to be sustained for long periods of time. This postulate is inferred from the various papers quoted which show return of function for a short period of time, observe transient growth of centrally derived nerve fibers into the cicatrix, or have not pursued studies on the drugs utilized. The numbers of nerve fibers in the regenerates have not been quantitatively determined, but in general they appear to be low. However, there is no data on the number or type of nerve fibers needed for successful return of function or the number of new fibers that could prove to be sufficient. Nevertheless, it is clear that nerve fibers can be induced to regenerate across the cicatrix.

SYNAPTIC RECONNECTIVITY AS AN INDEX OF MAMMALIAN SPINAL CORD REGENERATION

An important consideration in regeneration of the mammalian spinal cord is whether or not mammalian spinal neurons deafferentated by spinal cord injury are capable of forming new synaptic connections. In order to establish this fact, a model for synaptic reconnectivity in the mammalian spinal cord had to be established. The model proposed in the following studies is a hemisection in which the left half of the spinal cord is hemisected at the T1-T2 interface and the spinal cord rostral to the hemisection studied qualitatively and quantitatively with both light and electron microscopy (Fig. 4). Using this model, it was established with qualitative ultrastructural analysis that deafferentated motorneurons (by hemisection) in the ventral horn of the rat and monkey spinal cord showed a progressive formation of varicosities along their dendritic shafts (from terminal to proximal dendrite). It was also demonstrated that these varicosities could act as sites for axodendritic synapses (6,7,13). In addition, synaptic complexes appeared in abnormal profiles on the dendritic shaft of motorneurons and, on these grounds, were suspected to be, in part, new synaptic complexes.

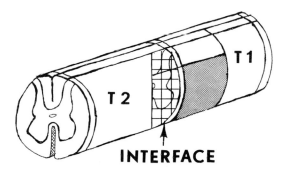

FIG. 4. Schematic of area of spinal cord hemisection *(grid)* in the rat and monkey spinal cord. The spinal cord for morphological (0–5 mm rostral, *shaded*) and for chemical analysis (segment rostral) were taken for analysis.

In the monkey, presynaptic boutons were observed to terminate over postsynaptic cisterns that may have been former postsynaptic sites. Also boutons were observed that were cup-shaped and had pre- and postsynaptic specializations consisting of presynaptic vesicles at the periphery of the cup-shaped terminal, a central enlarged synaptic space and a postsynaptic subsurface cistern (13). This was interpreted as the possible formation of new presynaptic boutons reinnervating a former postsynaptic site. The cup-shaped bouton was seen as an index of postsynaptic membrane reorganization and postsynaptic neuronal membrane supersensitivity (13). It appeared on the basis of these features, some of the presynaptic boutons observed after spinal hemisection were new.

Based on these studies, a series of experiments were carried out to determine if the synaptic profile of partially deafferentated, spinal neurons showed a process of synaptic renewal following spinal cord hemisection. The first segment rostral to the hemisection was chosen for analysis since, not only could the question of synaptic renewal be answered, but, in addition, a source of nerve fibers could be shown to be available for regeneration (Fig. 5). The absolute number of boutons was calculated on lamina IV neurons, lamina VII interneurons, and motorneurons in the ventral horn by counting the boutons revealed by the Rasmussen silver impregnation technique (55) for the demonstration of presynaptic boutons. An analysis of the data is presented in Figs. 5 to 7. The three types of neurons studied have several characteristics in common. In all cases studied the spinal neurons in the first segment rostral to a hemisection were partially deafferentated over the entire postoperative period (see "normal" in Figs. 5–7). The number of presynaptic boutons on the soma and primary dendrite were at a minimum 10 to 20 days after hemisection, reached a maximum at 30 days, and spontaneously decreased in number until 60 days after the operation. At 30 days the number of boutons on the dendrites of the cells returned to

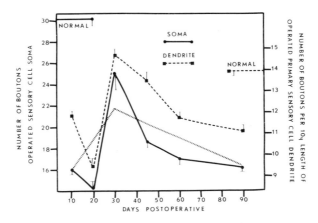

FIG. 5. Average number of boutons on soma and primary dendrite of lamina IV neurons one segment rostral to a spinal hemisection over postoperative days. The *dotted line* represents the curve derived from the polynomial regression of soma counts (11).

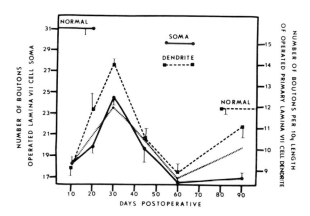

FIG. 6. Average number of boutons on soma and primary dendrite of lamina VII neurons one segment rostral to a spinal hemisection over postoperative days (11).

normal; however, the soma was always partially denervated after hemisection. The spontaneous loss of boutons from 30 to 60 days has been confirmed by electron microscopic observations which showed that boutons of various morphological configurations were degenerating at that time period (14). At 60 to 90 days after hemisection, the number of boutons on motorneuron soma increased again (Fig. 7). The rise in boutons from 60 to 90 days occurred on soma only, but was indicative of the cyclic nature of the change in the number of boutons on the neuron. In the case of motorneuron soma, there was a 30-day cyclic loss, increase, loss, and increase in boutons over a 90-day period. This cyclic loss and renewal in numbers of boutons is the result of a single hemisection (11).

Not only were there 30-day cyclic losses and gains of presynaptic boutons,

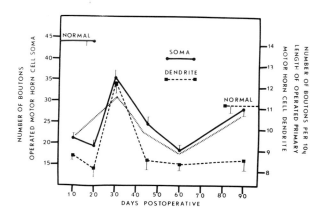

FIG. 7. Average number of boutons on soma and primary dendrite of α-motorneurons one segment rostral to a spinal hemisection over postoperative days (11).

but the ultrastructural morphology of the boutons revealed a consistent alteration and renewal in synaptic morphology of the presynaptic boutons on the soma of lamina VII interneurons (Fig. 8) and lamina IX motorneurons (Fig. 9). This is summarized in Fig. 10. These data were analyzed from counts on coded grids from hemisected spinal cords in which the frequency of the boutons was determined after all grids were counted (Fig. 4). The morphological types of presynaptic boutons counted were designated as S (spherical, clear synaptic vesicles) and F (flattened, clear synaptic vesicles). The counts were made on interneurons in lamina VII and on motorneuron soma in the first segment rostral to the site of spinal cord hemisection (Fig. 4). The data in the figure were normalized (8) so that a value of 1.0 indicates an occurrence equal to the normal frequency or number of the presynaptic boutons at that postoperative day.

The number of boutons on interneuron soma after hemisection showed that these neurons were chronically denervated (Fig. 8, A), and there was a loss of both S- and F-type presynaptic boutons. Normally, on interneurons (Fig. 8, A) there were more S- and F-types of boutons. For the first 45 days after hemisection, F presynaptic boutons were gained and S-types were lost. From 45 to 60 days this trend was reversed. Frequency analysis of the bouton types (Fig. 9, B) showed that there was a 45 day gain in the frequency of F- and loss in the frequency of S-type presynaptic boutons. The opposite was true for the motorneuron (Fig. 10, A), but the change in frequency was due solely to

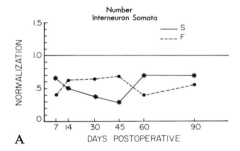

A

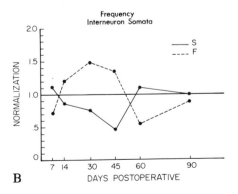

B

FIG. 8. Normalized number (A) and frequency (B) of S- and F-type presynaptic boutons on lamina VII neuron somata over days posthemisection (14).

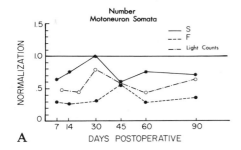

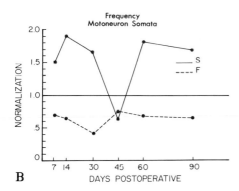

FIG. 9. Normalized number **(A)** and frequency **(B)** of S- and F-type presynaptic boutons on α-motorneuron somata over days posthemisection (14).

NORMALIZATION OF BOUTON FREQUENCY

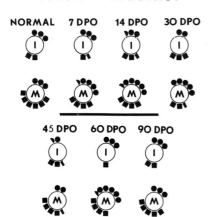

FIG. 10. Schematic of bouton frequency presented as percent normal (normalized) of S- *(circle)* and F-type *(squares)* boutons on lamina VII neurons (I) and α-motorneuron (M) somata over days posthemisection.

the gain and loss (45 days after the operation) in the frequency of S-type presynaptic boutons (Fig. 10, B). The frequency of F-type boutons remained relatively stable, although below normal. There was a critical difference between the reafferentation of the interneuron and motorneuron. Ninety days after hemisection, the frequency of the presynaptic bouton-types on interneurons returned to normal, whereas on motorneurons there were more S-types than normal. Normally there were more S- than F-type presynaptic boutons on interneurons and more F- than S-type presynaptic boutons on motorneurons (Fig. 10). On both of these neurons the dominant type of presynaptic bouton on the soma is stable and gains in frequency over nondominant presynaptic boutons.

It is interesting to note that in the rat and cat the motorneuron is exclusively innervated by the interneuron. The possible sources of the new presynaptic boutons are varied and can come from long tracts or from the segmental neurons. However, assuming that the major reinnervation is segmental (14) and the interneuronal pool sampled is a reflection of the interneurons reinnervating the motorneuron, then a gain of frequency of F presynaptic boutons on interneurons is correlated with a gain of S presynaptic boutons on motorneurons. The possibility exists that axonal sprouting or regeneration of a neuron is in part determined by the trophic influences on interneurons. This would result in the growth of axons with S vesicular boutons or perhaps the growth of such processes capable of producing neurons S vesicles from other axons, since it is not known if a regenerated or sprouted neuron can produce only one type of vesicle.

New synaptic complexes can be formed on partially deafferented neurons. The number of boutons on the neurons fluctuates over postoperative days with cyclic renewal of both numbers and types, suggesting that in mammals the system is dynamic with a source of axons in the segment rostral to the site of the spinal cord lesion. The presence of the nerve fibers was reflected by the fluctuation of presynaptic boutons on interneurons which normally receive local segmental, extended segmental, and long tract afferents and by motorneurons in the rat which receive local segmental and extended segmental afferents derived from interneurons. In terms of the regenerative capacity of the spinal cord, these findings are exciting. However, there is little successful regenerative growth even though nerve fibers are available.

It is our hypothesis that nerve fibers do not grow into the scar because local growth is achieved at the expense of regenerative growth in the mammalian spinal cord. It appears that the deafferentated neuron in the spinal cord accepts the afferents it has available. The process segregates the nerve fibers produced in the segment rostral to the injury since they terminate on a partially deafferentated neuron and the formation of a synaptic complex removes that nerve fiber from the regenerative pool. Control of the process of synapse formation by drugs or other means may release this source of nerve fibers in the segment which can be induced to grow into the distal stump of the spinal cord where experiments with lower vertebrates have shown that they can form synaptic complexes which, by morphological criteria, should be active.

AMINO ACID PRECURSOR INCORPORATION INTO PROTEIN AS A CORRELATE OF SPINAL CORD REGENERATION

The neurochemical analysis of spinal injury to date has largely been confined to experiments studying neurotransmitter alterations associated with the acute aspects of spinal cord injury (36,47,59). Few metabolic studies of brain and spinal cord tissue have been carried out over postoperative periods in which regenerative synaptic renewal and reorganization is known to occur. The following is a review of studies which have attempted to define some aspects of CNS protein and amino acid metabolism over time periods during which synaptic remodeling is known to occur after spinal cord hemisection.

There are alterations in amino acid incorporation into protein of the hemisected rat (39,65) and monkey spinal cord (12,64). An intraperitoneal injection of 200 μCi of ^{14}C-leucine (1 hr incorporation) into rats with a spinal hemisection at T1-T2 (Fig. 4) demonstrated a significant increase in the incorporation of radioactivity into trichloracetic acid (TCA)- precipitable protein in the lesioned and adjacent spinal cord segments 7 and 30 days after the operation (39). In the brain, significant increases in ^{14}C-leucine incorporation were also noted bilaterally in somatomotor cortex 30 days after the operation with the left somatomotor cortex decreasing to less than controls ($p < 0.05$) by 70 days. More recent studies (65) suggested that increases in ^{3}H-lysine incorporation (200 μCi, subcutaneous injection, 1 hr incorporation into TCA-precipitable protein and soluble fractions of the hemisected rat spinal cord occurred at earlier time intervals (Fig. 11). In addition, the overall levels of incorporation of ^{3}H-lysine into

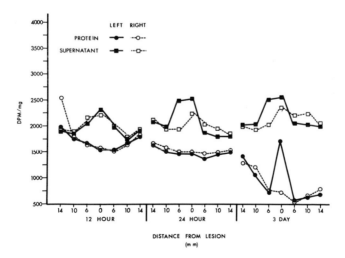

FIG. 11. ^{3}H-lysine incorporation (200 μCi subcutaneous injection, 1 hour) into TCA- precipitable and soluble fractions of rat (N = 5, per time period) spinal cord over time postoperative. Distance from the site of the lesion (0) both rostral and caudal to the site of hemisection was measured in mm on left and right side of the spinal cord. TCA- precipitable protein in DPM/mg protein and soluble fraction in DPM/mg dry weight (65).

both protein and soluble fractions of spinal cord were affected by the surgical procedure (stress response), as suggested in studies in the Cebus monkey (64) and general studies of amino acid incorporation into protein in brain following sensory stimulation and/or stress (56,61).

In the Cebus monkey (12,64), left spinal hemisection at the interface of the first and second thoracic vertebrae (Fig. 4) produced overall alterations in the uptake of label into TCA-precipitable protein and soluble fractions of brain and spinal cord and alterations in the uptake in local regions of spinal cord and brain. In the spinal cord (Fig. 12), the average uptake (overall spinal samples) of ^{3}H-lysine from a subcutaneous injection of 1.0 μCi (1 hr incorporation) into TCA-labeled protein was increased in a three-day sham-operated animal (dural incisure) compared with normals. In three-day hemisected animals, the average uptake of amino acid was higher in both TCA-precipitable and soluble fractions than in sham and normal animals. These overall increases in amino acid incorporation appeared to be related to surgical stress. This conclusion was supported by the fact that there was a decrease in the overall incorporation of amino acid into proteins in the spinal cord at six days postoperative. At 13 days postoperative, however, the overall levels of protein radioactivity had increased again to the 3-day levels. This secondary increase of ^{3}H-amino acid incorporation into protein was not consistent with the stress model proposed earlier. The nature of the secondary increase as a stress, regenerative, or injury reaction could not be evaluated since sham animals were not done at this time period. The average TCA-soluble fraction radioactivity of spinal cord samples for hemisected animals was constant over postoperative intervals, although it was statistically greater than that of normal- or sham-operated animals. This may suggest an alteration in the amino acid incorporation of brain and spinal cord protein in these animals; however, an altered time course of peripheral uptake cannot be ruled out. At the site of the lesion (Fig. 12), the radioactivity of protein increased progressively with time within that portion of the spinal cord that was injured, indicating that the scar area was metabolically very active. These local increases in protein radioactivity over time at the lesion site may be related to edema, gliosis, neuronal reaction, regenerative responses, and/or cells infiltrating from the periphery.

In brain (12), the overall levels of protein radioactivity over postoperative days were similar to those observed in spinal cord. Local areas of brain, including leg areas of motorcortex, occipital cortex, and superior colliculus, exhibited a greater incorporation into the left hemisphere than into the right hemisphere (L > R). The overall increases in brain and spinal cord appeared to be related to stress and unknown factors, perhaps blood-borne. Focal laterality differences in brain were correlated with synaptic depletion, blood flow alterations, axonal sprouting, and/or increased metabolic demand upon the intact side.

These experiments suggest that surgical procedures and spinal injury may affect overall CNS metabolism. However, injury-induced changes in nervous

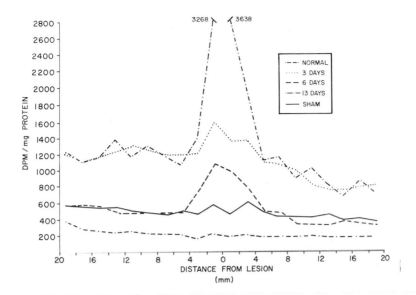

FIG. 12. ^{3}H-lysine incorporation (1.0 μCi, subcutaneous injection, 1 hour) into TCA precipitable protein of the hemisected side of the spinal cord in monkeys over postoperative time. TCA-precipitable protein radioactivity is expressed as DPM/mg over distance from the lesion (0). The average TCA-soluble fraction radioactivity for hemisected groups was constant over time, but statistically greater ($p < 0.05$) than normal or sham animals (64).

system metabolism may also arise from peripheral nerve injuries (66). In the rabbit (30) and mouse (44), injured peripheral nerves regenerate at a faster rate after two sequential lesions, i.e., an initial "priming" lesion separated by a two-week postoperative interval followed by a second lesion. The priming lesion effect has been attributed to a reorganization of the neuron's protein synthetic machinery for increased production of structural or growth related proteins (21,29,44). Priming lesion experiments with a similar design (66) carried out on rat sciatic nerve produce not only a faster rate of regeneration, but also differences in the average incorporation of lysine into the TCA-precipitable protein and soluble fractions of brain and spinal cord 1 hr following a subcutaneous injection of 200 μCi of ^{3}H-lysine (Fig. 13). These differences in CNS protein synthesis rates are attributable to the subsequent second lesion of the nerve, since on experimental and control animals, except for the interval between lesions, identical surgical procedures were performed.

Analysis of ^{3}H-lysine incorporation into protein following spinal injury revealed increased levels of incorporation throughout the brain and spinal cord. This increased incorporation was due to a stress response to surgical procedures as well as to specific CNS responses following injury during the regenerative process. In the spinal-hemisected monkey over the first 2 postoperative weeks, the overall levels of incorporation of amino acid followed a three-phase pattern:

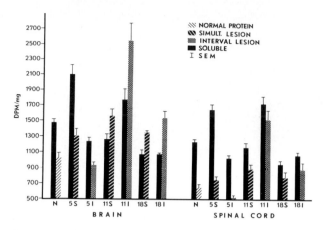

FIG. 13. Overall uptake of ³H-lysine (subcutaneous injection, 1 hour incorporation) into the TCA-precipitable protein and soluble fractions of rat brain and spinal cord after simultaneous (S) and interval (I) sciatic nerve lesions over postoperative days (5,11, and 18 days). TCA-precipitable protein radioactivity is in DPM/mg protein and soluble fraction radioactivity in DPM/mg dry weight.

an increase, decrease, and increase again at 3, 6, and 13 days after the operation, respectively. In the rat, general levels of amino acid incorporation increased within 6 hrs after surgery and declined progressively to 14 days (65). This suggests that there is an interspecies difference in the general response to the injury, a possibility supported by differences in incorporation at the site of injury in the rat and monkey. In the monkey, amino acid incorporation at the lesion, corrected for the average level of incorporation in the spinal cord, increased over the time period examined (64). In the rat, the local response at the site of injury peaked between 3 and 7 days (65) and subsequently declined. For both species the lesion site was very active metabolically. It is possible that the magnitude of the overall incorporation could mask some local selective reactions occurring soon after injury. Thus, the early regenerative phase is marked by the massive stress response.

Protein incorporation responses after injury may be correlated with subsequent morphological events in regeneration. More information as to the specific proteins involved in CNS changes at the lesion site as well as the stress and specific nervous system response might lead to more effective control of regeneration following injury. Control of certain aspects of the metabolic response to injury could be utilized to coordinate the growth of axons in the CNS and to maintain deafferented neurons in a synaptic receptive state.

ACKNOWLEDGMENTS

Supported in part by a grant from the National Institute of Health (NINCDS, NS-06164).

REFERENCES

1. Beggs, J. L., and Waggener, J. D. (1975): Vasogenic edema in the injured spinal cord: a method of evaluating the extent of blood-brain barrier alteration to horseradish peroxsidase. *Exp. Neurol.,* 49:86–96.
2. Bernstein, J. J. (1964): Relation of spinal cord regeneration to age in adult goldfish, *Exp. Neurol.,* 9:161–174.
3. Bernstein, J. J. (1970): Anatomy and physiology of the central nervous system. In: *Fish Physiology, Vol. 4,* edited by W. S. Hoar and D. J. Randall, pp. 1–90. Academic Press, New York.
4. Bernstein, J. J., and M. E. Bernstein (1967): Effect of glial-ependymal scar and teflon arrest on the regenerative capacity of goldfish spinal cord. *Exp. Neurol.,* 19:25–32.
5. Bernstein, J. J., and Bernstein, M. E. (1969): Ultrastructure of normal regeneration and loss of regenerative capacity following teflon blockage in goldfish spinal cord. *Exp. Neurol.,* 24:538–557.
6. Bernstein, J. J., and Bernstein, M. E. (1971): Axonal regeneration and formation of synapses proximal to the site of lesion following hemisection of the rat spinal cord. *Exp. Neurol.,* 30:336–351.
7. Bernstein, J. J., and Bernstein, M. E. (1973): Neuronal alteration and reinnervation following axonal regeneration and sprouting in the mammalian spinal cord. *Brain Behav. Evol.,* 8:135–161.
8. Bernstein, J. J., and Bernstein, M. E. (1976): Ventral horn synaptology in the rat. *J. Neurocytol.,* 5:109–123.
9. Bernstein, J. J., and Gelderd, J. B. (1970): Regeneration of the long spinal tracts in the goldfish. *Brain Res.,* 20:33–38.
10. Bernstein, J. J., and Gelderd, J. B. (1973): Synaptic reorganization following regeneration of goldfish spinal cord. *Exp. Neurol.,* 41:401–410.
11. Bernstein, J. J., Gelderd, J. B., and Bernstein, M. E. (1974): Alteration of neuronal synaptic complement during regeneration and axonal sprouting of rat spinal cord. *Exp. Neurol.,* 44:470–482.
12. Bernstein, J. J., and Wells, M. R. (1977): Amino acid incorporation in medulla, pons, midbrain and cortex following spinal cord hemisection in the Cebus monkey *(Cebus apella). Brain Res.,* 122: 475–483.
13. Bernstein, M. E., and Bernstein, J. J. (1973): Regeneration of axons and synaptic complex formation rostral to the site of hemisection in the spinal cord of the monkey. *Int. J. Neurosci.,* 5:15–26.
14. Bernstein, M. E., and Bernstein, J. J. (1977): Synaptic frequency alteration on rat ventral horn neurons in the first segment proximal to spinal cord hemisection: an ultrastructural statistical study of regenerative capacity. *J. Neurocytol.,* 6: 85–102.
15. Bjorklund, A., and Stenevi, U. (1972): Nerve growth factor: stimulation of regenerative growth of central noradrenergic neurons. *Science,* 175:1251–1253.
16. Brown, L. T. (1971): Projections and termination of the corticospinal tract in rodents. *Exp. Brain Res.,* 13:432–450.
17. Clemente, C. C. (1955): Structural regeneration in the mammalian central nervous system and the role of neuroglia and connective tissue. In: *Regeneration in the Central Nervous System,* edited by W. F. Windle, pp. 147–161. Charles C Thomas, Springfield, Ill.
18. Cockett, S. A., and Kiernan, J. A. (1973): Acceleration of peripheral nervous regeneration in the rat by exogenous triiodothyronine. *Exp. Neurol.,* 39:389–394.
19. Cook, R. A., and Kiernan, J. A. (1976): Effects of triiodothyronine on protein synthesis in regenerating peripheral neurons. *Exp. Neurol.,* 52:514–524.
20. Dorland (1959): *Medical Dictionary,* p. 1172, W. B. Saunders Co., Philadelphia and London.
21. Ducker, T. B., Kempe, L. G., and Hayes, C. J. (1969): The metabolic background for peripheral nerve surgery. *J. Neurosurg.,* 30:270–280.
22. Dunn, A. J., Iuvone, P. J., and Rees, H. D. (1976): Neurochemical responses of mice to ACTH and lysine vasopressin. *Pharm. Biochem. Behav.,* 5 (Suppl. 1):139–145.
23. Feringa, E. R., Johnson, R. D., and Wendt, J. S. (1975): Spinal cord regeneration in rats after immunosuppressive treatment. *Arch. Neurol.,* 32:676–683.
24. Fertig, A., Kiernan, J. A., and Seyan, S.S.A.S. (1971): Enhancement of axonal regeneration in the brain of the rat by corticotrophin and triiodothyronine. *Exp. Neurol.,* 33:372–385.

25. Freeman, L. W. (1955): Functional recovery in spinal rats. In: *Regeneration in the Central Nervous System,* edited by W. F. Windler, pp. 195–207. Charles C Thomas, Springfield, Ill.
26. Freeman, L. W., MacDougall, J., Turbes, C. A., and Bowman, D. E. (1960): The treatment of experimental lesions of the spinal cord of dogs with trypsin. *J. Neurosurg.,* 17:259–265.
27. Gelderd, J. B., and St. Onge, M. G. (1977): The effects of L-thyroxine and enzyme treatment following spinal cord transection in rats: a light microscopic study. *Anat. Rec.,* 187:586.
28. Goldberger, M. E., and Murray, M. (1974): Restitution of function and collateral sprouting in the rat spinal cord: the deafferented animal. *J. Comp. Neurol.,* 158:37–54.
29. Grafstein, B. (1975): The nerve cell body response to axotomy. *Exp. Neurol.,* 48:32–51.
30. Gutmann, E. (1942): Factors affecting recovery of motor function after nerve lesions. *J. Neurol. Psychiatr.,* 5:81–95.
31. Harvey, J. E., and Srebnik, H. H. (1967): Locomotor activity and axon regeneration following spinal cord compression in rats treated with L-thyroxine. *J. Neuropath. Exp. Neurol.,* 26:661–668.
32. Heinicke, E. (1977): Influence of exogenous triiodothyronine on axonal regeneration and wound healing in the brain of the rat. *J. Neurol. Sci.,* 31:293–305.
33. Henry, I. A. (1975): The response of adrenergic neurones to axotomy and nerve growth factor. *Brain Res.,* 94:87–97.
34. Kelly, P. T., and Luttges, M. W. (1975): Electrophoretic separation of nervous system proteins on exponential gradient polyacrylamide gels. *J. Neurochem.,* 24:1077–1079.
35. Klatzo, I., Miquel, J., and Ostenasek, R. (1962): The application of fluorescine labelled serum proteins to the study of vascular permeability in the brain. *Acta Neuropathol.,* 2:144–160.
36. Lewin, M. G. Hansebout, R. R., and Pappius, H. M. (1974): Chemical characteristics of traumatic spinal cord edema in cats: effect of steroids on potassium depletion. *J. Neurosurg.,* 40:65–75.
37. Litrell, J. L. (1955): Apparent functional restitution in Piromen treated spinal cats. In: *Regeneration in the Central Nervous System,* edited by W. F. Windler, pp. 219–228. Charles C Thomas, Springfield, Ill.
38. Levi-Montalcini, R., and Angeletti, P. U. (1968): Nerve Growth Factor. *Physiol. Rev.,* 48:534–569.
39. Luttge, W., Mannis, M., and Bernstein, J. J. (1975): Alterations of central nervous system protein synthesis in response to spinal cord hemisection. *J. Neurosci. Res.,* 1:77–82.
40. Lynch, G., and Cotman, C. W. (1975): The hippocampus as a model for studying anatomical plasticity in the adult brain. In: *The Hippocampus, Vol. 1:Structure and Development,* edited by R. L. Isaacson and K. H. Pribram, pp. 123–154. Plenum Press, New York.
41. Lynch, G., Stanfield, B., and Cotman, C. (1973): Developmental differences in postlesion axonal growth in the hippocampus. *Brain Res.,* 59:155–168.
42. Matinian, L. A., and Andreasian (1976): *Enzyme Therapy in Organic Lesions of Spinal Cord,* translated by E. Tanasecu, pp. 156. Brain Information Service (UCLA), Los Angeles.
43. McMasters, R. E. (1962): Regeneration of the spinal cord in the rat. Effects of Piromen and ACTH upon the regenerative capacity. *J. Comp. Neurol.,* 119:113–116.
44. McQuarrie, I. G., and Grafstein, B. (1973): Axon outgrowth enhanced by a previous nerve injury. *Arch. Neurol.,* 29:53–55.
45. Murray, M., and Goldberger, M. E. (1974): Restitution of function and collateral sprouting in the cat spinal cord: the partially hemisected animal. *J. Comp. Neurol.,* 158:19–36.
46. Nemceck, S., Petr, R., Suba, P., Roxzvial, V., and Melka, O. (1977): Longitudinal extension of oedema in experimental spinal cord injury. Evidence for two types of post traumatic oedema. *Acta Neurochirugica,* 37:7–16.
47. Osterholm, J. L. (1974): The pathophysiological response to spinal cord injury. The current status of related research. *J. Neurosurg.,* 40:5–33.
48. Piatt, J. (1955): Regeneration of the spinal cord of the salamander. *J. Exp. Zool.,* 129:177–207.
49. Prendergast, J., and Stelzner, D. J. (1976): Changes in the magnocellular portion of the red nucleus following thoracic hemisection in the neonatal and adult rat. *J. Comp. Neurol.,* 166:163–172.
50. Prendergast, J., and Stelzner, D. J. (1976): Increases in collateral axon growth rostral to a thoracic hemisection in neonatal and weanling rat. *J. Comp. Neurol.,* 166:145–162.
51. Puchala, E., and Windle, W. F. (1977): The possibility of structural and functional restitution after spinal cord injury. A review. *Exp. Neurol.,* 55:1–42.

52. Raisman, G. (1969): Neuronal plasticity in the septal nuclei of the adult rat. *Brain Res.,* 14:25–48.
53. Raisman, G., and Field, P. (1973): A quantitative investigation of the development of collateral reinnervation after partial deafferentation of the septal nuclei. *Brain Res.,* 50:241–264.
54. Ramón y Cajal, S. (1959): *Degeneration and Regeneration of the Nervous System,* edited by R. J. May, pp. 769, Hafner, New York.
55. Rasmussen, G. (1957): Selective silver impregnation of synaptic endings. In: *New Research Techniques of Neuroanatomy,* edited by W. F. Windler, pp. 27–39. Charles C Thomas, Springfield, Ill.
56. Rees, H. D., Brogan, L. L., Entingh, D. J., Dunn, A. J., Shinkman, P. G., Damstra-Entingh, T., Wilson, J. F., and Glassman, E. (1971): Effect of sensory stimulation on the uptake and incorporation of radioactive lysine into protein of mouse brain and liver. *Brain Res.,* 68:143–156.
57. Rhodes, A., Ford, D., and Rhines, R. (1964): Comparative uptake of D-L-Lysine-^{3}H by normal and regenerative hypoglossal nerve cells in euthyroid, hypothyroid and hyperthyroid male rats. *Exp. Neurol.,* 10:251–263.
58. Rustinoni, A., and Sotelo, C. (1974): Some effects of chronic deafferentation on the ultrastructure of the nucleus gracilis of the cat. *Brain Res.,* 73:527–533.
59. Schoultz, T. W., DeLuca, D. C., and Reding, D. (1976): Norepinephrine levels in traumatized spinal cord of catecholamine depleted cats. *Brain Res.,* 109:367–374.
60. Scott, D., and Liu, C. N. (1964): Factors promoting regeneration of spinal neurons: positive influence of nerve growth factor. *Prog. Brain Res.,* 13:127–150.
61. Seminginovsky, B., Jakoubek, B., Kraus, M., and Erdosova, R. (1974): Stress induced changes of the amino acid uptake and protein synthesis in the brain cortex slices of rats: effect of adrenalectomy. *Physiol. Bohemoslov.,* 23:503–510.
62. Stuart, E. G. (1955): Tissue reactions and possible mechanisms of Piromen and desoxycorticosterone acetate in central nervous system regeneration. In: *Regeneration in the Central Nervous System,* edited by W. F. Windler, pp. 162–170. Charles C Thomas, Springfield, Ill.
63. Valverde, F. (1966): The pyramidal tract in rodents. A study of its relations with the posterior column nuclei, dorsolateral reticular formation of the medulla oblongata, and cervical spinal cord. *Zeitsch. fur Zellforsch.,* 71:297–363.
64. Wells, M. R., and Bernstein, J. J. (1976): Early changes in protein synthesis following spinal cord hemisection in the Cebus monkey *(Cebus apella). Brain Res.,* 111:31–40.
65. Wells, M. R., and Bernstein, J. J. (1977): Amino acid uptake in the spinal cord and brain of the short term spinal hemisected rat. *Exp. Neurol.,* 57:900–912.
66. Wells, M. R., and Bernstein, J. J. (1977): Amino acid incorporation into rat spinal cord and brain after simultaneous and interval sciatic nerve lesions. *Brain Res. (in press).*
67. West, N. R., and Bunge, R. P. (1977): Observations on the role of the nerve growth factor (NGF) and Schwann cells in the chromatolytic response of sympathetic neurons. *Anat. Rec.,* 187:747.
68. Willenborg, D. O., Staten, E. A., and Eidelberg, E. (1977): Studies on cell-mediated hypersensitivity to neural antigens after experimental spinal cord injury. *Exp. Neurol.,* 54:383–392.

Neuronal Plasticity, edited by
Carl W. Cotman.
Raven Press, New York © 1978.

Recovery of Movement and Axonal Sprouting May Obey Some of the Same Laws

Michael E. Goldberger and Marion Murray

Department of Anatomy, The Medical College of Pennsylvania, Philadelphia, Pennsylvania 19129

IN RECOVERY, WHAT IS RECOVERED?

Recovery of motor behavior following lesions in the adult CNS may be accomplished either by the return of the function which was initially lost or by the substitution of other, residual functions. If lost functions return, then the resulting movement will presumably be performed in the same way as it is normally. If residual functions are substituted, then motor behavior will be produced in a manner different from the normal, but may be similar in appearance. The difference between movement produced in the normal way and that produced by substituted mechanisms can be used to define the permanent motor deficit due (a) to the failure of destroyed CNS pathways to regenerate and (b) to the failure of residual systems to mimic precisely the functions of the pathways that were destroyed. It is possible through combining the examination of both reflex and volitional movements to show that some residual functions may become enhanced during recovery. Cerebellar lesions disrupt the timing of movements in monkeys and produce tremor. During recovery from cerebellar lesions, functions which ordinarily depend upon somatosensory cortex, e.g., the positioning of limbs, acquire increased importance in the control of movement (16) and are able to mask or minimize the tremor. When, after recovery, the somatosensory cortex is ablated, the original cerebellar deficit, tremor, recurs and becomes permanent (14). Similarly, forced grasping is evoked by premotor cortex lesions. During recovery, the opposing reflex pattern, evasion, becomes enhanced. When the pathway which mediates evasion, the pyramidal tract, is secondarily destroyed, the initial impairment, forced grasping, returns and no further recovery is seen (13). Thus, the functions mediated by the pathways important to the recovery may become enhanced, and this enhancement may contribute to the mediation of a behavioral substitution underlying recovery. One way in which a pathway might enhance the potency of the functions it mediates is by increasing its terminal field, i.e., by the sprouting in new terminals.

Axonal Sprouting Occurs in the Adult, Sometimes

Sprouting in the adult central nervous system was first described by Liu and Chambers (34). They unilaterally removed all of the dorsal roots but one *(spared root preparation)* from the cat's spinal cord, and found that the spared root's projection had increased[1] when compared with that of the same dorsal root on the normal side of the cord. The functional significance of this increased projection was unknown. The pattern of the increased projection was similar

---

[1] The usual strategy used in testing for sprouting is to make a unilateral lesion and to allow a year or more for stainable degeneration to disappear. Then an acute, bilaterally symmetrical lesion *(test lesion)* is made and the degeneration stained by various modifications of the Nauta stain. Since, normally, the degeneration arising from symmetrical lesions is also symmetrical, bilaterally, any increase in density or extent of degeneration on the chronically lesioned side may be due to sprouting from the test system on that side.

to that of the normal dorsal root projection, but it had increased in amount. The mechanism of increasing the projection was assumed to be sprouting of new terminals and/or axon collaterals into areas partially denervated by the original lesion and was thus considered to be analogous to sprouting that occurs in the peripheral nervous system (12). Since that time, sprouting in the adult central nervous system has been demonstrated in the visual system (11,19), limbic system (53), red nucleus (50), and again in the spinal cord and dorsal column nuclei (15,17,18,47). It fails to occur in the trigeminal nucleus of the cat (27) or spinal cord of the rat (62). Thus sprouting occurs under some conditions or in some parts of the CNS but not others. The rules which govern the success and failure of sprouting are not at all clear at present.

DUAL ORGANIZATION OF DORSAL ROOT PROJECTIONS

The central projection of the dorsal roots of the cat (Fig. 1) have provided us with a system which lends itself to a consideration of the factors important to recovery of function and its possible relationship to sprouting following CNS lesions. The 34 pairs (28) of dorsal roots mediate the transmission of somatotopically organized somatosensory information, of reflex activity, and of topographic feedback from movement.

Each dorsal root projection manifests a dual organization: specific (or discrete)

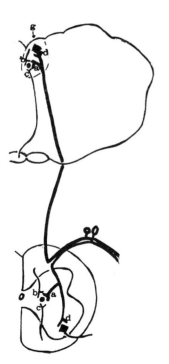

FIG. 1. Dorsal root projections to a spinal segment and, ascending, to the dorsal column nuclei of the medulla. d, Relatively non-overlapping, discrete projections to the spinal motor nuclei and to the cell cluster region of the nucleus gracilis (g). a, Another collateral projection to a "loosely organized" region: the zona intermedia (spinal cord) and base of the nucleus gracilis. This projection overlaps with b, dorsal root collaterals from other segments and c, collaterals from descending systems.

and generalized[2] The specific projections are characterized by maximal preservation of somatotopic localization, a relative lack of overlapping projection fields
of different dorsal roots with each other, and a lack of overlap of the dorsal
root fields with those of descending systems and the ascending nonprimary
afferents. Such specific projections are found in the cell clusters of the dorsal
column nuclei and in the monosynaptic projections to motor neurons. More
generalized projections show larger receptive fields, less strict somatotopic localization, and greater overlap of dorsal root projections with each other and, in
many cases, with the terminal fields of descending systems. The most generalized
projections are found in the base, and in the rostral reticular regions of the
gracile nucleus, and in the zona intermedia and base of the dorsal horn (laminae
V–VIII) in the spinal cord. The degree of somatotopic organization in the dorsal
horn (laminae II and III) and in Clarke's nucleus is probably intermediate
between these, although a direct comparison between these two areas and the
cluster regions of the dorsal column nuclei has not been made. Studies of animals
in which deafferentations have been performed reveal motor deficits which can
similarly be divided into (a) loss of specific motor responses and (b) loss of
generalized movement patterns (14,15,17,36,66,67,69). Although each dorsal
root shows both types of projection, there are also regional differences in the
patterns of central projections between dorsal roots of the limbs and those
supplying axial regions of the body. For example, the roots supplying the limbs
show a strictly unilateral projection, whereas roots supplying the trunk and
sacral regions project across the midline.

AFTER LESIONS, RECOVERY OF MOVEMENT AND OF AFFERENT INPUT ARE INCOMPLETE

Changes in Descending Systems' Function After Deafferentation

A cat's hindlimb can be completely deafferented by cutting all lumbar and
sacral dorsal roots between the ganglion and the spinal cord. If the lesion is
made extradurally, then damage to the spinal cord can be minimized or avoided
(33,71). If in addition the dorsal root ganglia are removed, afferent fibers that
travel in the ventral roots (8) are also destroyed. Because of the unique relationship of the dorsal roots to the periphery, no other system can mediate the
same topographic information to central targets. Therefore, when the lumbosacral dorsal roots are destroyed, the recovery which occurs must be due to the
ability of the nervous system to substitute different information mediated by
other structures.

Immediately following deafferentation, a complete flaccid paralysis of the
ipsilateral hindlimb occurs, despite the fact that a number of central pathways

---

[2] This interpretation of the anatomy is based on refs: 6, 7, 24, 26, 29, 31, 32, 36, 43, 54–57,
59, 60, 64, and 65.

to the hindlimb interneurons and motor neurons remain. The remaining systems include ipsilateral and contralateral descending motor systems, postural reflex systems of the trunk, and the crossed reflex pathways mediated by contralateral dorsal roots. Initially none of these systems is able to elicit movement in the deafferented hindlimb. This period may last for 1 or sometimes 2 days. The affected limb is dragged uselessly during locomotion. Active movement of the limb begins, usually on the second postoperative day, but it is uncontrolled and haphazard in its direction. The gait is wide-based, and the leg is not placed under the animal's center of gravity. If the locomotion is tested on boards of varying width, the cats can only negotiate the widest of them. The deafferented limb appears to be weak and capable of bearing very little weight. The inaccuracy of movements of the deafferented limb slow the animal's rate of locomotion considerably (Fig. 2). At this time the reflex movements of the deafferented leg can be elicited by stimulation of the intact systems. This is the period of recovery of generalized movements; movement has returned, but accuracy in the placement of the limb is absent.

During the second week postoperatively, several events occur which herald a dramatic change in motor ability. Certain extensor responses, including the vestibular placing response (extension of the limb during vertical drop) and the tilt responses, become hyperactive. The scratch reflex, a flexor response at all joints of the deafferented limb to stimulation of the ipsilateral ear, also becomes hyperactive. These are reflexes mediated exclusively by ipsilateral descending systems. In addition the animals now appear to use cues from the trunk, i.e., body posture and changes in center of gravity, to guide the hindlimb to more accurate placement. Now for the first time performance of a conditioned

LUMBOSACRAL   HEMI—DEAFFERENTATION

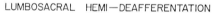
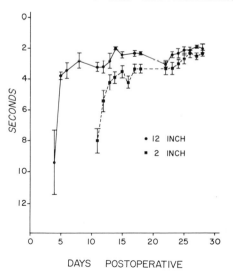

FIG. 2. Graph showing the rate of recovery of locomotion on a 12-inch wide runway and a 2-inch wide runway *(broken line)* in a unilaterally hindlimb-deafferented cat. Each crossing of the 9-foot runways was timed; each *point* on the graph represents the mean time for 10 crossings. The increase in speed of crossing the 12-inch runway occurs before the animals recover accurate placement of the limb which permits crossing of the 2-inch runway.

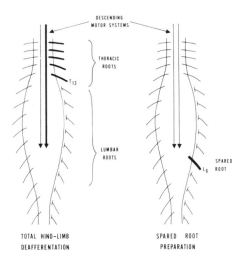

FIG. 3. These diagrams are intended to show which remaining systems increase in importance after total and partial deafferentation. The systems important for recovery are drawn in *thicker lines*. After removal of all dorsal roots (a) the ipsilateral descending systems (and to a lesser degree, the postural reflexes of the trunk, mediated in part by thoracic dorsal roots) mediate recovery. After partial deafferentation (b), recovery is mediated primarily by the spared root.

locomotor task shows that the cats can cross a runway only 2 inches in width (Fig. 2). The hindlimb is accurately placed on the narrow board without the use of vision, and of course, without somatotopic feedback from movement. Recovery is not affected by the presence or absence of the ventral root afferents and is also independent of preoperative training (15) (Fig. 3).

CHANGES IN DESCENDING SYSTEMS' PROJECTION AFTER DEAFFERENTATION

In order to explore the possible relationship between recovery and sprouting, behavioral observations can be used to suggest the anatomical pathways in which an increased projection might be anticipated. The increase in reflex activity during recovery was found only in reflexes mediated by ipsilateral descending supra- and propriospinal pathways (e.g., vestibular placing, scratch reflex). When the distribution of the totality of descending systems of the two sides was compared 1 year after hindlimb deafferentation (17), there was an increase in density and a spread of these projections on the previously deafferented side in all (deafferented) segments caudal to the deafferentation (L_1). The location of these increased projections was confined to some but not all of the normal projection fields of the descending systems. Certain parts of the gray matter partially denervated by the deafferentation, namely laminae I, II, and III of the dorsal horn and the motor nuclei of the ventral horn, received no compensatory projections from the descending systems. There was considerable sprouting into Clarke's nucleus which appeared on light microscopic examination to receive no direct descending projection on the control side. The fact that a direct descending projection was revealed by electron microscopy (Fig. 4) showed that Clarke's nucleus is no exception to the general rule that in the adult sprouting increases an already existing projection rather than creating a new and therefore aberrant

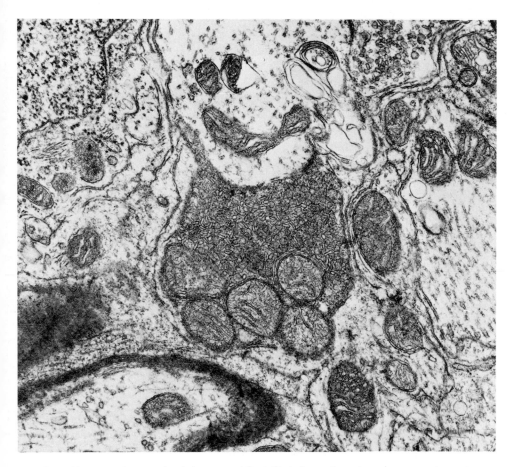

FIG. 4. Electron micrograph of the neurophil of Clarke's nucleus, L_3 segment, 4 days after ipsilateral lower thoracic hemisection (sparing the dorsal column). A number of dark, presumably degenerating terminals were found, only on the side of the lesion. They had flat and pleomorphic vesicles. This demonstrates the presence of a descending proprio- or supra-spinal projection to Clarke's nucleus which could not be detected in previous light microscopic studies (17).

projection. The sprouting of descending systems in response to deafferentation was therefore confined to laminae IV to VIII, regions of already existing overlap of the sensory and motor projections.

The Lowest Remaining Root Also Sprouts

The other behavioral observation relevant to the anatomical considerations is that of the increased importance of postural cues during recovery from hind-limb deafferentation. The increased reliance on postural reflexes for limb movements suggests the possibility of a greater use of information from the sensory nerves of the trunk; the importance of these reflexes in recovery would presumably be enhanced if the central processes of the dorsal roots of trunk nerves were to sprout. Therefore projections of the lowest remaining thoracic root (T_{13}) were examined in chronically hindlimb-deafferented cats. The ipsilateral T_{13} root had increased its projection during the postoperative year but in a rather limited and apparently specific fashion. The intraspinal projection had increased only locally, that is, in the segment of entry (T_{13}) and the immediately adjacent segments $(L_1$ and $T_{12})$. Furthermore, the increase was restricted to the ventral horn and zona intermedia. The ascending and descending spinal projections of the T_{13} root appeared to be symmetrical on the two sides, and the degeneration in Clarke's nucleus and dorsal horn was not increased. The ascending projection to nucleus gracilis also showed an apparently restricted increase, for the greater density and spread of degeneration was limited to the base of the nucleus at caudal levels and, less so, in the rostral reticular zone. The projection to the cell nest region was similar on the two sides. Thus after hindlimb deafferentation, evidence for sprouting from two systems was obtained: the lowest remaining thoracic root increased its input locally while caudal to this level the descending systems increased their projection field.

It is not possible to examine directly, with the available methods, the effect of sprouting upon recovery. It is possible, however, to examine the structures and mechanisms on which the recovery of locomotion and, in particular, accurate locomotion depend and further to ask whether the pathways that have sprouted are of particular importance for the recovered behavior. This can be answered in part by demonstrating decompensation due to a second lesion made in the animal that has recovered from hindlimb deafferentation. If decompensation takes place and the animals then recompensate to the previously recovered state, then the second lesion has presumably removed structures which were important for the behavior, without necessarily destroying the specific pathway(s) mediating the recovery. If the recompensation is less or fails to occur altogether after the second lesion, then presumably, the second lesion destroyed a system essential to maximal recovery. A lesion (hemisection) destroying the ipsilateral descending system in the deafferented, recovered animal abolished not only the recovery but all locomotion in the affected hindlimb. [Hemisection alone produces a relatively mild, temporary, locomotor deficit, (47).] In addition, the hyperactivity of ipsilateral descending reflexes (vestibular placing, tilt reflexes, scratch reflex) is also abolished. All of these effects are permanent. The contralateral descending systems and dorsal roots are unable to mediate locomotion in the deafferented, hemisected hindlimb. Thus the mediation of recovery is not equally distributed among all the remaining systems (Table 1).

ROLE OF TRUNK-POSTURAL REFLEXES IN LOCOMOTION AND IN RECOVERY FROM HINDLIMB DEAFFERENTATION

The postural reflexes of the trunk appeared to be important in the recovery

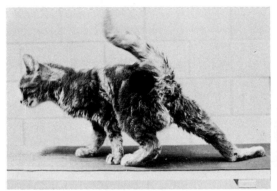
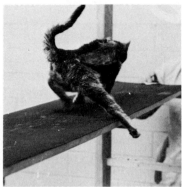

FIG. 5. Two cats with lower thoracic (T_5–T_{13}) deafferentations on the right side, showing the tonic bending of the trunk to the opposite side and the abnormal posture of the hindlimbs.

of accurate guidance of the deafferented hindlimb to appropriate destinations during locomotion. It is difficult if not impossible to destroy selectively central systems that control trunk-posture mechanisms but not phasic-limb movements. It is, however, possible to interfere with and imbalance the postural reflexes of the trunk by destroying their afferent input. Thus the lower thoracic roots (T_5–T_{13}) were cut unilaterally in otherwise normal animals. The early effects of this lesion are bizzare (Fig. 5). There is initially a loss of righting on the side of the lesion and the trunk is sharply twisted away from the side of the lesion. Fixation of the pelvis during locomotion is greatly impaired so that the hindquarters sway rather violently with each step. The posture of the hindlimbs is, acutely, frozen in ipsilateral flexion, contralateral extension. There is, as a result of this abnormal posture of the limbs, a suppression of placing and hopping reflexes. The fundamental deficit appears to be related to the loss of body-contact righting reflexes (41,52) from one side, with a consequent, unopposed and therefore relative overactivity of that same system from the intact side. Therefore, unilateral trunk deafferentation produces a deficit qualitatively and obviously different from unilateral hindlimb deafferentation. Both groups of animals are initially unable to walk, albeit for different reasons, but the time course of recovery of uncontrolled movement and recovery of accurate locomotion are very similar in the two groups. The degree of recovery (speed on narrow runways) is also similar.

The importance of lower thoracic roots and their postural reflexes for normal locomotion was surprising. Presumably, they would be even more important for locomotion of the deafferented hindlimb. This would be manifested as a decrease in recovery when the two deafferentations were combined. The recovery from the hindlimb deafferentation in those animals whose thoracic roots had been cut several months previously was indeed less than after simple hindlimb deafferentation. The time course and pattern of recovery was similar between

TABLE 1. Locomotor recovery

Lesion	Impairment	Recovery	Reflexes important for recovery	Anatomical observation
Hindlimb deafferentation	Severe	Of accurate locomotion	Postural (trunk) Ipsilateral descending	Sprouting from lowest remaining root (T_{13}), sprouting of ipsilateral descending system
Thoracic deafferentation	Severe	Of accurate locomotion	Hindlimb reflexes	Sprouting of ascending collaterals of lumbosacral dorsal roots
Hindlimb deafferentation and ipsilateral hemisection	Complete (no locomotion)	None	—	No sprouting of contralateral dorsal roots
Spared root preparation (L_6 spared–all other lumbosacral roots cut)	Mild	Almost "complete"	Segmental reflexes of spared root	Sprouting of spared root, no sprouting from descending systems
Hemisection (alone)	Mild	Of accurate locomotion	Segmental reflexes (ipsilateral)	Sprouting of ipsilateral dorsal root

the lumbosacral deafferented animals and those in whom thoracic roots had previously been removed; general locomotor movements performed on wide runways began to recover on the second day postoperatively, whereas accurate locomotion took place beginning in the second week. The movements never became as accurate in the absence of thoracic roots, and therefore the animals were permanently slower in the locomotor test. Thus the ipsilateral thoracic dorsal roots play a role in recovery from hindlimb deafferentation, but their presence, when ipsilateral descending systems are destroyed (by hemisection), is ineffective in providing any recovery whatsoever. This implies that the contribution of thoracic roots to recovery from lumbosacral deafferentation is mediated through the ipsilateral descending systems and that these descending systems are essential for recovery in the deafferented hindlimb. Cues for posture mediated by ipsilateral thoracic dorsal roots will be used for recovery, if present, but in the absence of the thoracic roots the descending systems can use other cues in guiding the limb to accurate placements during locomotion (Table 1).

RECOVERY AND SPROUTING ARE REGULATED, PERHAPS HIER-ARCHICALLY: THE SPARED ROOT PREPARATION

Thoracic dorsal roots and ipsilateral descending systems both contribute to the mediation of recovery from hindlimb deafferentation, but they are not equally important (Table 1). These observations suggest the possibility of a hierarchical regulation of recovery mechanisms. This can be explored further by examining the spared root preparation. In the spared root preparation, all the lumbar and sacral dorsal roots but one (usually L_6) are cut. In these animals the locomotor deficits are quantitatively different from deficits following deafferentation. Recovey occurs more quickly and is more nearly complete, and there are no indications that the ipsilateral descending systems contribute to the mediation of that recovery. There is, first, considerable sparing of function. The affected hindlimb is used for locomotion soon after the lesion. If the root spared is one which innervates the foot, the animals recover enough accuracy by the third or fourth postoperative day, so that they can successfully walk along the narrow (2 inch) runway. If the root spared is one which innervates only the proximal parts of the limb, there is somewhat less sparing of locomotor function, and accurate movements do not return until the second week. The sparing of placing and hopping reflexes underlies the greater sparing of locomotion. Placing reactions are performed, crudely, early in the postoperative period. The receptive zone for eliciting placing depends on the peripheral distribution of the root which was spared. This reflexogenous zone does not change postoperatively. The placing response, however, becomes more easily elicited and more accurately performed during the second week. If the spared root innervates the foot, then hopping will also be present. Other characteristics of recovery are also different in the totally and partially (spared root) deafferented hindlimbs. Abnormal patterns for locomotion, e.g., 3-legged locomotion, used at times by the deafferented animal, never occurs. The reflex activity of the ipsilateral descending system, e.g., scratch reflex and vestibular reflexes, are never depressed but, more significantly, at no time do they become hyperactive. In contrast, the segmental reflexes mediated by the spared root, e.g., tendon reflexes, become considerably stronger during the recovery period. (Fig. 3).

If the anatomical experiments which revealed increased descending projections in the deafferented animals are repeated in spared root preparations, there is a striking difference (Table 2) in the results. The test lesion, spinal transection, in the deafferented cat demonstrated an increase in descending projection on the experimental side. This is not the case in the spared root preparation. The same acute lesion in the chronic spared root preparation yields a normal and comparable distribution of degeneration on both sides. The presence of the spared root apparently prevented the increase in descending projections that occurs when all the roots are cut. If, instead, the spared root and its equivalent on the contralateral, control side of the cord are cut acutely one year after the partial deafferentiation, the distribution of the intraspinal degeneration demonstrates an increase in the projection of the spared root. This was demonstrated first by Liu and Chambers (34). The increased projection was found in all cord segments to which the spared root normally projected and in the nucleus gracilis. As in other preparations, these increased projections were not found in all partially denervated areas. There was an increased density of dorsal root degeneration in the zona intermedia and in Clarke's nucleus in most spinal segments examined. Most dramatic, however, was the increased density and lateral spread of the projection within the dorsal horn by the spared dorsal root (Fig. 6). In contrast, the projection to the motor neuron pools of lamina IX was not increased, although these regions were certainly partly denervated by the original lesion. In the nucleus gracilis, there is also an increase in the spared root's projection and, once again, the increase in selective. In the cell nest (cluster) region, there is no increase; whereas in the base of the nucleus, at the same rostrocaudal levels, and rostrally, in the reticular zone of the nucleus, there is an increased projection (Fig. 7).

Spared Root Versus Lowest Remaining Root

Both a spared root (all roots cut above and below L_6 or L_5, the intact one) and a lowest remaining root (T_{13}, all lumbosacral roots cut) can increase their projections. The pattern and amount of increase is not the same, however, and these differences cannot be explained simply by differences in amount of denervation in the two experimental paradigms. Differences in patterns of dorsal root sprouting in the spared root (L_6) preparation and the lowest remaining root (T_{13}) preparation are qualitative as well as quantitative. In the projection to nucleus gracilis, the localization of the increased projection is similar in the two cases; it occurs in the base and in the rostral reticular regions but not in the cell nest region. In the spinal cord, in both preparations, the projection

TABLE 2. *Distribution of sprouting*

System tested	Chronic lesion	Test lesion	Presence and location of sprouting
Ipsilateral descending systems	Lumbosacral deafferentation	Transection at T_{13}–L_1	Laminae IV–VIII below L_1
Lowest remaining root (T_{13})	Lumbosacral deafferentation	Bilateral section of T_{13} roots	Nucleus gracilis base (not cell nests); ventral horn in segments T_{13}, T_{12}, L_1 and zona intermedia
Ipsilateral descending systems	Spared root preparation (lumbosacral deafferentation sparing L_6)	Transection at T_{13}–L_1	No sprouting of descending systems seen
Spared root (L_6)	Spared root preparation (lumbosacral deafferentation sparing L_6)	Bilateral section of L_6 roots	Nucleus gracilis base (not in cell nests) and reticular region; dorsal horn, zona intermedia and Clarke's nucleus of spinal cord

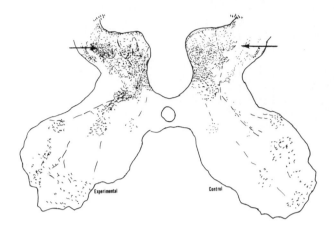

FIG. 6. Tracing of L_6 spinal segment of a cat (spared root preparation) in which the dorsal roots of one side, sparing L_6, were cut. One year later L_6 was cut on both sides. Four days later the animal was killed and the spinal cord stained by Nauta and Fink-Heimer techniques. The figure shows the L_6 projections on the **experimental** and **control** sides. The degeneration around the motoneurons of the ventral horn appears similar on the two sides. The **experimental side** shows an increase in the projection within the lateral part of the dorsal horn and in the zona intermedia. The increased degeneration presumably reflects sprouting of terminals and/ or axon collaterals into some of the denervated regions at some time during the postoperative year.

to the zona intermedia is increased. They differ, however, in that the spared root's projection to the dorsal horn and Clarke's nucleus is increased, whereas the projection of the lowest remaining root is increased in the ventral horn. Furthermore, the lowest remaining root increases its projection only locally, e.g., in its segment of entry (T_{13}) and the immediately adjacent segments (L_1 and T_{12}). Caudal to this, an increase in descending system degeneration is found. The spared root projection is increased in all segments to which it projects normally, and at the same time, sprouting from descending systems is apparently absent in those segments. Furthermore, the increase in the projection of the lowest remaining T_{13} root is much less than that of the spared root. The reason for this difference is not clear. The pattern of increase suggests several trends that can be examined experimentally: (a) The increase is found in those regions in which the normal projection is greatest. Thoracic roots have a relatively small projection to the dorsal horn and Clarke's nucleus, but a large one to the ventral horn where the increase occurs. The spared lumbar root increases its projection in the regions in which its normal input is greatest; the dorsal horn and Clarke's nucleus. Perhaps a critical density and number of normal terminals in a projection is required for sprouting of the projection to be demonstrable. (b) The original denervation is different quantitatively and qualitatively in the two preparations. The amount of surrounding denervation of the spared root's terminal field is greater than that of the lowest remaining root. The greater denervation might elicit more sprouting but should not determine its differential distribution. (c) The spared root (L_6), representing the hindlimb,

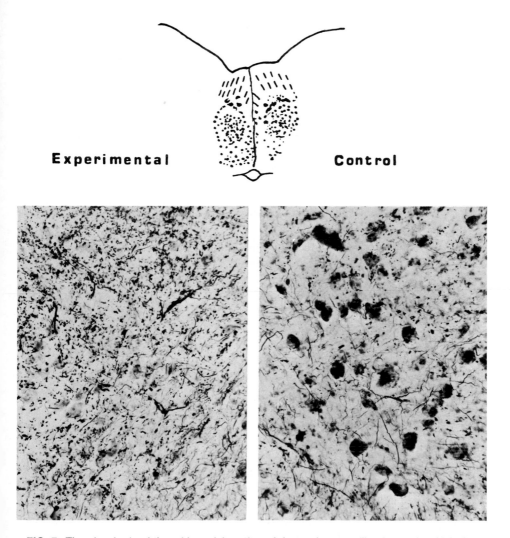

FIG. 7. The *drawing* is of the mid-caudal portion of the nucleus gracilis of a cat in which the dorsal roots on one side, sparing L_6, were cut (same preparation as Fig. 6). The *diagram* shows the L_6 projections on the **experimental** (previously deafferented) and **control** sides. The projection is equal in the cell cluster region but increased in the ventral part (base) of the nucleus. A photomicrograph of the base region of the two sides shows this increase on the experimental sides.

is asked to sprout into space normally occupied by other hindlimb roots (homonymous sprouting). T_{13}, however, represents the trunk, and may replace hindlimb afferents (heteronymous sprouting) with greater difficulty suggesting that the functional and anatomical organization of dorsal roots and their central targets may determine the capacity to sprout into denervated territory and to subserve recovery of function.

RULES FOR RECOVERY: OVERLAP HELPS

Several factors appear to determine the ability of remaining systems to mediate recovery of locomotion after dorsal roots are removed. If one hindlimb dorsal root remains when the rest have been destroyed, the local segmental information from its single dermatone-myotome appears to be the most effective cue in guiding movements of the hindlimb and, therefore, in substituting for the loss of peripheral segmental information from the rest of the limb segments. It is important to note here that there is no recovery of the function of the destroyed dorsal roots; the reflex activity which they mediated preoperatively does not return. Thus, the tendon reflexes are abolished except for those one or two which the spared root normally mediates. The same is true for the placing and hopping responses. There is no postoperative spread of reflexogenous zone and no change in the number of reflexes evoked by peripheral stimulation. Only the residual reflexes become more potent over time and more effective in guiding movements of the deafferented parts of the limb. In these spared root animals, there is no perceptible change in the use of postural (trunk) reflexes, no appearance of abnormal motor patterns, and no increase in descending reflex activity. In the absence of the spared lumbar root (complete hindlimb deafferentation), reflexes from more rostral spinal segments, i.e., those of the trunk, contribute to locomotor recovery. It is not clear whether the trunk righting reflexes themselves are used as cues for accurate limb position or the righting reflexes and other postural cues for deafferented limb movements are simply mediated by the same structures. Imbalance of the body righting reflexes and disturbance of postural cues for movement produced by cutting the dorsal roots of one side of the trunk causes: (a) A severe locomotor impairment which shows amelioration in two or three weeks, and (b) a permanent reduction in the amount of recovery which is possible after hindlimb deafferentation. Control of deafferented hindlimb movements, however, does not require reflexes mediated by thoracic roots, since in their absence incomplete recovery of normal locomotor patterns takes place *pari passu* with the use of abnormal (3-legged) locomotor patterns and increasing activity of descending reflexes. In contrast, in the absence of the ipsilateral descending reflex system no recovery occurs, and the affected hindlimb is never used again in locomotion. The inability of the contralateral reflex systems to take over the mediation of these hindlimb movements has no obvious explanation. It has been shown that neither descending systems nor dorsal roots are required for locomotion (20–22,39) elicited by treadmills, brainstem stimulation, or drugs. Apparently the contingencies are different for the production of voluntary, overground locomotion.

Control of Systems Which Mediate Recovery; Overlap is not Enough

It appears that the process by which one system is substituted for another in the mediation of locomotor function obeys certain laws. The residual function most similar to those destroyed, i.e., that mediated by a spared lumbar root, is most efficient and provides the most nearly complete recovery. The spared root also prevents the appearance of exaggerated postural and descending reflex activity which follows complete deafferentation. The trunk reflexes are less capable of mediating the return of near-normal locomotion. This postural reflex system appears to utilize a supraspinal pathway since the trunk dorsal roots are ineffective in mediating recovery unless the descending systems are also present. Recovery mediated by the descending systems is qualitatively different from that seen when one root is spared. The substitution of nontopographic feedback is certainly less efficient than the topographic input mediated by dorsal roots in guiding accurate limb movements. Transmission to the spinal cord of the nontopographic information depends on the integrity of only the ipsilateral descending systems, not of all remaining systems. The contralateral reflex systems alone cannot confer "voluntary" locomotion upon a hindlimb. Apparently, substitution has not only relative but also absolute limits.

Recovery Occurs in Stages

In the preparations examined so far (hindlimb deafferentation, trunk deafferentation, spared root preparation, hemisection) the recovery of reflexes and locomotion appeared to take place in stages. Regardless of the lesion, there is always a period, lasting one or two days, in which little or no movement is elicited by activation of intact reflex systems, or by the animal itself. This of course is the period of spinal shock (58) or diaschesis (45). Hyperpolarization of motor neurons (2) could be the basis of the hypo- or areflexia, although the reason for the hyperpolarization is unknown. The first signs of recovery are characterized by (a) the reemergence of reflex activity, and (b) the appearance of "voluntary" but poorly controlled movements. This is the time in which previously "silent synapses" have become effective in driving partially denervated cells (3,44,70) and also the time in which denervation supersensitivity might be expected to begin (61). During the second postoperative week, a more specific change is superimposed upon the pattern of generalized activity. Reflex hyperactivity attributable to one of the residual systems develops, and accurate movement returns. This is the period in which, on the basis of a number of observations (9,10,37,40,42), sprouting of new terminals might be expected to become important.

RULES FOR SPROUTING: OVERLAP AND PROXIMITY ARE NOT ENOUGH

Organization of the Postsynaptic Cell Group

An increased projection due, presumably, to sprouting, has been demonstrated in the same anatomical pathways which contribute to recovery after partial or total hindlimb deafferentation; a spared lumbar dorsal root, a lowest remaining thoracic root, and the ipsilateral descending systems. Just as the recovered behavior was never exactly the same as the behavior that had been lost, so the increased projections do not appear to restore the normal amount of afferent input. Thus, some structures that were partially denervated do not seem to receive a replacement for the lost system. For example, sprouting into the cell nest region of the nucleus gracilis has not been seen, nor has it been found among the motor nuclei of the spinal cord. Increased projections to immediately adjacent nuclear groups *have* been revealed by degeneration methods; the base of the gracilis, the zona intermedia (lamina VII) of the spinal cord. The major differences between the former regions in which no substituted projection appears, and the latter, in which sprouting can be shown, is the degree of "tightness" of organization (cf. 14).

The cell nest region of the dorsal column nuclei and the spinal motor nuclei receive restricted, highly topographical afferent input, and this type of organization characterizes their output as well. The factors which originally determined this exclusiveness of input during development may still operate in the adult state and may prevent sprouting from occurring in regions organized in a restricted and topographic way. The failure of sprouting to occur in the lateral geniculate nucleus (23) and the failure of cervical roots to sprout into trigeminal territory (27) would be consistent with this interpretation. This does not preclude the possibility that new terminals attempt reinnervation of denervated sites. It does suggest that they may be unsuccessful in certain parts of the nervous system and that the laws determining original synaptic organization persist after loss of an afferent system.

Proximity: Sprouting Occurs Within the Confines of the Original Projection and Denervation

Not only do some CNS regions seem to be resistant to sprouting but, when sprouting does occur, the sprouting fibers appear to fail to grow beyond the confines of their original projection field in the spinal cord. Whether the denervation is maximal, as in the dorsal horn of the deafferented animal, or less severe, as in the case of the motor neurons in the same preparation, the descending systems, which sprout into adjacent laminae, stop short of extending beyond their original projection at least as far as can be determined by degeneration methods with the light microscope. Two factors may be active here; distance and some specific relationship between a presynaptic terminal and a postsynaptic site, i.e., "neural specificity." Studies of sprouting made with the electron microscope show that sprouted terminals may extend along a dendrite or from a dendrite to the soma (50,53). In the adult, these sprouts may not be able to grow from cell to cell or into adjacent nuclei, even though in the infant such growth is easily demonstrated (25,38,48,49). The effect of specificity is much more difficult to evaluate. Our own results suggest that overlap, although a requirement for sprouting in the adult, is not enough; neural specificity may play a role, probably restraining, in establishing the success or failure of sprouting.

Competition May Also Be Important

Neural specificity may also act as a relative rather than an absolute restraint. When two different but overlapping systems are given access to the same denervated space, one may succeed in forming permanent sprouts at the expense of the other. For example, at the end of 1 year sprouting by descending tracts can be demonstrated by degeneration methods after total deafferentation but not when one root is spared. This is apparently the lasting anatomical change. These methods tell us nothing of the dynamic events (cf. 4) which occur during that year. It is possible that the descending tract axons do form sprouts in both the totally and partially (spared root) deafferented preparations. In fact, one can imagine that in the initial postlesion period sprouting may be a property of all terminals in the immediate vicinity, but that not all of these sprouts persist. Some sprouts appear to make competent synapses (50,53). Others, unsuccessful, may degenerate or be resorbed. Why one group of sprouts is successful and another is not may have a simple answer. Perhaps persisting sprouts are those which normally occupy sites on the membrane nearest to the denervated spaces, or it may be the postsynaptic receptor which has a mechanism for accepting some sprouting terminals and rejecting others.

A FEW LAWS WHICH SPROUTING MAY OBEY

Strict definitions of neural specificity, like strict notions of functional localization, will account for some of our observations of collateral sprouting or recovery of function but not others. The fact that dorsal roots can be induced to increase their projections even in the adult cat, implies that the rules which govern the establishment and maintenance of synaptic contacts in the CNS are subject to modification. It is equally important to recognize, however, that sprouting is limited; it does not occur randomly and can be demonstrated only under certain conditions.

Our observations suggest conditions which are important for the demonstration of sprouting. These conditions include: (a) Proximity or overlap of the destroyed and sprouting projection systems; (b) the nature of the functional organization of the postsynaptic structures; and, (c) the competition between the overlapping projection systems which remain.

Proximity and Overlap

In the damaged adult nervous system, neurons do not appear to make aberrant connections. Axonal growth then does not seem to occur outside of the normal projection field. Increased projections are therefore limited to areas in close proximity to the original projection of the sprouting system, which overlaps the one that was destroyed.

Organization of the Postsynaptic Cell Group

The presence of proximate or overlapping projections, however, is not sufficient for the demonstration of sprouting. The nature of the synaptic organization also seems to be important. Sprouting is less easily demonstrated in areas of strict somatotopic organization. Whether this reflects minimal convergence at the cellular level in strictly somatotopic organization, or other factors (e.g., receptor specificity) is not known.

Competition

The demonstration of sprouting will also depend upon which systems remain, indicating that not all remaining systems are equipotential in the formation of persisting sprouts.

UNKNOWN LAWS

Other factors regulating sprouting cannot be examined by the methods we have used to examine the distribution of projection systems. For example, the role of interneurons merits consideration. Sprouting by local neurons certainly cannot be excluded, but our methods cannot reveal the presence of such sprouting. Significant sprouting by interneurons, however, might restrict sprouting by long tracts. Second, the limited patterns of sprouting we have described represent the anatomical changes which persist a year or more after the original experimental lesion. It is clearly possible that many or most sprouts do not survive very long. The factors responsible for the survival of some of these sprouts, but not others, would determine in part the final projection pattern which is reestablished. Third, the final projection pattern may be affected by mechanical factors if they facilitate growth of sprouts in some directions and prevent it in others. Glial cells represent a candidate for this process, since they are mobilized to phagocytize the degenerating axons produced by the initial lesion and are therefore present in locally significant numbers at the time and place where sprouting occurs. The processes of glial cells do not necessarily present a barrier to axonal growth (cf. 51). Furthermore, glia seem to aid in regeneration of some systems rather than to block it (46), and they may similarly aid in the direction of sprouting terminals. Finally, following axotomy, glial processes intervene between the axotomized cell and its presynaptic terminals (63). When regeneration takes place, the processes are apparently retracted, and synaptic contact is reestablished. The glia are therefore also capable of considerable plasticity.

It is interesting that in parts of the nervous system in which shrinkage and gliosis are maximal, e.g., in the dorsal horn after complete deafferentation (17) and cell clusters of the Nucleus gracilis, evidence of sprouting was not seen. When, in the spared root preparation, sprouting occurred in the dorsal horn, the amount of shrinkage was greatly reduced *(unpublished observations)*. Conceivably, sprouting aids in the maintenance of more normal morphology. Alternatively, very dense gliosis and marked shrinkage may, in some cases, act as a barrier to sprouting.

SPECIFIC FUNCTIONS DO NOT RECOVER; SYSTEMS DESTROYED DO NOT REGENERATE

The recovery of movement following partial or complete hindlimb deafferentation is mediated by some of the remaining spinal systems. There is no evidence that these systems alter their reflex functions during recovery or mediate functions which they did not already subserve preoperatively. There is some evidence that these functions increase in strength and/or that they exert a greater control over limb movements than in the normal animal. The abolished reflexes never return. This would explain the observation that the recovered movements are always somewhat different, at least in their details, from the normal ones, although they may achieve the same ends. The recovery is not mediated equally by the remaining systems; some are more important than others, as demonstrated by the degree of decompensation and later recompensation due to the second lesion. The systems shown to be important or essential for recovery are also shown to increase their projection fields at some time during the recovery period due presumably to sprouting. The increased projection may be responsible for the increased activity of the reflexes mediated by the sprouting system. If the normal amount of reflex activity in these systems is inadequate to mediate recovery, this would explain the failure of recovery to occur sooner. The substitution of one reflex system for another, i.e., the one initially lost, does not occur immediately; its effects are seen on the 8th to 10th day. The changes in a system which underlie the observed increase in its activity and which occur during that period are unknown. The evidence that sprouting is involved in this process is thus purely circumstantial. It is our hypothesis, however, that the failure of recovery of accurate movement to occur before the second week demonstrates that the undamaged systems do not simply "take over" the missing functions until there is some change in these systems. We suggest that enhancement of the normal function of a remaining system is part of the process by which this function is substituted for the one lost, thus providing recovery of movement, and furthermore, that sprouting of new terminals from this same system could mediate the enhancement of its normal function.

Lesions which interrupt projections to the spinal cord are followed by an impairment in general usage of the limbs and a loss of specific motor patterns (1,15,17,30,47,68). Many specific motor patterns are permanently lost although similar movements can often be retrieved by the use of conditioning procedures (5,13,35,66). A considerable degree of recovery is seen, however, in the generalized usage of the limbs (14). Collateral sprouting is more readily demonstrated in areas of generalized, overlapping projections than in the more specifically somatotopically organized regions (15,17,18,47). The greater sprouting in areas of generalized projections may underlie the greater recovery of generalized movements.

ACKNOWLEDGMENTS

The help of the following people is greatly appreciated: Edith Coleman, Barbara Nance, George Grigonis, Lynn Prendergast, and Dianne Struse. Supported by the National Institutes of Health grant NS11919.

REFERENCES

1. Bard, P. (1938): Studies on the cortical representation of somatic sensibility. *Bull. N.Y. Acad. Med.,* 555–605.
2. Barnes, C. D., Joynt, R. J., and Schottelius, B. A. (1962): Motoneuron resting potentials in spinal shock. *Am. J. Physiol.,* 203:1113–116.
3. Basbaum, A. I., and Wall, P. D. (1976): Chronic changes in the response of cells in adult cat dorsal horn following partial deafferentation. *Brain Res.,* 116:181–207.
4. Bernstein, J. J., Geldred, J. B., and Bernstein, M. E. (1974): Alteration of neuronal synaptic contact during regeneration and axonal sprouting of rat spinal cord. *Exp. Neurol.,* 44:470–482.
5. Chambers, W. W., and Kozart, D. (1965): Conditional tactile discrimination in monkey with corticospinal or pyramidal tract lesions. *Anat. Rec.,* 151:499.
6. Chambers, W. W., and Liu, C. N. (1957): Corticospinal tract in the cat. *J. Comp. Neurol.,* 198:23–55.
7. Chambers, W. W., and Liu, C. N. (1958): Corticospinal tract in the monkey. *Fed. Proc.,* 17:24.
8. Coggeshall, R. E., Coulter, J. D., and Willis, W. D. (1974): Unmyelinated axons in the ventral roots of the cat lumbosacral enlargement. *J. Comp. Neurol.,* 153:39–58.
9. Cotman, C. W., Matthews, D. A., Taylor, D., and Lynch, G. (1973): Synaptic rearrangement in dentate gyrus. *Proc. Natl. Acad. Sci. U.S.A.,* 70:3473–3477.
10. Cotman, C. W., and Lynch, G. S. (1976): Reactive synaptogenesis in the adult nervous system. In: *Neuronal Recognition,* edited by S. H. Barondes. Plenum Press, New York.
11. Cunningham, T. J. (1972): Sprouting of the optic projections after cortical lesions. *Anat. Rec.,* 172:288.
12. Edds, M. V., Jr. (1953): Collateral nerve regeneration. *Quart. Rev. Biol.,* 28:260–276.
13. Goldberger, M. E. (1972): Restitution of function in the CNS: the pathological grasp reflex. *Exp. Brain Res.,* 15:79–96.
14. Goldberger, M. E. (1974): Recovery of movement following lesions of the motor systems in monkeys. In: *Recovery of Function after Brain Damage,* edited by D. G. Stein. Academic Press, New York.
15. Goldberger, M. E. (1977): Locomotor recovery after unilateral hindlimb deafferentation in cats. *Brain Res.,* 123:59–74.
16. Goldberger, M. E., and Growden, J. H. (1973): Pattern of recovery following cerebellar deep nuclear lesions in monkeys. *Exp. Neurol.,* 39:307–322.
17. Goldberger, M. E., and Murray, M. (1974): Restitution of function and collateral sprouting in the cat spinal cord: the deafferented animal. *J. Comp. Neurol.,* 158:37–54.
18. Goldberger, M. E., and Murray, M. (1976): Lack of collateral sprouting and its presence after spinal lesions in the adult cat. *Neuroscience II* (2):814.

19. Goodman, D. G., and Horel, J. A. (1966): Sprouting of the optic tract projections in the brain stem of the rat. *J. Comp. Neurol.*, 127:71–83.
20. Grillner, S. (1975): Locomotion in vertebrates: central mechanisms and reflex interaction. *Physiol. Rev.*, 55:247–364.
21. Grillner, S., and Zangger, P. (1974): Locomotor movements generated by the deafferented spinal cord. *Acta Physiol. Scand.*, 91:387–394.
22. Grillner, S., and Zangger, P. (1975): How detailed is the central pattern for locomotion? *Brain Res.*, 88:367–371.
23. Guillery, R. W. (1972): Experiments to determine whether retino geniculate axons can form translaminar collateral sprouts in the dorsal lateral geniculate of the cat. *J. Comp. Neurol.*, 146:407–419.
24. Hand, P. (1966): Lumbosacral dorsal root terminations in the nucleus gracilis of the cat. Some observations of terminal degeneration in other medullary sensory nuclei. *J. Comp. Neurol.*, 126:137–156.
25. Hicks, S. P., and D'Amato, C. J. (1970): Motor-sensory and visual behavior after hemispherectomy in newborn and mature rats. *Exp. Neurol.*, 29:416–438.
26. Hultborn, H. (1972): Convergence on interneurons in the reciprocal Ia pathway to motoneurons. *Acta Physiol. Scand. (Suppl.)*, 375:1–42.
27. Kerr, F. W. L. (1972): The potential of cervical primary afferents to sprout into the spinal nucleus of V following long term trigeminal denervation. *Brain Res.*, 43:547–560.
28. Krieg, W. J. S., and Groat, R. A. (1944): Topography of the spinal cord and vertebral column of the cat. *Quart. Bull. Northwestern Univ. Med. Sch.*, 18:265–268.
29. Kruger, L., Siminoff, R., and Witkovsky, P. (1961): Single unit analysis of dorsal column nuclei and spinal nucleus of trigeminal in cat. *J. Neurophysiol.*, 24:353–349.
30. Kuypers, H. G. J. M. (1964): The descending pathways to the spinal cord, their anatomy and function. In: Organization of the Spinal Cord. *Prog. Brain Res.*, 11:178–203.
31. Kuypers, H. G. J. M., and Tuerk, J. D. (1964): The distribution of cortical fibers within the nuclei cuneatus and gracilis in the cat. *J. Anat.*, 98:143–162.
32. Liu, C. N. (1956): Afferent nerves to Clarke's and the lateral cuneate nuclei in the cat. *Arch. Neurol.*, 75:67–77.
33. Liu, C. N. (1977): *Personal Communication.*
34. Liu, C. N., and Chambers, W. W. (1958): Intraspinal sprouting of dorsal root axons. *Arch. Neurol. Psychiatr.* 79:46–61.
35. Liu, C. N., and Chambers, W. W. (1962): Conditioned tactual responses and discrete movements in monkeys with pyramidal lesions. *Fed. Proc.*, 21:376.
36. Liu, C. N., and Chambers, W. W. (1971): A study of cerebellar dyskinesia in the bilaterally deafferented forelimbs of the monkey. *Acta Neurobiol. Exp.*, 31:263–289.
37. Loeser, J. D., and Ward, A. A. (1967): Some effects of deafferentation on neurons of the cat spinal cord. *Arch. Neurol.*, 17:629–636.
38. Lund, R. D., and Lund, J. S. (1971): Synaptic adjustment after deafferentation of the superior colliculus of the rat. *Science*, 171:804–807.
39. Lundberg, A., (1966): Integration in the reflex pathway. In: *Muscular Afferents and Motor Control*, edited by R. Granit, pp. 275–307. Wiley, New York.
40. Lynch, G. S., and Cotman, C. W. (1975): The hippocampus as a model for studying anatomical plasticity in the adult brain. In: *The Hippocampus, Vol. I.*, edited by R. I. Isaccson and R. H. Pribram, pp. 123–151. Plenum, New York.
41. Magnus, R. (1926): Studies on the physiology of posture. *Lancet*, 2:531–536.
42. McCouch, G. P., Austin, G. M., Liu, C. N., and Liu, C. Y. (1958): Sprouting as a cause of spasticity. *J. Neurophysiol.*, 21:205–216.
43. Millar, J., and Basbaum, A. I. (1975): Topography of the body surface of the cat to cuneate and gracile nuclei. *Exp. Neurol.*, 49:287–290.
44. Millar, J., Basbaum, A. I., and Wall, P. D. (1976): Restructuring of the somatotopic map and appearance of abnormal neuronal activity in the gracile nucleus after partial deafferentation. *Exp. Neurol.*, 50:658–672.
45. Monakow, C. von (1914): Die Lokalisation in grosshern und der albou der funktion durch kortikale hinde. Wiesbaden, J. F. Bergmann.
46. Murray, M. (1976): Regeneration of retinal axons into the goldfish optic tectum. *J. Comp. Neurol.*, 168:175–196.

47. Murray, M., and Goldberger, M. E. (1974): Restitution of function and collateral sprouting in the cat spinal cord: The partially hemisected animal. *J. Comp. Neurol.,* 155:19–36.
48. Nah, S. H., and Leong, S. K. (1976a): An ultrastructural study of the anomalous corticorubral projection following neonatal lesions in the albino rat. *Brain Res.,* 111:162–166.
49. Nah, S. H., and Leong, S. K. (1976b): Bilateral corticofugal projection to the red nucleus after neonatal lesions in the albino rat. *Brain Res.,* 197:433–436.
50. Nakamura, Y., Mizunn, N., Koniski, A., and Sato, M. (1974): Synaptic reorganization of the red nucleus after chronic deafferentation from cerebellorubral fibers. *Brain Res.,* 82:293–301.
51. Prendergast, J., and Stelzner, D. J. (1976): Increases in collateral axonal growth rostral to a thoracic hemisection in neonatal and weanling rat. *J. Comp. Neurol.,* 166:145–162.
52. Rademaker, A. (1931): *Das Stehen* translated and summarized by A. Mussen, *Arch. Neurol.,* 28:141–163.
53. Raisman, G. (1969): Neuronal plasticity in the septal nuclei of the adult rat. *Brain Res.,* 14:25–48.
54. Rustioni, A. (1973): Non-primary afferents to the nucleus gracilis from the lumbar cord of the cat. *Brain Res.,* 52:81–95.
55. Rustioni, A., and Macchi, G. (1968): Distribution of dorsal root fibers in the medulla oblongata of the cat. *J. Comp. Neurol.,* 134:113–126.
56. Rustioni, A., and Molenaar, I. (1975): Dorsal column nuclei afferents in the lateral funiculus of the cat: distribution pattern and absence of sprouting after chronic deafferentation. *Exp. Brain Res.,* 23:1–12.
57. Rustioni, A., and Sotelo, C. (1974): Synaptic organization of the nucleus gracilis of the cat. Experimental identification of dorsal root fibers and cortical afferents. *J. Comp. Neurol.,* 155:441–468.
58. Sherrington, C. S. (1899): On the spinal animal. *Med-chiro. Trans.,* 82:449–477.
59. Sprague, J. M. (1958): The distribution of dorsal root fibers on motor cells in the lumbosacral spinal cord of the cat, and the site of excitatory and inhibitory terminals in monosynaptic pathways. *Proc. Roy. Soc. B.,* 149:534–556.
60. Sprague, J. M., and Ha, H. (1964): The terminal fields of dorsal root fibers in the lumbosacral spinal cord of the cat, and the dendritic organization of the motor nuclei. *Prog. Brain Res.,* 11:120–154.
61. Stavraki, G. W. (1961): *Supersensitivity Following Lesions of the Nervous System.* Univ. of Toronto Press. Toronto, Canada, p. 205.
62. Stelzner, D. J., and Weber, E. (1974): A lack of dorsal root sprouting found after spinal hemisection in neonatal or weanling rat. *Society for Neuroscience Program and Abstracts,* pp. 437.
63. Sumner, B. E. H., and Sutherland, F. I. (1973): Quantitative electron microscopy on the injured hypoglossal nucleus in the rat. *J. Neurocytol.,* 2:315–328.
64. Szenthagethei, J. (1963): Neuronal and synaptic arrangement in the substantia gelatinosa rolandi. *J. Comp. Neurol.*
65. Szenthegothai, J., and Kiss, T. (1949): Projection of dermatomes on the substantia gelatinosa. *Arch. Neurol.,* 62:734–744.
66. Taub, E. (1977): Movement in non-human primates deprived of somatosensory feedback. *Exercise and Sport Sci. Rev.,* 4:335–374.
67. Taub, E., and Berman, A. J. (1968): Movement and learning in the absence of sensory feedback. In: *The Neuropsychology of Spatially Oriented Behavior,* pp. 173–192. Dorsey, Homewood, Illinois.
68. Tower, S. S. (1935): The dissociation of cortical excitation from cortical inhibition by pyramid section and the syndrome of that lesion in the cat. *Brain,* 58:238–255.
69. Twitchell, I. E. (1954): Sensory factors in purposive movement. *J. Neurophysiol.,* 17:239–252.
70. Wall, P. D., and Egger, M. D. (1971): Formation of new connections in adult rat brains after partial deafferentation. *Nature (Lond.),* 232:542–545.
71. Wiesendanger, M. (1964): Rigidity produced by deafferentation. *Acta Physiol. Scand.,* 62:160–168.

Neuronal Plasticity, edited by
Carl W. Cotman.
Raven Press, New York © 1978.

Plasticity of Connection in the Adult Nervous System

E. G. Merrill and P. D. Wall

Cerebral Functions Research Group, Department of Anatomy, University College London, London WC1E 6BT, England

In a series of different types of experiments on the somatosensory system in adult rat and cat, we have established that when cells lose their normal afferent input, they may begin to respond to a novel input. Here we review the evidence for this switching of inputs and then proceed to discuss the mechanisms by which the changes might occur. There are six classes of mechanisms which might explain the switch (see Fig. 1): (1) denervated cells atrophy and normally innervated cells migrate into the shrunken region; (2) intact afferents sprout to occupy the evacuated sites; (3) disinhibition of existing afferents; (4) disinhibition of polysynaptic alternative drives; (5) disinhibition via transsynaptic denervation atrophy of inhibitory cells; (6) the appearance of activity in normally silent cells.

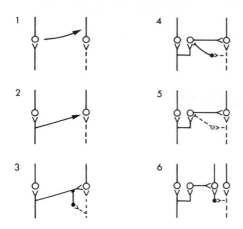

FIG. 1. Six mechanisms by which cells may respond to novel inputs following loss of normal input. *Filled in* and *stippled cells* are inhibitory interneurones (see text). Dashed axons on the *lower right* of each part represent the interrupted afferent input.

THE PHENOMENON OF CELLS RESPONDING TO A NEW INPUT FOLLOWING LOSS OF THEIR NORMAL AFFERENT DRIVE

We chose to examine thalamus, dorsal column nuclei, and spinal cord since these three structures all contain detailed somatotopic maps of the body surface. This means that cells in a particular location of the structure have highly predictable locations of their receptive fields on the body surface. Therefore the appearance of cells with unusual receptive fields distant from the expected region of skin is significant and a clear indication of some plasticity of connections.

Adult Rat Thalamus

Chronic

The thalamus contains a ventral posterior lateral nucleus (VPL) in which the body surface is mapped. Its major input comes by way of the medial lemniscus from the cuneate nucleus, subserving the arms, and the gracile nucleus, subserving the legs. The intact rat VPL was mapped by us and by others, and it was shown that the arm is represented in the medial two-thirds of the nucleus and that the leg occupies the lateral third (Fig. 2). There is an abrupt transition from leg to arm areas. One nucleus gracilis was surgically removed, thereby abolishing the input to the leg area. The nucleus VPL was mapped at various times after the destruction of nucleus gracilis, and the map was compared with the map obtained on the intact opposite nucleus VPL. In animals examined from 1 to 17 weeks after the lesion, the arm area had expanded to occupy two-thirds of the area previously responding to stimulation of the leg (Fig. 3). The beginning of this expansion was first noted at 3 days after the lesion and was complete by 7 days. If the nucleus gracilis was left intact, but its input was cut by section of the thoracic dorsal column, there was no expansion of the arm area.

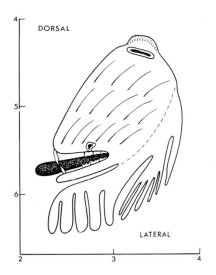

DORSAL

LATERAL

FIG. 2. Somatotopic map of the rat in the ventral posterior lateral and medial nuclei of the thalamus. The data were obtained by recording with metal microelectrodes at 100 μm intervals throughout a cross-section of the nucleus in animals under urethane anesthesia. The stimuli used were brushing on the body surface. The numbers on the horizontal scale represent length in mm from the midline and on the vertical scale represent length in mm below the cortical surface.

Acute

In these preparations, deeply anesthetized with urethane, natural stimulation failed to evoke any responses in the leg area of VPL immediately after removal of the nucleus gracilis, and similar negative results were obtained during the succeeding 48 hours (Fig. 4). During this period, ongoing activity was recorded from cells in the leg area while other parts of the nucleus and the opposite intact nucleus responded normally. We did not test the apparently silent part of the nucleus using electrical peripheral stimuli or different anesthetic conditions to discover if weak inputs existed.

Adult Cat Dorsal Column Nuclei

Chronic

We first obtained a more detailed map of the normal intact gracile and cuneate nuclei (15). We then studied the maps 8 or more months after the nucleus gracilis had been partially deafferented by cutting all but one of the dorsal roots serving one hind leg. Using a regular grid of mapping points, we found almost no nonresponsive areas in these chronically deafferented nuclei. The most obvious change in the map was that the area of nucleus gracilis which served the abdomen and thorax had risen from the normal area of 17 to 47%. In addition to the absence of a silent area and the exaggeration of the trunk area, abnormally responding cells were detected that had two clearly separated receptive fields, each supplied by an innervated region of skin. Such cells were quite common in these animals but are almost never seen in the intact animal.

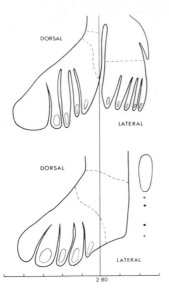

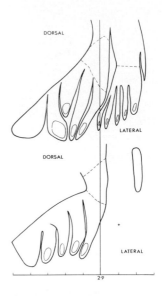

FIG. 3. Transverse map of distribution of receptive fields in intact VPL *(above)* and the map produced by continuing the mapping place across the midline into the opposite VPL studied 7 weeks after destruction of the nucleus gracilis which projected to this nucleus *(below)*. The *vertical line* marks an electrode track 2.8 mm from the midline which samples a similar region of the thalamus on the intact side to the vertical line shown in Fig. 3. The thalamus on the medial side of the line contains a similar map on both the intact and deafferented side. But the region representing the arm, especially the lower arm, has expanded on the operated side to invade a region which responds to leg on the intact side. At the lateral edge of the nucleus four cells were encountered which responded to body or leg stimulation, but most cells in this region failed to respond to any peripheral stimuli. (Reprinted from ref. 20.)

FIG. 4. Transverse map of distribution of receptive fields in the ventral posterior lateral (VPL) nucleus of the thalamus in rat 1 day after destruction of nucleus gracilis on one side. The map *(above)* shows the distribution in the thalamus supplied by the intact dorsal column nuclei with the forelimb representation medial, leg lateral, and body dorsolateral. The *dotted lines* mark the elbow and wrist on arm and the ankle on leg. The face area is not mapped. The map *(below)* shows the result of continuing the transverse search plane directly across the midline to the opposite thalamus that is not receiving an input from nucleus gracilis. The arm-hand-finger is similar in both maps. The leg area contained no responding cells in this plane with one exception marked by a *cross*. The *horizontal axis* marks 200-μm intervals in the mediolateral direction. The *vertical line* marks electrode tracks 2.9 mm from the midline penetrating both left and right thalamic maps. These tracks passed through the lateral arm region in each thalamus and show how similar the two arm regions are. (Reprinted from ref. 20.)

Acute

In acute preparations, all roots but one from the hind leg were cut in one series of experiments, and in a later series, all roots from the hind leg were cut. Then the normal intact nuclei on one side were compared with the acutely deafferented nuclei on the other (Fig. 5). As expected, large areas of the nucleus

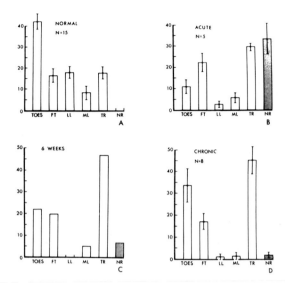

FIG. 5. Graphs of the percentage distribution of different body regions in a transverse "map" across the caudal gracile nucleus. For each map, the size of a particular region was calculated from the number of grid points where cells had receptive fields within the region. These grid point totals were then converted to percentages and then averages were calculated from a series of maps in different animals. For **A, B,** and **D,** the number of maps from which the graphs have been calculated is indicated as *N*. **C** is taken from a single map. The height of the bar representing a particular region indicates the mean percentage size (and SD) of this region in the nucleus (in the *plane* of the map). Regions are indicated on the ordinate: TOES includes all grid points where cells with receptive fields on individual toes or the foot pad were found. FT, foot and heel. LL, entire anterolateral leg. ML, posteromedial leg, perineum and groin. TR, trunk as far as the caudal borders of the rib cage. TH, thorax rostral to this level. NR, spontaneously active but nondrivable cells (see text). **A,** normal, intact gracile. **B,** immediately after all dorsal roots caudal to L4 except S1 had been cut. **C,** a single animal with S1 intact 6 weeks after rhizotomy. **D,** S1 or L7 intact and surviving at least 8 months between operation and mapping. (Reprinted from ref. 16.)

gracilis failed to respond to peripheral natural stimuli. This contrasted with the chronic condition where almost the entire region contained cells that responded to peripheral stimulation. In the intact nucleus, 10.9% of the area contains cells responding to abdominal stimulation, but after section of all hind leg dorsal roots, this number rose to 22.9%. As with the chronic animals, certain normally rare responses became more common immediately after root section. These included double receptive fields, habituating cells, cells requiring a flick of hair rather than gentle movement, and cells with distant inhibitory zones.

Instantaneous

Since we observed changes of input to be apparent in the hours immediately after root section, we decided to investigate the effect on single cells followed throughout a period of complete blockade of dorsal columns. Forty cells in the lateral nucleus gracilis were selected, and their receptive fields were investi-

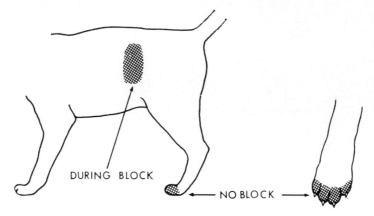

FIG. 6. An example of the receptive field of a unit with and without cold block of the cord at L4. During the block the receptive field on the toes was lost and a receptive field on the lateral abdomen appeared. (Reprinted from ref. 5.)

gated in the intact state. Then the entire dorsal columns at L4 were cold blocked. Nineteen cells that had their receptive fields on the leg became unresponsive to peripheral stimuli during the cold block and then returned to normal when the cold block was removed. This, of course, is the expected effect and showed no signs of switching of input. Similarly two cells began with their receptive fields on the abdomen and remained unchanged during the block. Eight cells in the intact state had receptive fields which included both abdomen and upper leg. These cells lost the leg part of their receptive field (RF) but retained the abdominal responsiveness. Thus 29 of the 40 cells showed the expected rigid effect of abolishing afferent drive to the cells. However, 11 cells switched their receptive fields when the afferents from the normal field were cold blocked. Each cell had a single receptive field on the leg, foot, or toes. Repeated, careful, strong stimulation outside their normal excitatory RF completely failed to excite these cells. Subsequently, the cord was cold blocked at L4. As the block took effect, a new brush field appeared on the abdomen and remained throughout the period of blockade of the afferents from the leg (Fig. 6). The new RF was novel since it had been stimulated repeatedly before the block. The new RFs had definite edges and responded to brush of the hair. Stimulating electrodes were installed in the new RF. When the block was removed, the RF disappeared, the cell failed to respond to either natural or electrical stimuli in the area, and the original receptive field on the hind limb reappeared.

Adult Cat Spinal Cord

Chronic

One side of the lumbar enlargement in adult cats was partially deafferented by cutting all dorsal roots, but one, and in a further series, all dorsal roots were cut. By 1 week and complete by 6 weeks, cells began to appear with RFs in unusual locations and with a series of unusual properties. The "new" receptive fields included some with unusually small areas and abrupt edges. Some cells habituated, and many more than usual had widely separated, double-receptive field cells.

Acute

Unlike the situation in the dorsal column nuclei, we have been unable to discover cells which switch their receptive fields in the first min or hr after cutting or blocking of the afferent fibers. Instead we find that cells lose all or part of their peripheral receptive field as dorsal roots or peripheral nerves are blocked.

POSSIBLE MECHANISMS

Could the "Newly" Connected Cells Be Transposed Normal Cells?

We can definitely dispose of this proposal. It might be suggested that with the cutting of afferent fibers there is a shrinkage of the deafferented cells and a migration of normal cells into the shrunken region. In this situation there would be no new connection, only a new location of normally connected cells.

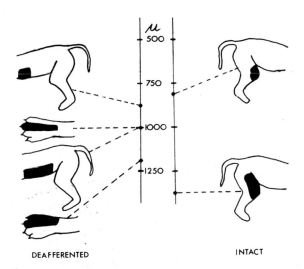

FIG. 7. Examples of the receptive fields and location of cells on the deafferented side and intact side of dorsal horn in the junction of the L4-5 segments. Cells with abdominal, distal foot, and combined double fields were found midway between the medial and lateral edges of the dorsal horn. On the intact side, cells in this region have receptive fields on the upper leg. These cells were recorded from an animal 32 weeks after root section. (Reprinted from ref. 1.)

We have excluded this possibility in the rat thalamus experiments (20) by showing that the map of the body surface in the S1 area of sensory cortex also shows a great expansion of the arm area just as is seen in the VPL. If there had been no new connections and simply a migration of arm cells into the previous leg area, the axons from the disconnected cells would still project to the cortex and there would be no change of the cortical map. In the dorsal column nuclei there were immediate changes which obviously cannot be explained by shrinkage. It is true that in the chronic animals there were a greater number of switched cells, and there was a 16% shrinkage of the cross-sectional area of the deafferented nucleus (16). However, this is hardly large enough to explain the substantial changes of the nuclear map. Again, in spinal cord there was a 23% shrinkage in transverse area of the deafferented dorsal horn (1), but here it would be necessary for cells to have migrated more than 1 cm in a longitudinal direction where there was no evidence of shrinkage.

Could Sprouting of Intact Afferents Explain the Responses of Deafferent Cells to a Novel Input?

Clearly this suggestion could not explain the shift of response in those dorsal column nuclei cells which changed their input immediately after deafferentation. However, even in the gracile nucleus there was an exaggeration of the change taking some weeks to complete. In rat thalamus we saw changes occurring only after 2 to 3 days and in cat cord after 7 days. With these more chronic changes we must obviously consider seriously the possibility of sprouting. Anatomical evidence for sprouting has been provided in rat septal nuclei (17) and in the rat hippocampus (11) (see also Cotman and Nadler, *this volume*). One of the earliest pieces of evidence for central sprouting came from work on partially deafferented spinal cord in which it was suggested that intact afferents spread very vigorously (10). More recent work using labeled amino acid transport has supported this although the expansion shown was very much less dramatic than in the earlier papers (7) (see also Goldberger and Murray, *this volume*). A problem has arisen with this spinal cord work in which, as we shall see, there is later work showing that the afferents already exist. It may therefore be the case that the changes which were previously interpreted as sprouting are in fact changes in staining or transport properties of existing fibers. We need to be careful in our definition of the word "sprouting" since it could be used to apply to some long distance extension of a completely new axon or, at the other extreme, to apply to some swelling of an existing bouton or proliferation of a final terminal arborization. Because of the near proximity of afferent intact fibers and of the dendrites of the cells whose responses change, we do not know the distance over which it would be necessary for new sprouts to stretch. The timing of the beginning of our chronic changes may be somewhat shorter than the beginning of central sprouting changes. If sprouting occurred, it would be necessary to show that the new connections are monosynaptic, a subject to which we shall return.

Could the New Responses Result from the Unmasking of Existing Afferents?

Unmasking might occur by one of three processes: (a) disinhibition of presynaptic inhibition; (b) transsynaptic atrophy of tonic inhibitory cells; (c) denervation hypersensitivity. For these unmasking possibilities to be considered it would be necessary first to show that afferents exist which could be unmasked and then to show physiologically that the new connections are monosynaptic.

Is There Anatomical Evidence for the Existence of Afferents Which Could Be Responsible for the Newly Effective Connections?

We are asking the question about whether distant afferent nerve fibers have been shown to terminate in regions where cells switch their responses if they lose the nearby afferents. In the dorsal column nuclei, two studies have shown anatomical evidence for anomalous afferent endings from the ipsilateral forelimb and the contralateral hind limb in the gracile nuclei (8,18). In spinal cord degeneration, studies show that L4 dorsal root terminating at least as far as segments T11 to S1 (9). In a study using microelectrode stimulation we have shown afferents extending caudally from the L2 dorsal root at least as far as the S1 segment, i.e. six to seven segments in the caudal direction (22). Therefore it is possible that there are candidate axons which extend into the region of the switched cells. Now we must ask if there is genuine evidence that these axons are in fact normally ineffective, and secondly, if the newly responding cells react monosynaptically to their new input.

Are the Long-Range Afferents Ineffective in the Intact Animal?

The answer to this question is complex and indefinite and must be answered in a series of stages.

First, very small numbers of cells in normal intact cord have large proximal receptive fields which extend over many segments rostral and caudal to the segment within which the cell lies. Devor and Wall (3) searched the L7-S1 dorsal horn of 22 cats and located 120 cells whose excitatory receptive field included the upper leg. All of them lay in the most dorsolateral part of the dorsal horn. Of the 120, 24 had large receptive fields extending over many segmental dermatomes from the base of the tail to mid abdomen and a variable distance down the leg. If such cells lost the bulk of their leg afferents, they would seem to have only abdominal RFs. However, we do not believe that the existence of such cells in the intact animal explains the appearance of all the cells responding to abdominal stimulation in the deafferented animal. In the intact animal such cells were rare, one cell discovered per animal on average;

whereas they were discovered at each recording station in lamina 4 and 5 in the chronic deafferented animal. Furthermore, in the intact animal these cells were entirely located in the extreme lateral dorsal part of the dorsal horn, whereas in the deafferented animal they were scattered throughout the dorsal horn.

Second, electrical stimulation of a distant dorsal root evokes firing of cells in intact cord that do not respond to natural stimuli applied to the dermatome of the distant dorsal root. Merrill and Wall (13) showed that the afferents transmitting impulses from the natural stimulus receptive field to a particular type of lamina 4 cell all ran in one fraction of a dorsal root. When these axons were cut or blocked, it was still possible to stimulate the cell monosynaptically by electrical stimulation of the neighboring root. This suggested that a group of afferents converged on a cell that were incapable of firing the cell unless the impulses from them arrived in synchrony. A search was therefore made to discover if electrical stimulation of more distant dorsal roots would also stimulate cells in intact cord (4). Two hundred eighty-four cells were located in L7-S1 that responded to electrical stimulation of L3-L4 dorsal roots. Only 20 of these cells had natural receptive fields that approached the dermatomes of L3 or L4. These cells which responded to electrical stimulation of distant dorsal roots might be considered a particularly excitable fraction of cells that receive an input from distant roots. It would then be predicted that a much larger number would show excitatory postsynaptic potentials if intracellular recordings were made with stimulation applied to distant roots or dermatomes. This study has now been completed (12) and shows that many cells do indeed have excitatory inputs from distant roots or dermatomes; however, it also shows that most of these are very delayed, follow high frequency stimulation very poorly, and that in intact cord there is a subliminal fringe of excitatory inputs that converge on a cell from far beyond the region of the naturally evoked receptive field of the cell.

Third, the obvious question is "why do these distant inputs not fire the cell when natural stimuli are used?" One answer is that they produce too small a depolarization of the cell to reach firing threshold unless they are synchronized by electrical stimulation. We have only considered, however, excitatory influences. Distant stimuli often produce inhibition with or without an admixture of excitation (12).

There is some evidence that the effect of distant afferents may be particularly subject to segmental inhibition. We have also investigated cells that respond to natural and electrical stimulation within their own dermatome but only to electrical stimulation and not to natural stimulation of a distant dermatome. If the hair outside the natural RF for these cells is gently rubbed, there is no effect on ongoing activity or on response from the RF. However, this stimulus turns off the response of many cells to electrical stimulation of a distant dermatome (14). This suggests that there are peculiarly effective inhibitions that have a selective inhibition on long-range inputs while leaving intact the intrinsic and segmental circuits affecting the cell.

Fourth, are the distant excitatory inputs excitatory in a monosynaptic fashion in the intact cord? The definition of monosynaptic is easy in words, but not in experimental terms (2). The first problem is that one must know the conduction velocity in long-running fine central axons so as to know the time of delivery of the impulses on the cell surface. Second, one must know the time course of the rise of the excitatory postsynaptic potential (which can itself be variable). An assumed correlate of monosynaptic transmission is a high safety factor with high frequency following of stimuli. It is evident that a small number of distal synapses could produce monosynaptic excitation with long delays and low reliability, but these would be impossible to differentiate from powerful polysynaptic excitation. Therefore, we can only be certain that some low latency-highly reliable responses are in fact monosynaptic and can make no statement about later, less reliable responses. Using these criteria, only 3.5% of the 284 cells in one segment that responded to roots three to four segments away could be certainly labeled as responding monosynaptically. Intracellular recording does not suggest that there are many more cells with short latency-high reliability EPSPs evoked by distant root or dermatome stimulation than is apparent by recording evoked spikes by extracellular recording.

Do Long-Range Afferents Become Effective Monosynaptically After Deafferentation?

It is evident that cells in deafferented regions begin to respond to inputs to which they did not previously respond. Is there evidence that the new input travels over the same number of neurons as the input that has been destroyed? In rat thalamus the normal pathway is long and passes at least one synapse in the dorsal column nuclei. No latency difference could be detected between the normal unaffected arm cells and the "newly" connected arm cells (20), but the normal scatter of latencies does not allow a positive identification of slow monosynaptic connections versus fast polysynaptic pathways. In the dorsal column nuclei of cat, the response latency of 61 cells subserving abdomen in intact animals exactly matched the latencies of 61 such cells in the deafferented animals, many of which were in abnormal parts of the nucleus (5). Again, a superficial interpretation is that the "new" connection had, on average, the same latency as the intact connections; but to be critical, a more careful interpretation would maintain that the figures had too wide a scatter to decide that the new connections had the same latency as the intact connections and were therefore monosynaptic. In the deafferented spinal cord, the cells in question are at some distance from the entry point of the afferent nerve fibers which excite them. Since the conduction time within the cord of the afferent impulses in these long range axons is not known, it is difficult to assess the significance of latency. Ten "newly" connected cells at a distance of 40 mm from the root entry site responded in 1.5 to 1.8 msec to root stimulation (1). This is in a reasonable range of monosynaptic connection, but it is impossible to prove that another synapse might not have intruded. Similarly, we argue that latency, ability to follow high frequency stimulation, and stability of response latency are consistent with these "new" connections being monosynaptic, but we cannot rule out that they are not the result of fast, powerful polysynaptic connections.

Thus far we have suggested that the experimental evidence cannot differentiate between the exaggeration of existing monosynaptic connections or the opening of new polysynaptic connections. Recent intracellular spinal cord interneuron recording suggests a development in the deafferented animal of fast, secure excitation of cells by distant inputs of a type that are rarely if ever recorded in the normal, intact animal (12). The intracellular recording technique is difficult in that only small numbers of cells can be examined in any one animal. Therefore there is a considerable danger of sampling bias, particularly after deafferentation atrophy. In spite of this, our tentative conclusion (12) is that in the intact animal the great majority of cells that show an excitatory postsynaptic potential from a distant input are responding by way of polysynaptic, insecure inputs. By contrast, after local deafferentation, cells commonly respond to distant inputs with low latency and high security. Therefore the present evidence does not support the suggestion that the "new" responses are simply an exaggeration of normally existing direct monosynaptic excitations of cells.

Could the New Responses Result from the Unmasking of Polysynaptic Pathways?

The experimental difficulty in differentiating between mono- and polysynaptic routes has been discussed. The next problem is whether a cell is being excited monosynaptically by a slowly conducted weak excitation on distal dendrites or by a secure polysynaptic pathway that impinges close to the cell body. For example, cells in the cat intact gracile nucleus respond to stimulation of the ipsilateral foot in 9 to 20 msec. However, some of these cells also respond at a shorter latency to electrical stimulation of the forepaw, and some respond to contralateral foot stimulation with a latency at least 1 msec longer than their response to the ipsilateral foot (6). Can we attribute these anomalous connections to polysynaptic pathways or to monosynaptic connections? These arguments are vacuous in the present state of our experimental abilities, and we must leave open both possibilities. This is particularly true in relation to natural stimuli, which are the events with which we should be practically concerned. If a nerve cell fires, the next nerve cell does not know if the impulse it receives has been evoked by mono- or polysynaptic excitation. The question fascinates neurophysiologists (but not the cell which receives the evoked impulse). The "new" response of a cell in nucleus gracilis which appears after cold block of afferents from the lumbar enlargement has a considerably longer latency than that produced from the "normal intact" receptive field. It is reasonable to propose that the novel receptive field is activated by an unmasked polysynaptic afferent input. In our present state of knowledge, we should not choose between the two possibilities. Either mono- or polysynaptic connections may be opened by the destruction of the normally active afferent input. Indeed, there is no reason to decide in the present state of our knowledge that both may not be true. Results show that new responses occur but do not differentiate between the mechanisms by which the switch is produced.

Could the New Responses Result from Some Chronic Process Which Unmasks Indirect Connections?

Whether the newly effective connections are direct or indirect, it is clear that there is some relatively prolonged process involved in their maturation. This could be the time taken for the growth of collateral sprouts, but we have discussed reasons both for and against this above. We know that shrinkage develops in the deafferented structures, and this atrophy could involve tonically active inhibitory neurons that slowly fail to inhibit normal ineffective linkages. Finally, it has been suggested that denervation hypersensitivity develops in the deafferented cord, although the evidence is indirect (19). This process could also lead to the switching on of inputs that were normally ineffective.

Could the New Responses Occur in Normally Silent Cells?

Under certain conditions, many nerve cells appear to be strongly inhibited and fail to fire to stimuli that excite other cells in the region. In the freely moving rat, dorsal horn cells may remain silent until switched on by a change of descending control (21). However, we and many other workers have examined spinal cord under conditions of maximal excitability with descending control cut and with antihibitory drugs such as bicuculline, strychnine, and picrotoxin. Under these conditions of extreme excitability, we have not detected cells either with very large receptive fields or with distant receptive fields. Clearly, in the case of the dorsal column nuclei where we followed single cells during the blockade of their inputs and the switching of their receptive fields, it was evident that the same cell had two potential inputs. We cannot prove that the cells observed with distant inputs in the chronic preparations were the same cells as those which had lost their afferents. However, these switched cells are so frequently observed that it would be necessary to postulate a very large population of entirely silent cells in the intact animal.

CONCLUSION

There is an immediate development of new receptive fields when some types of cells lose their normal afferent drive. The explanation for this immediate shift could be the disinhibition of indirect polysynaptic inputs to the cell. As days and weeks pass after deafferentation, in all three examined areas more and more cells develop novel inputs. We still have no definite explanation of the mechanism of this chronic change. Intracellular recording in these cells suggests that powerful inputs have developed that are rarely seen in the intact animal. In the intact animal the equipment exists for development of new responses following deafferentation; that is to say, there are long range axons, and there are rare monosynaptic and more common polysynaptic inputs from distant regions. After chronic partial deafferentation, cells begin to respond to natural stimuli applied to distant areas. These new responses are common, rapid, and secure. Possibly these new responses are simply an exaggeration of what already exists in the intact animal, but new growth cannot be ruled out.

REFERENCES

1. Basbaum, A. I., and Wall, P. M. (1976): Chronic changes in the response of cells in adult cat dorsal horn following partial deafferentation: the appearance of responding cells in a previously non-responsive region. *Brain Res.,* 116:181–204.
2. Berry, M. S., and Pentreath, V. W. (1976): Criteria for distinguishing between monosynaptic and polysynaptic transmission. *Brain Res.,* 105:1–20.
3. Devor, M., and Wall, P. D. (1976): Dorsal horn cells with proximal cutaneous receptive fields. *Brain Res.,* 118:325–328.
4. Devor, M., Merrill, E. G. and Wall, P. D. (1977): Dorsal horn cells that respond to stimulation of distant dorsal roots. *J. Physiol.,* 270:519–531.
5. Dostrovsky, J. O., Millar, J., and Wall, P. D. (1976): The immediate shift of afferent drive of dorsal column nucleus cells following deafferentation: a comparison of acute and chronic deafferentation in gracile nucleus and spinal cord. *Exp. Neurol.,* 52:480–495.
6. Dostrovsky, J. O., Jabbur, J., and Millar, J. (1977): Anomalous connexions in cat gracile nuclei. *J. Physiol. (in press).*
7. Goldberger, M. E., and Murray, M. (1974): Restitution of function and collateral sprouting in the cat spinal cord. *J. Comp. Neurol.,* 158:37–54.
8. Hand, P. J. (1966): Lumbosacral dorsal root terminations in the nucleus gracilis of the cat. *J. Comp. Neurol.,* 126:137–156.
9. Imai, Y., and Kusama, T. (1969): Distribution of the dorsal root fibres in the cat. An experimental study with the Nauta method. *Brain Res.,* 13:338–359.
10. Liu, C. N., and Chambers, W. W. (1958): Intraspinal sprouting of dorsal root axons. *Arch. Neurol. Psychiatry,* 79:46–61.
11. Lynch, G., and Cotman, C. W. (1975) The hippocampus as a model for studying anatomical plasticity in the adult brain. In: *The Hippocampus, Vol. 1,* edited by R. L. Isaacson and K. H. Pribram. pp. 123–155. Plenum, New York.
12. Mendell, L. M., Sassoon, E. M., and Wall, P. D. (1977): Properties of synaptic linkage from "distant" afferents onto dorsal horn neurons in normal and chronically deafferented cats. *J. Physiol. (in press).*
13. Merrill, E. G., and Wall, P. D. (1972): Factors forming the edge of a receptive field. The presence of relatively ineffective afferents. *J. Physiol.,* 226:825–846.
14. Merrill, E. G., and Wall, P. D. (1977): Selective inhibition of distant afferent input to cat dorsal horn cells. *J. Physiol. (in press).*
15. Millar, J., and Basbaum, A. I. (1975): Topography of the projection of the body surface of the cat to cuneate and gracile nuclei. *Exp. Neurol.,* 49:281–290.
16. Millar, J., Basbaum, A. I., and Wall, P. D. (1976): Restructuring of the somatotopic map and appearance of abnormal neuronal activity in the gracile nucleus after partial deafferentation. *Exp. Neurol.,* 50:658–672.
17. Raisman, G., and Field, P. M. (1973): A quantitative investigation of the development of collateral reinnervation of the septal nuclei. *Brain Res.,* 50:241–264.

18. Rustioni, A., and Macchi, G. (1968): Distribution of dorsal root fibers in the medulla oblongata of the cat. *J. Comp. Neurol.,* 134:113–126.
19. Treasdale, R. D., and Stavraky, G. W. (1953): Responses of deafferented spinal neurons to corticospinal impulses. *J. Neurophysiol.,* 16:367–375.
20. Wall, P. D., and Egger, M. D. (1971): Formation of new connections in adult rat brains after partial deafferentation. *Nature,* 232:542–545.
21. Wall, P. D., Freeman, J., and Major, D. (1967): Dorsal horn cells in spinal and freely moving rats. *Exp. Neurol.,* 19:519–529.
22. Wall, P. D., and Werman, R. (1976): The physiology anatomy of long ranging afferent fibres within the spinal cord. *J. Physiol.,* 255:321–334.

Neuronal Plasticity, edited by
Carl W. Cotman.
Raven Press, New York © 1978.

Synaptic Plasticity in the Red Nucleus

N. Tsukahara

*Department of Biophysical Engineering, Faculty of Engineering Science, Osaka University,
Toyonaka, Osaka, Japan*

Critical experimental evidence for the formation of new synapses in the adult mammalian central nervous system is largely of recent origin. Although Liu and Chambers (14) demonstrated quite early in 1958 that, based on light microscopic observation, the dorsal root fibers can sprout in the cat spinal cord, it is the more recent work by Raisman (31) and Raisman and Field (32) with the adult rat septum that seems to have had the greatest impact in this field. In a series of studies, Raisman and Field provided dramatic microscopic evidence of compensatory synaptic formation on septal neurons after interruption of either the fimbrial or medial forebrain bundle inputs. Similar results were reported by Moore et al. (23), who followed the reaction of catecholaminergic fibers by fluorescence histochemistry. Over the past 5 or 6 years these findings have been extended to several regions of the central nervous system by numerous investigators. In sum, sprouting in response to lesions of the central nervous system has now been firmly established by a variety of histological techniques (6).

In further efforts to identify the properties of these sprouted fibers, the physiological effectiveness and detailed physiological properties of newly formed synapses have received some consideration. For example, Lynch et al. (17) and Steward et al. (41,42) have reported both morphological and electrophysiological evidence that new synapses which form on hippocampal granule cells after partial denervation are physiologically effective. The physiology of these synapses clearly must be investigated in greater detail, and the present article is addressed to this problem.

In studying problems of synaptic plasticity, neurons of the red nucleus (RN) provide an excellent substrate. They are easily accessible to microelectrode manipulation because of their large size, and there exists an ample body of histological and physiological literature on the synaptic organization in this region and the properties of intrinsic cell membranes (2). Of particular importance for the present purpose is the discrete lamination of their two major synaptic inputs. That from the nucleus interpositus (IP) of the cerebellum terminates on the somatic portion of the cell membrane (43,48,49), whereas that from the sensorimotor cortex (SM) forms synapses on the distal dendrites (48,49). This synaptic arrangement has allowed us to characterize the postsynaptic potentials produced by activation of these afferents (48,49).

Analysis of the spatial characteristics of synaptic potentials has been greatly aided by recent advances in neuronal modeling made possible by recent advances in computer technology. One of the most important achievements of the latter is the analysis of the detailed electrical properties of dendrites with complex geometry by mathematical modeling. Most notably, Rall and associates (33–36) developed a model of the dendritic membrane consisting of a cascade of lumped compartments. With this model, it became possible to analyze the complex spatial and temporal features of synaptic activity generated at various loci on the soma-dendritic membrane. This model has been successfully applied to the synaptic excitation of motoneurons by large muscle spindle afferents and has helped to disclose the detailed location of their synapses on the motoneuron membrane (35).

CHANGING PROPERTIES OF POSTSYNAPTIC POTENTIALS AS A TOOL FOR INVESTIGATING AXON SPROUTING

The first question that arises in regard to physiological studies of newly formed synapses is how to demonstrate physiological efficacy. The most straightforward way would be to show the appearance of new synaptic potentials. Unfortunately, addition of synaptic potentials of the same nature is extremely difficult to demonstrate in the mammalian central nervous system where convergence of many presynaptic fibers onto a single neuron is the general rule. An increase in amplitude of the postsynaptic potential cannot be a reliable measure for this, because the amplitude of the postsynaptic potential is very much dependent on the resting membrane potential and the membrane conductance, which vary considerably with the recording conditions. Denervation supersensitivity, which might well occur after denervation, is also a complicating factor.

Time Course of the Excitatory Postsynaptic Potentials

If fibers form new synapses at sites different from normal, one could approach the question of physiological efficacy by examining the time course of the excitatory postsynaptic potentials (EPSPs), since this depends on the distance of the synapses from the soma. A change in location of a synaptic population relative to the soma produces a corresponding change in the electrotonic distortion of the waveform and the latency of its detection at the soma. Thus, various descriptive and theoretical accounts of the cable properties of neurons and the location of synapses (33,34,37,48,49) are the important bases for this approach. A wealth of anatomical and physiological data on the RN neurons (2) has greatly facilitated the recent physiological investigation of collateral sprouting and formation of physiologically effective synapses from the cerebrum on RN cells after destruction of the IP nucleus of the cerebellum (Tsukahara et al., 45–47). Of particular importance is the finding that the time to peak of the EPSPs induced by stimulation of the sensorimotor cortex or the corticorubral pathway at the cerebral peduncle (CP) decreased 2 or more weeks after a lesion of the IP nucleus as illustrated in Fig. 1A. This was taken to indicate that new corticorubral synapses formed on the proximal portion of the soma-dendritic membrane of RN cells. This interpretation was based on the simple assumption that the cable properties

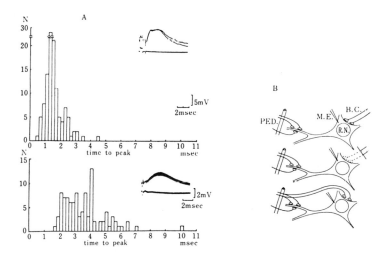

FIG. 1. Rise time of the corticorubral EPSPs induced by stimulating the cerebral peduncle (CP) after lesion of the interpositus nucleus (IP). **A:** Frequency distribution of the time to peak of the CP-EPSPs in operated cats *(upper histogram)* and in normal cats *(lower histogram)*. Specimen records of the intracellular and corresponding extracellular records are shown in the inset of each histogram. **B:** Diagram of the experimental arrangement. R.N., red nucleus neuron. B.C., input from IP through brachium conjunctivum. PED., input from cerebrum through cerebral peduncle. M.E., microelectrode. (Modified from ref. 47.)

of dendrites of RN neurons do not change drastically after interruption of their input, and this, of course, poses a big problem for the physiological test.

Cable Properties of RN Neurons Before and After Partial Denervation

In order to rule out the possibility that a change in the cable properties of the soma-dendritic membrane of RN neurons was responsible for the above-mentioned change in time to peak of the EPSPs, we had to devise a method of measuring the cable properties of dendrites and then determine the effect on the time to peak of the EPSP of a given change in these properties. Fortunately, there are both theoretical and experimental foundations for handling this problem. Rall (34) has shown that the electrotonic length of the neuron, one of the most important parameters of cable properties, can be estimated from the analysis of the membrane potential change produced by applying current stepwise through the intrasomatic microelectrode according to the following equation:

$$L = \frac{\pi}{\sqrt{\tau_0 / \tau_1 - 1}} \tag{1}$$

where L is the electrotonic length of a neuron and τ_0, τ_1 are the passive membrane time constant and the largest equalizing time constant, respectively.

This equation has been applied to the cat motoneuron by several authors (4,16,30). Lux et al. (16) have concluded that Rall's mathematical constraint of the dendritic branching pattern for deriving the above-mentioned equation, i.e., the sum of the 3/2 power of all branch diameters at any particular electrotonic distance remains constant, indeed holds true for motoneurons. However, Barrett and Crill (3) reexamined this constraint by injecting fluorescent procion yellow dye into motoneurons and then reconstructing their geometry. Their study did not support the equivalent cylinder approximation for these neurons.

In applying these models to the "real neuron," it thus appears important to know whether the specific assumptions used for the model are fulfilled. For this, it is important to have a theoretical prediction of the model which can be tested directly by both electrophysiological and histological methods. Sato and myself (37) obtained a theoretical relation by using Rall's compartmental neuron model:

$$E_1/E_0 = (1 + \cos \pi/n)\tau_1/\tau_0 \tag{2}$$

where n is the number of compartments employed, τ_0 and τ_1 are the passive membrane time constant and the largest equalizing time constant of a neuron, respectively, and E_0 and E_1 are amplitudes of these exponential components.

This theoretical relation was used to test the applicability of the compartment model to RN neurons. Tsukahara et al. (49) found by studying transient response of RN neuronal membrane to current steps that the relation of Eq. 2 holds approximately true for RN neurons.

After establishing the applicability of the model to RN neurons, the electrotonic length of the individual neurons was calculated, and the mean value *(L)* was 1.1. A similar measurement was made in cats with chronic destruction of the IP nucleus. The electrotonic length of the RN neurons thus obtained was 1.05 ± 0.1 as compared to 1.1 ± 0.15 in unoperated cats. This indicates a slight, but probably insignificant, reduction of the electrotonic length of RN neurons after IP lesions.

The next step was to estimate the change in the time to peak of the EPSPs produced by the above-mentioned change in the electrotonic length of RN neurons. Based on the compartmental neuron model and using parameters obtained experimentally, theoretical EPSPs were computed giving the same conductance increase at each compartment of the five compartment model as schematically illustrated in the inset of Fig. 2A. By assuming that the corticorubral fibers in normal cats terminate at the most distal portion of the dendritic branches (the most distal compartment) (see Tsukahara et al., 49), it is possible to estimate how large would be the reduction of the time to peak of the corticorubral EPSPs produced by the slight reduction of the electrotonic length of RN neurons which occurs after IP lesions. The graph of Fig. 2A illustrates the relation of electrotonic length to the time to peak of the theoretical EPSPs. From this

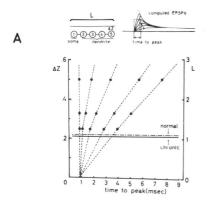

A

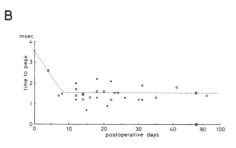

B

FIG. 2. **A:** Estimation of the location of the fast rising component of the CP-EPSP in operated cats based on the compartmental model of Rall (33). The *inset diagram* illustrates a chain of five equal compartments having the same electrical parameters. The pulse-shaped conductance increase of 0.9-msec duration *(dotted line in the inset diagram)* occurs in each one of these compartments and the resultant potential changes at the first compartment *(soma)* are called the computed EPSPs. The times to peak of these computed EPSPs are plotted against electronic length (L) or increment of electrotonic length (ΔZ). The computation was performed at three different values of ΔZ. The resultant times to peak of these computed EPSPs are plotted as *filled circles*. The normal corticorubral EPSP is considered to be initiated at the *fifth compartment* (49). *Dashed line* shows the electrotonic length of normal cats (average of 25 RN cells). The *solid line* shows that of chronic (operated) cats (average of 11 RN cells). **B:** Time course of the change of the rise time of the CP-EPSPs after IP lesion. *Open circles*, the mean time to peak of CP-EPSPs of more than six RN cells per animal. *Filled circles*, the mean time to peak of the CP-EPSPs of two to five RN cells per animal. *Cross* on the ordinate indicates the mean time to peak of the CP-EPSPs of 100 RN cells in normal cats. (From ref. 47.)

relation, it becomes apparent that the reduction of the electrotonic length observed experimentally accounts for only a minor portion (less than 5%) of the observed decrease of the time to peak of corticorubral EPSPs after IP lesion.

Other Sources of Errors

Having established that the altered time course of the corticorubral EPSPs after IP lesion is not due to a change in the cable properties of RN neurons, other possible mechanisms were considered. One possibility is that the earlier potential is a dendritic spike and not an EPSP. In hippocampal pyramidal cells (38) and alligator Purkinje cells (15), dendritic spike potentials have been investigated in detail. The possibility, therefore, had to be considered that the fast rising component of the corticorubral response which appeared after chronic destruction of the IP could have been a dendritic spike. This possibility was tested by analyzing responses to membrane potential displacement. The postsynaptic potential could be reversed in sign by depolarization. Furthermore, the time course of the potential is characterized by a rapid rise and slow exponential decline resembling an EPSP. Finally, the potential could be graded by changing the stimulus intensity. For these reasons the potential was considered to be an EPSP.

Another factor which must be considered is the possible development of denervation supersensitivity to the chemical transmitter. Partial denervation may increase the sensitivity of the postsynaptic membrane to transmitter substances, as demonstrated after complete denervation of muscle fibers (22). Such hypersensitivity could possibly account for an increase in the amplitude of the corticorubral EPSPs but not for the decrease in rise time of the EPSPs.

In summary, it must be concluded that the changing time course of the corticorubral EPSPs was not due to changes in cable properties, development of dendritic spikes, or denervation supersensitivity, but rather most likely resulted from formation of physiologically effective synapses on the RN neurons. This is supported by the responses of the new EPSPs to membrane potential displacement, as will be shown below, and also by an electron microscopic study by Nakamura et al. (29).

PROPERTIES OF TRANSMISSION AT THE NEWLY FORMED CORTICORUBRAL SYNAPSES

The hypothesis that new corticorubral synapses were formed after an IP lesion was further supported by more detailed physiological studies. We first examined the compound corticorubral EPSP, in which EPSPs of old and new synapses are intermingled (45–47). By following the change in the compound EPSP, we determined the time course of sprouting after the destruction of IP. Figure 2B illustrates the relationship between the average time to peak of the corticorubral EPSPs and the number of days after IP lesion for each experimental animal. Four days after the lesion, there was already a significant shortening of the time to peak. After 10 days the shortening reached its maximum and remained at this value for at least 3 months.

In order to characterize the physiological properties of the newly formed synapses more completely, it was necessary to separate the EPSPs produced by the sprouted synapses from those of the old ones. For this reason, unitary EPSPs were analyzed in some detail (20).

The unitary EPSPs in cats with an IP lesion fell into two groups: corticorubral unitary EPSPs with shorter time to peak and larger amplitude than normal (Fig. 3A) and those of normal range (Fig. 3B). Figure 3C shows the relation between time to peak of the unitary EPSPs and their amplitudes. Filled circles represent EPSPs in normal cats and open circles those in operated cats. Note that the EPSPs in normal cats typically had a longer time to peak and smaller amplitudes than those in operated cats. Furthermore, there was a tendency for the larger unitary EPSPs to rise faster. This tendency is predicted from calculation of the theoretical EPSPs generated at each compartment of the five compartment model as schematically illustrated in the inset of Fig. 3C. Times to peak and amplitudes of these theoretical EPSPs are plotted on the larger graph (large circles labeled 1–5). Parameters used to compute the data

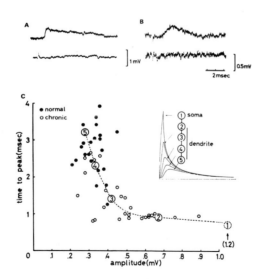

FIG. 3. Corticorubral unitary EPSPs. **A,B:** Intracellular EPSP evoked by stimulation of sensorimotor cortex at a rate of 1/sec in a cat with IP lesion 27 days before acute experiment **(A)** and in a normal cat **(B)**. *Upper traces,* intracellular potentials. *Lower traces,* extracellular field corresponding to the upper traces. **C:** Relation between time to peak and amplitude of the unitary EPSPs. *Open circles* represent unitary EPSPs of operated cats and *filled circles* represent those of normal cats. *Large open circles* represent times to peak and amplitudes of theoretical EPSPs derived by Rall's compartmental model initiated at each compartment of a five-compartment chain. The time course of the theoretical EPSPs generated in these compartments is diagrammatically shown in the *inset* of the figure. (Modified from ref. 26.)

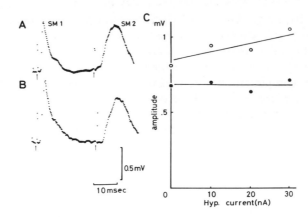

FIG. 4. Sensitivity of amplitude of the EPSPs to membrane polarization. **A:** Fast rising (SM1) and slowly rising (SM2) corticorubral EPSP recorded in the same cell by stimulating different points of sensorimotor cortex in an operated cat. **B:** Same as **A** but the EPSPs were recorded during hyperpolarization produced by injecting current through a microelectrode. *Upward arrows* indicate the onset of stimulation. **C:** Relation between amplitude of EPSP and injected current. *Open circles* correspond to the fast rising EPSPs and *closed circles* to slowly rising ones. (Modified from ref. 26.)

in Fig. 2 were also used here (47,49). A good agreement of the theoretical curve with the experimental points strongly supports the hypothesis that new synapses were formed on the proximal portion of the soma-dendritic membrane of RN cells after an IP lesion.

Frequently both fast and slowly rising EPSPs could be recorded in the same cell by stimulating different loci within the sensorimotor cortex of operated cats as illustrated in Fig. 4A. When the membrane was hyperpolarized as shown in Fig. 4B, the amplitude of the fast rising EPSPs increased, whereas the amplitude of the slowly rising EPSPs remained almost unchanged. Figure 4C shows the relation between the amplitudes of the EPSPs (open circles for fast rising EPSPs and filled circles for slowly rising ones) and the amount of injected current. This finding indicates that the synapses responsible for the fast rising EPSPs are located more proximally to the soma than those which produce the slowly rising EPSPs. Therefore, the fast rising unitary EPSPs are produced by activity of the newly formed synapses (26).

Frequency Facilitation and Posttetanic Potentiation at the Newly Formed Synapses

The behavior of the postsynaptic potentials during and after repetitive stimuli characterizes physiological properties of synapses (5). Two phenomena are well known. Firstly, when a pair of stimuli are presented, the EPSP produced by the second stimulus is larger than that produced by the first as shown for the corticorubral synapse in Fig. 5A,B. This is referred to as "facilitation" or "frequency facilitation" (18,24). Secondly, after prolonged tetanic stimulation, a test pulse induces a larger response than normal for a period lasting from seconds to minutes. This is the well known phenomenon of posttetanic potentiation (PTP) (5).

The degree and time course of facilitation at newly formed corticorubral synapses (Fig. 5D) were not significantly different from those at the old synapses (Fig. 5E). The mean facilitation decayed more slowly in the case of new synapses when interstimulus intervals of 10 msec or less were used, but thereafter the facilitation decayed with similar time courses. The time courses could be fitted by two exponential functions as shown in the semilogarithmic plot of Figs. 5D and 5E. For the newly formed synapses the time constants were 44 and 6 msec, and for the old synapses, 54 and 3 msec.

Posttetanic potentiation was observed at newly formed, as well as old, corticorubral synapses. Maximal potentiation of the EPSP was attained immediately after the tetanic stimulation and then declined slowly over several min. Since

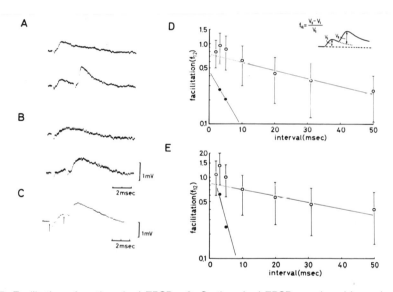

FIG. 5. Facilitation of corticorubral EPSPs. **A:** Corticorubral EPSPs produced by a single CP stimulation *(upper trace)* and those produced by a pair of stimuli of the same intensity *(lower trace)* in an operated cat. **B:** Same as **A** but in a normal cat. Responses exemplified in **B** were averaged by a computer (30 traces) and displayed in **C**. *Arrows* indicate the onset of stimuli. **D, E:** Time course of facilitation of the EPSPs. *Ordinate,* the degree of facilitation expressed as shown in the inset diagram on a logarithmic scale. *Abscissa,* interval between two CP stimuli. Each point is the average of 14 EPSPs in operated cats **(D)** and 12 EPSPs in normal cats **(E)**. The plotted points *(open circles)* could be fitted by a straight line except for interstimulus intervals of 10 msec. The slope of the straight lines give time constants of 44 msec and 54 msec, respectively, for **D** and **E**. The differences between the experimentally obtained values *(open circles)* and the extrapolated straight line *(dotted lines)* were replotted on the same graphs *(filled circles)*. These values could be fitted by straight lines with time constants of 6 and 3 msec for **D** and **E**, respectively. (Modified from ref. 27.)

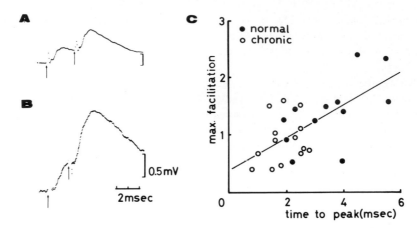

FIG. 6. A relation between the degree of facilitation and the time to peak of the EPSPs. **A:** Fast rising corticorubral EPSPs in response to two successive stimuli to CP. **B:** Same as **A** but for slowly rising corticorubral EPSPs. *Upward arrows* indicate onset of stimuli. **C:** The relation between the maximal degree of facilitation (measured at the peak of the facilitation curve) and time to peak of the EPSP. *Filled circles* for normal cats and *open circles* for operated cats. (Modified from ref. 27.)

there was no appreciable change in the resting membrane potential and resting membrane conductance, as measured by passing current pulses, these potentiations must have represented classical PTP. The degree of the potentiation was generally larger at newly formed synapses.

One of the conspicuous features of synaptic transmission at the newly formed synapses was a tendency for the rapidly rising EPSPs to facilitate less readily than the slowly rising ones, as illustrated in Fig. 6A,B. Figure 6C shows the relation between the maximal degree of facilitation and the time peak of the EPSPs. Note the positive correlation ($p < 0.005$) between these parameters. There is much physiological evidence indicating that a presynaptic mechanism underlies facilitation (5,18,24). Furthermore, it is also known that the rise time of the corticorubral unitary EPSP is associated with the location of these synapses on the soma-dendritic membrane. Therefore, this correlation suggests the most interesting possibility that the location of the synapse relative to the cell body in some way regulates its ability to facilitate. This relationship might be of functional significance in view of the marked reduction in amplitude of the EPSPs initiated at the distal dendrites during their electrotonic propagation toward the soma. The greater facilitation of EPSPs generated on the more distally located dendrites would compensate for their relatively greater electrotonic attenuation.

SYNAPTOGENESIS AFTER CROSS-INNERVATION OF THE PERIPHERAL NERVES

Although much evidence has been provided that synaptogenesis can and does take place after denervation in the mammalian central nervous system, we still have little idea of what triggers this process. For example, does the presence of degenerating fibers initiate the process of synaptogenesis? In this context, we might ask to what extent synaptogenesis occurs in circumstances other than denervation.

Published attempts to use the controlled cross-innervation of peripheral nerves for the purpose of investigating central reorganization are quite old. The most comprehensive review of this appeared in 1945 (40). Sperry investigated the functional compensation of movement disorders which followed cross-innervation of nerves innervating flexor and extensor muscles in various species of mammals. He found in monkeys that motor reeducation occurs by inhibiting the reversed action and by learning the correct and smooth coordinated movements (39). This has never been observed in similar experiments on rats (40).

Eccles et al. (7) investigated possible changes in synaptic connections of spinal motoneurons after cross-innervation of flexor and extensor nerves of hindlimbs. Although they found evidence suggesting the formation of new synapses on motoneurons after cross-innervation, this was restricted to the group of motoneurons whose axons were severed. Thus the extent of this reorganization was very limited. Subsequent investigation by Mendell and Scott (21) in motoneurons after crossing nerves to synergistic muscles failed to show synaptic reorganization.

It is important to note that in Sperry's experiment on monkeys the learning to flex or to extend the elbow in one situation did not necessarily become generalized for other performances. This indicates that the neuronal readjustment was not localized solely in the spinal centers, but involved reorganization at the supraspinal level. If the learning process involved rearrangements in the relationship of the primary or secondary neurons in the spinal cord, one would expect a complete transfer of learning from one performance to all.

Motivated with these considerations, we performed cross-innervation experiments to determine whether synaptic reorganization occurred at the supraspinal level. The corticorubrospinal system is one of the major motor outflows from the cerebrum to the spinal cord. Therefore, if synaptic reorganization (at the supraspinal level) should occur after cross-innervation, the corticorubrospinal system might well be affected. If so, we should be able to detect the changes by techniques similar to those described in the previous sections.

For cross-innervation of the forelimb nerves, the musculocutaneous, median, radial, and ulnar nerves were cut at the axillary region, and central stumps of the musculocutaneous, median, and ulnar nerves were united to the peripheral stump of the radial nerve by suturing the nerve sheath. A similar procedure was applied to the central stump of the radial nerve which was united to the peripheral stumps of the musculocutaneous, median, and ulnar nerves. All operations were performed under aseptic conditions. After a postoperative period varying from 2 to 6 months, the cats were prepared for intracellular recording from RN neurons contralateral to the cross-innervated muscles. In order to determine whether the muscles had been reinnervated and by which nerves, the distal tendons of the muscles of triceps and biceps muscles were cut, and the distal portion of each muscle was freed of surrounding structures. The cut tendon was attached to a tension transducer in order to measure isometric tension induced by direct as well as prejunctional stimulation. The degree of functional reinnervation was roughly evaluated from the ratio of the maximal tension obtained by nerve stimulation relative to that produced by direct stimulation of the muscle.

For self-union of the forelimb nerves, the above-mentioned nerves were sectioned and reunited without crossing by suturing the nerve sheath. The degree of reinnervation was also monitored as in the cross-union preparation.

These studies showed that 2 to 6 months after cross-innervation the rising time course of the corticorubral EPSPs induced by stimulation of the cerebral peduncle (CP) became shorter than that of normal cats. The typical slow EPSPs evoked by stimulating the CP in a normal cat are illustrated in the lower inset of Fig. 7A. In contrast, the EPSPs shown in Fig. 7 (left inset) from a cat with cross-innervation of the forelimb nerves innervating the upper spinal segment (C-cell) had a much faster rise time than in normal cats. In these experiments, C-cells were identified by the antidromic excitation produced by stimulating the C_1 spinal segment.

The frequency distribution of the times to peak of the CP-EPSPs of C-cells in cross-innervated cats is shown in Fig. 8A. The mean time to peak of the CP-EPSPs of C-cells in cross-innervated cats was significantly shorter than that of the normal cats (3.6 ± 1.4 msec, $n = 100$). On the contrary, the CP-

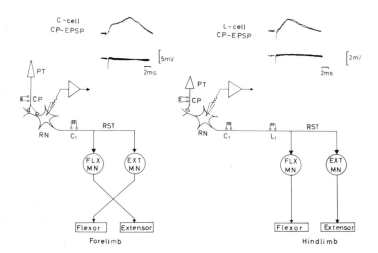

FIG. 7. Corticorubral EPSPs in cross-innervated cats. *Upper traces* are intracellular responses in RN neurons, whereas *lower traces* are corresponding extracellular fields. *Left traces* are from C-cell in a cat cross-innervated 133 days previously. *Right traces* are from an L-cell in a cat cross-innervated 87 days previously. *Lower schematic diagrams* illustrate the experimental arrangements. PT, pyramidal tract cell. CP, cerebral peduncle. RN, red nucleus cell. RST, rubrospinal tract. FLX MN, flexor motoneuron. EXT MN, extensor motoneuron. C_1, C_1 spinal segment. L_1, L_1 spinal segment.

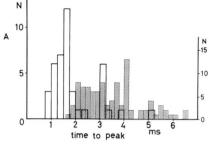

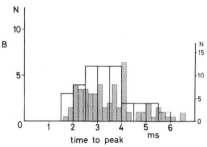

FIG. 8. The frequency distribution of time to peak of CP-EPSPs in cross-innervated cats. **A:** C-cells. **B:** L-cells. Number of cells is shown on the *ordinate* and the time to peak of CP-EPSPs in msec on the *abscissa*. The *shaded columns* in **A** and **B** illustrate the frequency distribution of time to peak in normal cats drawn from data given in ref. 47. The *right-hand ordinate scales* apply to normal cats and the *left-hand scales* for cross-innervated cats. (From ref. 44.)

EPSPs of the RN cells innervating the lower spinal segment (L-cell) had a much slower rise time than those of C-cells as shown in the right inset trace of Fig. 7. These RN cells could be antidromically excited by both C_1 and L_1 stimulation. The slower times to peak of CP-EPSPs in L-cells were also found in the histogram of Fig. 8B.

By analogy with the previous experiments, it was suggested that new synapses were formed at the proximal portion of the soma-dendritic membrane of RN cells by corticorubral fibers which normally terminate on the distal dendrites.

In order to investigate the time course of the change of CP-EPSPs after cross-innervation of the forelimb nerves, acute experiments were performed at various intervals after cross-innervation. Figure 9 illustrates the relation of the average time to peak of the CP-EPSPs and the postoperative survival period. In this study CP-EPSPs were categorized into two groups, those having times to peak of less than 3 msec (filled circles in Fig. 9), and those with times to peak equal to or greater than 3 msec (open circles in Fig. 9). It was noted that after about 2 months the time to peak of the CP-EPSPs reached a minimum and remained at that interval for more than 6 months.

Experiments were also performed in cats with self-union of the forelimb nerves. Even 84 days after self-union surgery, the time to peak of the majority of CP-EPSPs in C-cells was in the normal range, although occasional fast rising CP-EPSPs were observed.

Next we investigated the behavior of cats with cross-innervation of the forelimb nerves. It was not intended to explore in full quantitative detail the capacity for readjustment under such conditions. This would be a tremendous task, requir-

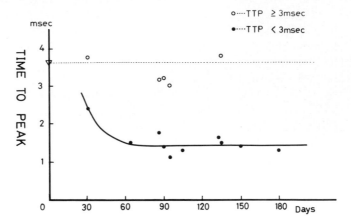

FIG. 9. Time course of the change of the rise time of the CP-EPSPs after cross-innervation of the forelimb nerves. *Open circles*, the mean time to peak of the CP-EPSPs equal or more than 3 msec. *Filled circles*, mean time to peak of the CP-EPSPs less than 3 msec. *Ordinate*, time to peak of the CP-EPSPs. *Abscissa*, days after cross-innervation. *Triangle*, mean time to peak of 100 CP-EPSPs in normal cats. (From Tsukahara et al., *unpublished.*)

ing a thorough analysis of normal kinesiology. The objective was rather to detect, if possible, any differences in a limited aspect of the motor behavior. Fortunately, the kinesiological analysis of quadripetal locomotion in the cat is available. It was hoped to find some evidence of relearning during quadripetal locomotion.

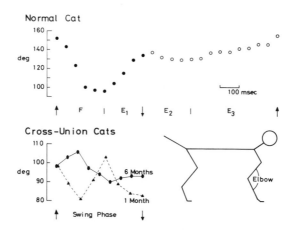

FIG. 10. Changes of forelimb movements during quadripedal locomotion in normal cats and after cross-innervation of the forelimb nerves. Elbow joint angles are illustrated during one step cycle of locomotion. F, flexion phase. E_1, E_2, E_3 phases, extension phase. *Upward arrow* indicates the onset of swing phase and *downward arrow* indicates the cessation of the swing phase. *Filled circles* of the cross-union cats indicate data from a cat cross-innervated 6 months previously. *Filled triangles* indicate those of a cat cross-innervated 1 month previously. See further explanation in text. (From Tsukahara et al., *unpublished.*)

The elbow joints during quadripetal locomotion were observed by a television monitor system, and the angles of the elbow joints of the normal cat, those studied 1 month after cross-innervation, and those studied 6 months after cross-innervation were compared. As in the intact walking cats previously reported (9,12,50), one cycle of locomotion could be divided into four phases: F, E_1, E_2, and E_3 phases (Fig. 10). At 1 month after cross-innervation, the elbow joint exhibited a short period of flexion followed by a large extension in the F phase, in sharp contrast to the flexion shown by normal cats during this phase. After 6 months, however, the elbow joint showed an initial short period of extension followed by a long flexion; thus, the overall movement was close to that of normal cats, except for the initial short extension period. This result suggests a partial recovery of normal movement.

DISCUSSION

There is considerable evidence indicating that collateral sprouting (8) occurs onto septal (23,31,32), hippocampal (17,41,42), tectal (11), and red nucleus neurons (29,45–47) after interruption of one of the convergent synaptic inputs to these neurons. We have addressed ourselves to the question of whether these sprouted synapses are functionally effective. For this purpose, we took advantages of the cable properties of dendrites of RN cells and their laminar synaptic organization: fibers from the nucleus interpositus of the cerebellum terminate on the soma and those from the cerebral sensorimotor cortex on the remote dendritic membrane (48,49).

Physiological investigation of collateral sprouting onto RN neurons has shown that the sprouted corticorubral synapses are functionally effective and exhibit physiological properties similar to those of the original corticorubral synapses as demonstrated by tests of facilitation and posttetanic potentiation (25–27).

The present investigation has supplied evidence that central synaptogenesis also takes place after cross-innervation of peripheral nerves (44). This is important for understanding the mechanisms of the initiation of sprouting. Until recently it has been believed that degeneration of nerve terminals might be required for the initiation of sprouting. If so, sprouting is merely a pathological reaction to damage. However, there are already two apparent exceptions to this rule. One is the cross-innervation experiment reported here. There is assumed to be no large-scale death of IP neurons after cross-innervation of peripheral nerves. Therefore, the postulated sprouting of corticorubral synapses after cross-innervation must occur in the absence of degeneration. The other is the finding reported by Aguilar et al. (1) that after mere interruption of axoplasmic transport in a peripheral nerve of the salamander, sprouting of adjacent peripheral nerves occurs in the absence of degeneration. The question therefore becomes: What factors determine whether the corticorubral fibers shall undergo collateral sprouting and by what means? At least in these cases, it seems unlikely that degenerating elements are essential.

A more functional view might be a competitive interaction among different kinds of inputs for the synaptic territory. One of the examples of this competition is that reported by Mark at the neuromuscular junction of lower vertebrates (19). Mark suggested that individual muscle fibers which accepted innervation from both original and foreign nerves after interruption of the nerve innervating that muscle suppressed transmission from the foreign nerve. Although this process of suppression did not occur in mammalian muscle (10), it was confirmed in adult newt muscle (51). During ontogenesis of the mammalian central nervous system, competitive interactions were suggested to occur. For example, Nah and Leong (28) have reported that unilateral lesion of the sensorimotor cortex in the rat during the first 3 days of birth induces a heavy anomalous corticorubral projection to cross the midline and ramify in the contralateral red nucleus. The density of this anomalous projection did not differ much in animals that had received their initial lesion within the first 3 days after birth, was only slightly less in animals operated at 5 days after birth, but was barely noticeable in animals operated on day 10 and thereafter. A similar competitive interaction at the early developmental stages was also reported for the cerebellorubral projection in rats (13).

Perhaps such a competitive interaction occurs even in adults. If the function of one of the synaptic inputs to RN is disorganized, the other input might make new connections which take over the synaptic territory held by the disorganized synapses. Thus what can be done surgically by lesions of the IP is considered to be only an exaggerated instance of a more general phenomenon encompassing disorders of IP input. From the functional viewpoint, this postulated sprouting of corticorubral synapses onto the proximal portion of the dendrites would mean a switching of control on RN neurons from cerebellar to cerebral predominance. In normal cats the interpositorubral synapses provide the main synaptic drive to RN neurons because of their somatic localization. After cross-innervation, or after lesion of IP, corticorubral synapses move closer to the neuronal trigger zone by sprouting new synapses, thus increasing their synaptic drive.

It is too soon to say for sure that synaptogenesis did take place in compensation for peripheral cross-innervation. Much more investigation is obviously needed. However, it is sufficient to say for the present purpose that there is reason to suppose that in adult cats, new synapses can be formed on RN neurons in the absence of damage to their afferent and efferent fibers.

REFERENCES

1. Aguiar, C. E., Bisby, M. A., Cooper, E., and Diamond, J. (1973): Evidence that axoplasmic transport of trophic factors is involved in the regulation of peripheral nerve fields in salamanders. *J. Physiol.*, 234:449–464.
2. Allen, G. I., and Tsukahara, N. (1974): Cerebrocerebellar communication systems. *Physiol. Rev.*, 54:957–1006.
3. Barrett, J. N., and Crill, W. E. (1974): Specific membrane properties of cat motoneurones. *J. Physiol.*, 239:301–324.

4. Burke, R. E., and Bruggencate, C. N. (1971): Electrotonic characteristics of alpha motoneurones of varying size. *J. Physiol.*, 212:1–20.
5. Eccles, J. C. (1964): *The Physiology of Synapses.* Springer-Verlag, Berlin, Heidelberg, New York.
6. Eccles, J. C. (1976): The plasticity of the mammalian central nervous system with special reference to new growths in response to lesions. *Naturwissenschaften,* 63:8–15.
7. Eccles, J. C., Eccles, R. M., Shealy, C. N., and Willis, W. D. (1962): Experiments utilizing monosynaptic excitatory action on motoneurons for testing hypothesis relating to specificity of neuronal connection. *J. Neurophysiol.*, 25:559–579.
8. Edds, Jr., M. V. (1953): Collateral nerve regeneration. *Q. Rev. Biol.*, 28:260–276.
9. Engberg, I., and Lundberg, A. (1969): An electromyographic analysis of muscular activity in the hindlimb of the cat during unrestrained locomotion. *Acta Physiol. Scand.*, 75:614–630.
10. Frank, E., Jansen, J. K. S., Lømo, T., and Westgaard, E. (1975): The interaction between foreign and original motor nerves innervating the soleus muscle of rats. *J. Physiol.*, 247:725–743.
11. Goodman, D. C. and Horel, J. A. (1967): Sprouting of optic tract projections in the brain stem of the rat. *J. Comp. Neurol.*, 127:71–88.
12. Goslow, G. E., Reinking, R. M., and Stuart, D. G. (1973): The cat step cycle: hindlimb joint angles and muscle lengths during unrestrained locomotion. *J. Morphol.*, 141:1–42.
13. Lim, K. H., and Leong, S. K. (1975): Aberrant bilateral projections from dentate and interposed nuclei in albino rats after neonatal lesions. *Brain Res.*, 96:306–309.
14. Liu, C. M., and Chambers, W. W. (1958): Intraspinal sprouting of dorsal root axons. *Arch. Neurol.*, 79:46–61.
15. Llinas, R., and Nicholson, C. (1971): Electrophysiological properties of dendrites and somata in alligator Purkinje cells. *J. Neurophysiol.*, 34:532–551.
16. Lux, H. D., Schubert, P., and Kreutzberg, G. W. (1970): Direct matching of morphological and electrophysiological data in cat spinal motoneurones. In: *Excitatory Synaptic Mechanisms,* edited by P. Andersen and J. K. S. Jansen. Universitetsforlaget, Oslo.
17. Lynch, G., Deadwyler, S., and Cotman, C. (1973): Postlesion axonal growth produces permanent functional connections. *Science,* 180:1364–1366.
18. Mallert, A., and Martin, A. R. (1967): An analysis of facilitation of transmitter release at the neuromuscular junction of the frog. *J. Physiol.*, 193:679–694.
19. Mark, R. (1974): *Memory and Nerve Cell Connections. Criticisms and Contributions from Developmental Neurobiology.* Clarendon Press, Oxford.
20. Martin, A. R. (1955): A further study of the statistical composition of the end-plate potential. *J. Physiol.*, 130:114–122.
21. Mendell, L. M., and Scott, J. G. (1975): The effect of peripheral nerve cross-union on connections of single Ia fibers to motoneurons. *Exp. Brain Res.*, 22:221–234.
22. Miledi, R. (1960): The acetylcholine sensitivity of frog muscle fibres after complete or partial denervation. *J. Physiol.*, 151:1–23.
23. Moore, R. Y., Björklund, A., and Stenevi, U. (1971): Plastic changes in the adrenergic innervation of rat septal area in response to denervation. *Brain Res.*, 33:13–35.
24. Muir, R. B., and Porter, R. (1973): The effect of preceding stimulus on temporal facilitation at cortico-motoneuronal synapses. *J. Physiol.*, 228:749–763.
25. Murakami, F., Fujito, Y., and Tsukahara, N. (1976): Physiological properties of the newly formed cortico-rubral synapses of red nucleus neurons due to collateral sprouting. *Brain Res.*, 103:146–151.
26. Murakami, F., Tsukahara, N., and Fujito, Y. (1977): Analysis of unitary EPSPs mediated by the newly-formed cortico-rubral synapses after lesion of the interpositus nucleus. *Exp. Brain Res.*, 30:233–243.
27. Murakami, F., Tsukahara, N., and Fujito, Y. (1978): Properties of synaptic transmission of the newly formed cortico-rubral synapses after lesion of the nucleus interpositus of the cerebellum. *Exp. Brain Res.*, 30:245–258.
28. Nah, S. H., and Leong, S. K. (1976): Bilateral corticofugal projection to the red nucleus after neonatal lesions in the albino rat. *Brain Res.*, 107:433–436.
29. Nakamura, Y., Mizuno, N., Konishi, A., and Sato, M. (1974): Synaptic reorganization of the red nucleus after chronic deafferentation from cerebellorubral fibers: an electron-microscopic study in the cat. *Brain Res.*, 82:298–301.

30. Nelson, P. G., and Lux, H. D. (1970): Some electrical measurements of motoneuron parameters. *Biophys. J.,* 10:55–73.
31. Raisman, G. (1969): Neuronal plasticity in the septal nuclei of the adult rat. *Brain Res.,* 14:25–48.
32. Raisman, G., and Field, P. M. (1973): A quantitative investigation of the development of collateral reinnervation after partial deafferentation of the septal nuclei. *Brain Res.,* 50:241–264.
33. Rall, W. (1964): Theoretical significance of dendritic trees for neuronal input-output relations. In: *Neural Theory and Modeling,* edited by R. F. Reiss, pp. 73–97. Stanford University Press, Stanford.
34. Rall, W. (1969): Time constants and electrotonic length of membrane cylinders and neurons. *Biophys. J.,* 9:1483–1508.
35. Rall, W., Burke, R. E., Smith, T. G., Nelson. P. G., and Frank, K. (1967): Dendritic location of synapses and possible mechanisms for the monosynaptic EPSP in motoneurons. *J. Neurophysiol.,* 30:1169–1193.
36. Rall, W., and Rinzel, J. (1973): Branch input resistance and steady attenuation for input to one branch of a dendritic neuron model. *Biophys. J.,* 13:648–688.
37. Sato, S., and Tsukahara, N. (1976): Some properties of the theoretical membrane transients in Rall's neuron model. *J. Theor. Biol.,* 63:151–163.
38. Spencer, W. A. and Kandel, E. R. (1961): Electrophysiology of hippocampal neurons. IV. Fast prepotentials. *J. Neurophysiol.,* 24:272–285.
39. Sperry, R. W. (1947): Effect of crossing nerves to antagonistic limb muscles in the monkey. *Arch. Neurol. Psychiatry,* 58:452–473.
40. Sperry, R. W. (1945): The problem of central nervous reorganization after nerve regeneration and muscle transposition. *Quart. Rev. Biol.,* 20:311–369.
41. Steward, O., Cotman, C. W., and Lynch, G. S. (1974): Growth of a new fiber projection in the brain of adult rats: reinnervation of the dentate gyrus by contralateral entorhinal cortex following ipsilateral entorhinal lesions. *Exp. Brain Res.,* 20:45–66.
42. Steward, O., White, W. F., Cotman, C. W., and Lynch, G. (1976): Potentiation of excitatory synaptic transmission in the normal and in the reinnervated dentate gyrus of the rat. *Exp. Brain Res.,* 26:423–441.
43. Toyama, K., Tsukahara, N., Kosaka, K., and Matsunami, K. (1970): Synaptic excitation of red nucleus neurons by fibers from interpositus nucleus. *Exp. Brain Res.,* 11:187–198.
44. Tsukahara, N., and Fujito, Y. (1976): Physiological evidence of formation of new synapses from cerebrum in the red nucleus neurons following cross-union of forelimb nerves. *Brain Res.,* 106:184–188.
45. Tsukahara, N., Hultborn, H., and Murakami, F. (1974): Sprouting of cortico-rubral synapses in red nucleus neurons after destruction of the nucleus interpositus of the cerebellum. *Experientia (Basel)* 30:57–58.
46. Tsukahara, N., Hultborn, H., Murakami, F., and Fujito, Y. (1975a): Physiological evidences of collateral sprouting and formation of new synapses in the red nucleus following partial denervation. In: *Golgi Centennial Symposium Proceedings,* edited by M. Santini, pp. 299–303. Raven Press, New York.
47. Tsukahara, N., Hultborn, H., Murakami, F., and Fujito, Y. (1975b): Electrophysiological study of formation of new synapses and collateral sprouting in red nucleus neurons after partial denervation. *J. Neurophysiol.,* 38:1359–1372.
48. Tsukahara, N., and Kosaka, K. (1968): The mode of cerebral excitation of red nucleus neurons. *Exp. Brain Res.,* 5:102–117.
49. Tsukahara, N., Murakami, F., and Hultborn, H. (1975c): Electrical constants of neurons of the red nucleus. *Exp. Brain Res.,* 23:49–64.
50. Udo, M., Oda, Y., Tanaka, K., and Hirokawa, J. (1976): Cerebellar control of locomotion investigated in cats: discharges from Deiter's neurons, EMG and limb movements during local cooling of the cerebellar cortex. In: *Understanding the Stretch Reflex,* edited by S. Homma. *Prog. Brain Res.,* 44:445–459.
51. Yip, J. W., and Dennis, M. J. (1976): Suppression of transmission at foreign synapses in adult newt muscle involves reduction in quantal content. *Nature,* 260:350–352.

Neuronal Plasticity, edited by
Carl W. Cotman.
Raven Press, New York © 1978.

The Olfactory System: A Model for the Study of Neurogenesis and Axon Regeneration in Mammals

P. P. C. Graziadei and G. A. Monti Graziadei

Department of Biological Science, Florida State University, Tallahassee, Florida 32306

The olfactory system of mammals has seldom been used for studies related to neuron dynamics and plasticity (18,19). However, we now have experimental evidence that this system may be very suitable for such studies (28,30,45). In this chapter we will discuss neuron dynamics and plasticity in two parts of the olfactory system, the olfactory epithelium and the olfactory bulb.

Recent studies have shown that the remarkable capacity of neurogenesis persists in the olfactory neuroepithelium of adult mammals. The primary olfactory neurons, in fact, undergo a continuous turnover which in turn is paralleled by a continuous renewal of their synaptic endings in the olfactory bulb glomeruli. Furthermore, this part of the olfactory system is amenable to experimental manipulation as a result of the anatomical accessibility and simple organization of the bulb, the discreteness of input and output within the bulb, and the well known and simple pattern of the receptor sheat. The presence of a specific marker protein, manufactured in the perikaria of the primary neurons and identified in the axons and axon terminals in the bulb (42,45), offers a further experimental advantage for the tracing and recognition of the regenerating neurons.

ANATOMY OF THE SYSTEM

The primary sensory neurons of the olfactory system are located peripherally in the *regio olfactoria* of the nasal cavity. The neuroepithelium of this region has been described by many authors (for a review see refs. 22,36) as being composed of basal cells, primary neurons, and supporting cells. The primary

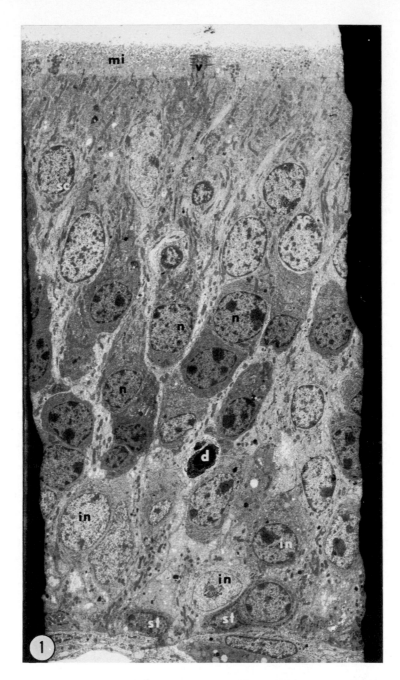

FIG. 1. Electron micrograph of the normal olfactory mucosa of rat. The free surface of the neuroepithelium is covered by a bushy layer of microvilli (mi) that belong to the supporting cells (sc). The olfactory vesicles (v) of the receptors can be seen in this layer. The supporting cells' nuclei form a layer close to the surface and discrete from the neuron nuclei (n). In proximity to the basal lamina of the neuroepithelium there are the stem cells (st) of the neurons (so-called basal cells), and above these lie the young immature neurons (in). A degenerating neuron fragment is seen at (d). ×1,900.

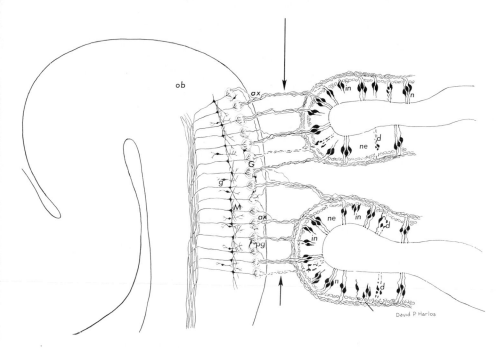

FIG. 2. The figure illustrates the connections of the olfactory neuroepithelium (ne) with the olfactory bulb (ob). In the olfactory neuroepithelium there are groups of mature neurons (n), young neurons (in), and degenerating neurons (d). The dendrite of the young neurons has not yet reached the surface of the epithelium, and the axons have not extended to the olfactory bulb. The two *arrows* indicate the structure of the lamina cribrosa, where the axotomy was performed. In the olfactory bulb the sensory axons (ax) branch in the glomeruli (G), where they synapse with the mitral cells' (M) dendrites and the periglomerular cells (pg). The granule cells (g) have also been indicated.

neurons are bipolar elements characterized by a unique, unbranched dendrite that reaches the surface of the epithelium and expands in a bulbous terminal provided with cilia (the olfactory vesicle of van der Stricht) (Fig. 1). These neurons have unmyelinated axons which in mammals form discrete bundles, called the *fila olfactoria*. The axons travel through the *lamina cribrosa* of the ethmoidal bone and reach the glomerular layer of the olfactory bulb (Fig. 2), where they synapse on the apical dendrite of the mitral cell (14). The mitral cell axons are the only efferent pathway from the olfactory bulb. Interneurons, both at the level of the glomeruli (the periglomerular cells) and at the level of the mitral cells (the granule cells), establish local connections, as previously described by Cajal (14) and, more recently, as studied at the ultrastructural level by many authors (5,7,31,34,52–56,59,60).

NEUROGENESIS IN THE OLFACTORY NEUROEPITHELIUM OF ADULT MAMMALS

The primary olfactory neurons originate, outside the neural tube, directly from the olfactory placode, a thickening of the cranial ectoderm (8,13,20,49,51).

Their axons secondarily grow to the telencephalic vesicle where they initiate the development of the olfactory bulb (32,50,51). While it has been generally held that neurons in the nervous system of adult mammals do not increase in number and cannot be replaced (11,12,40,41,43), there have been controversial reports in the literature claiming that neurogenesis can persist in the olfactory epithelium of adult mammals and that olfactory neurons can be replaced after injury (for a review see ref. 58).

During the past several years in our laboratory we have conducted studies designed to explore the possibility that neurogenesis may indeed occur in the olfactory neuroepithelium. Evidence in favor of this hypothesis has been collected from morphological, autoradiographic, and experimental studies. The results of these studies are summarized below.

With the use of colchicine it was possible at first to show the presence of mitotic figures collected in the basal layer of the olfactory neuroepithelium. These findings supported the observations of Andres (6,7), who described mitotic figures in the olfactory mucosa of young mammals and interpreted them as belonging to "blastoma cells" of the neurons. Since then, combined morphological and autoradiographic data have delineated the many different stages of maturation of the olfactory neurons (Figs. 3,4, and 5) and have provided an insight into the temporal pattern of their differentiation (22,23,25–28). In animals sacrificed at short survival times (from 1 to 24 hrs, following ^{3}H thymidine injection), the labeled elements are confined to the basal layer of the neuroepithelium

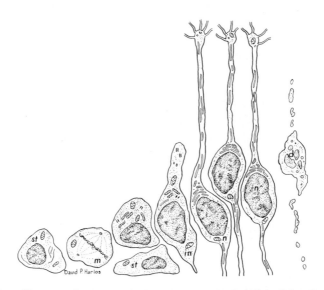

FIG. 3. The figure illustrates the stages of differentiation and maturation of the olfactory neurons as observed in the normal olfactory mucosa. Staminal cells (st) frequently divide (m) and differentiate into immature neurons (in). In n are indicated the mature neurons and in d the debris of a degenerated neuron.

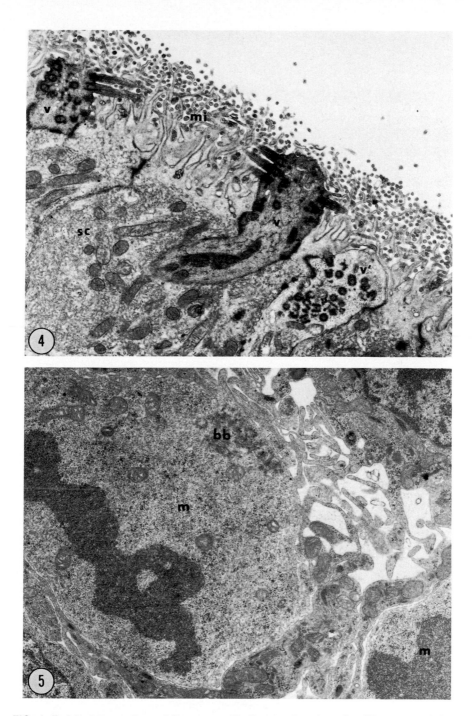

FIG. 4. Detail of the surface of the neuroepithelium to show how the different morphology of the olfactory vesicles (v) relates to the stages of maturation of the neurons. The olfactory vesicle (v′) belongs to a developing neuron and is characterized by a clear cytoplasm and many basal bodies (bb). ×20,500.

FIG. 5. The mitotic figure (m) at the base of the neuroepithelium is already characterized by many basal bodies (bb) which are a typical feature of the neurons. ×20,000.

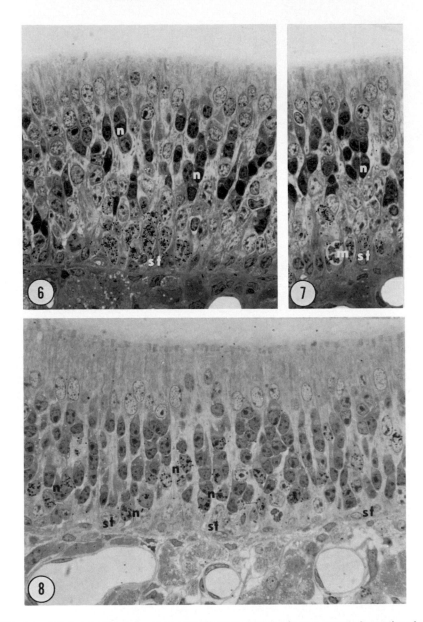

FIGS. 6 and 7. Autoradiographs of normal olfactory mucosa from a mouse 6 months of age. The animal was given three pulses of ³H-thymidine (5 μC/gm body weight) at 24, 18, and 12 hr before sacrifice. A group of basal cells (st) shows intense label; in Fig. 7, there are a mitotic figure (m) and other labeled basal cells (st). X750.

FIG. 8. Autoradiograph of normal olfactory mucosa of mouse, 6 months of age. The animal was injected with 3 pulses of ³H-thymidine for 3 days and sacrificed 11 days after the beginning of the experiment. All the labeled elements are mature neurons (n), some of them close to the basal lamina (n′). Basal cells (st) do not have label. X750.

(Figs. 6 and 7); after 7 days of survival the label is concentrated in the young developing neurons, and from 10 to 20 days in the mature cells (Fig. 8). The labeled elements have all migrated from the neuroepithelium when the animals are allowed to survive for 35 days after ^{3}H thymidine injection.

It has been suggested that the supportive epithelial cells that are secretory might be the ones to originate from the basal cells (23,47). However, the observation of mitotic figures in the upper third of the epithelium and of labeled elements, appearing at short survival time after pulse labeling and remaining unchanged for a period of over 35 days, indicates that the supporting cells divide *in situ* (upper third of the epithelium) and that their rate of turnover is slower than that of the neurons (28,46).

TURNOVER OF SYNAPSES IN THE NORMAL OLFACTORY BULB

If olfactory neurons in the sensory neuroepithelium turnover, then there must be a corresponding turnover of synaptic terminals in the olfactory bulb glomeruli where the olfactory nerves synapse with the glomerular cells. Ultrastructural observations in our laboratory have shown that in the normal glomerulus there exist, at any time, a number of terminals undergoing degeneration. The degenerating terminals can be recognized by the increased electron density of their cytoplasm and by the swelling of their synaptic vesicles. We have occasionally observed terminals with electron-lucent cytoplasm and large, clear vesicles, not clumped near the synaptic membrane. We interpret these as terminals in the early stages of degeneration. The glia, usually inconspicuous within the glomerular neuropile, expand in large profiles that surround the degenerating terminals (Fig. 9). The terminals become secondarily engulfed in the glial cells that resemble the phagosomes, previously described by Estable-Puig and deEstable (21) and Berger (9,10) in studies on degeneration of the bulb.

The recognition of newly established synaptic terminals in the normal glomerulus is morphologically more difficult due to their apparent close resemblance to mature terminals.

DEGENERATION AND REGENERATION IN THE OLFACTORY NEUROEPITHELIUM

In order to further explore the dynamic characteristics of the olfactory neuroepithelium, we severed the axons of the olfactory neurons at the level of the lamina cribrosa in rats and mice (Fig. 2). This resulted not only in the terminal degeneration of the axons and their synaptic endings in the bulb glomeruli, but also in the retrograde degeneration of the perikaria in the neuroepithelium (Fig. 10). With this procedure we demonstrated that retrograde degeneration of the olfactory perikaria was already apparent 24 hr after surgery and was completed by the 10th day. The neuroepithelium after 10 days contained only

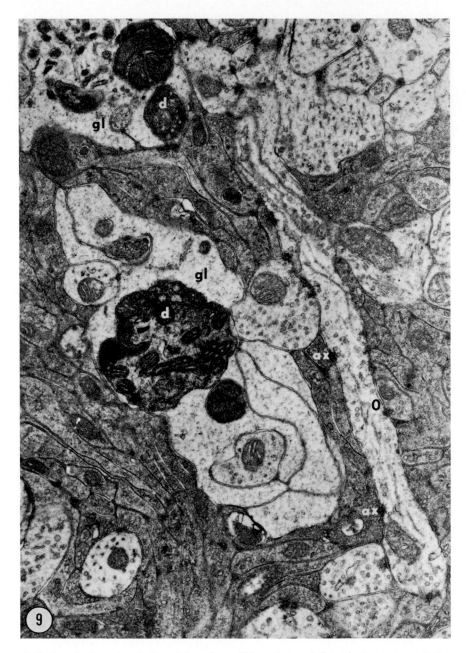

FIG. 9. Detail of a normal glomerulus of rat. The endings of the primary neurons (ax) are clearly seen for their dense appearance and the presence of vesicles clumped close to the synaptic membrane. Degenerating terminals (d) are engulfed in the glia profiles (gl). ×12,500.

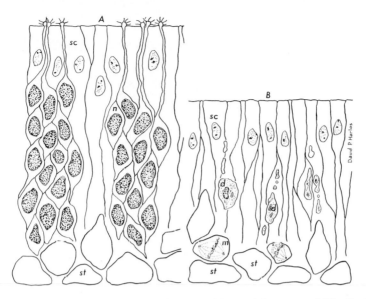

FIG. 10. A diagramatical representation of the normal **(A)** and degenerated **(B)** olfactory neuroepithelium. In **B** the neurons have totally disappeared. Remnants of degenerated elements are indicated at d. Basal cells (st) and mitotic figures (m) are illustrated at the base of the epithelium.

the supporting cells, the basal cells, and the immature neurons whose axons did not yet extend into the lamina cribrosa and therefore escaped damage during surgery (Figs. 11–13). Coincident to and following the degenerative process, an increased mitotic activity of the basal cells occurs in the neuroepithelium (28). This phenomenon can be documented both morphologically and autoradiographically. Differentiation of the basal cells into neurons follows the period of mitotic activity and by the 30th day the epithelium has regained a normal morphological organization, with the typical layers of basal cells, neurons, and supporting cells (Figs. 13,14)! We did not observe any substantial changes in the supporting cells during the degenerative and regenerative phases of the neuronal components of the neuroepithelium.

DEGENERATION AND REGENERATION OF AXONS IN THE OLFACTORY BULB

Following the surgical section of the axons, there ensues terminal degeneration of their centripetal portion. This degenerative process, which is restricted to the peripheral nerve layer and to the glomerular layer of the olfactory bulb, is clearly observed even at the light microscope level 44 hr after surgery. At this early time, electron micrographs show that the glial processes are dramatically hypertrophied and filled with degenerated terminals (compare Figs. 15 and 16 with Figs. 17 and 18). By the 10th day after surgery, the terminals

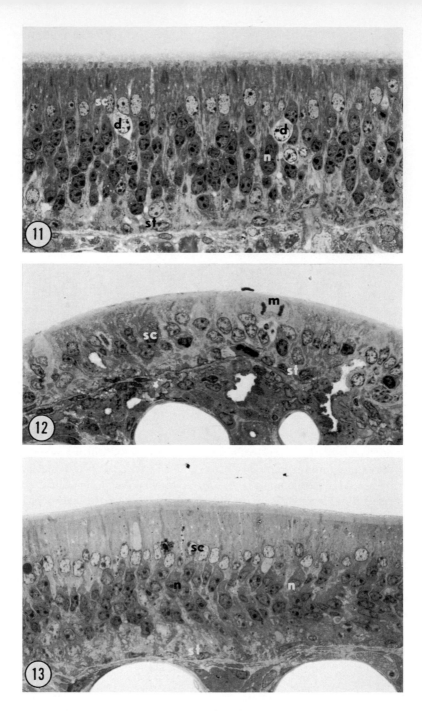

FIG. 11. Normal olfactory epithelium of rodent. Supporting cells (sc), neurons (n), and stem cells (st) can be clearly identified. Two degenerating neurons (d) are seen in the upper portion of the neuron layer. X750.

FIG. 12. Olfactory neuroepithelium 8 days after axotomy. The neuronal layer has practically disappeared, due to the retrograde degeneration of all the mature neurons. Supporting cells (sc) and basal cells (st) can be recognized. A mitotic figure (m) in the upper third of the epithelium belongs to a supporting cell. X750.

FIG. 13. Olfactory neuroepithelium of rodent 33 days after axotomy. The neuroepithelium has regained an organization similar to controls after the reappearance of the neurons (n). X750.

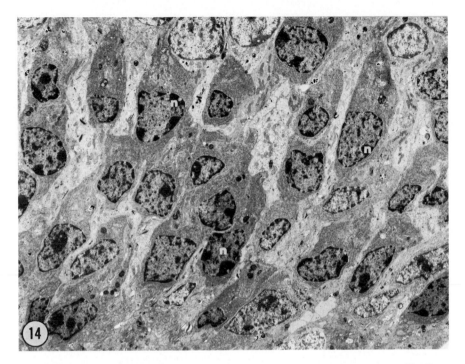

FIG. 14. Electron micrograph of the neuroepithelium of rat 33 days after axotomy. The illustration shows the neuron layer (n). The structural pattern of the neurons is characteristically homogeneous due to their synchronous development. In the normal neuroepithelia neurons are normally found at different stages of maturation. X2,600.

engulfed by the glia have disappeared and the thick glial processes again become inconspicuous. At 20 days the glomeruli, now containing only dendritic profiles of the periglomerular and mitral cells, show a reduction in their diameter to approxomately two-thirds their usual size (Fig. 19). At this time, however, the axons of the reconstituted neurons begin to reappear in the peripheral nerve layer. These axons are of small diameter, contain numerous microtubules, and run either singularly or in small groups in pockets of glial cells (Fig. 20). Many typical growth cones are seen in the distal tips of the growing axons (Fig. 21). At this early stage of regeneration the glomerular neuropile is still free of the sensory axons terminals. After 30 days these sensory endings can be recognized inside the glomerular neuropile (Figs. 22,23) where they establish synaptic contacts with the glomerular dendrites.

We have observed that the degenerative phenomenon follows a slightly different time course in different parts of the bulb. The rostroventral portion, which is closer to the lamina cribrosa, is the first to be affected by the degenerative process. It is in this region, even 44 hr following surgery, that most terminals are already in the final phases of degeneration. In the dorsocaudal portion 3

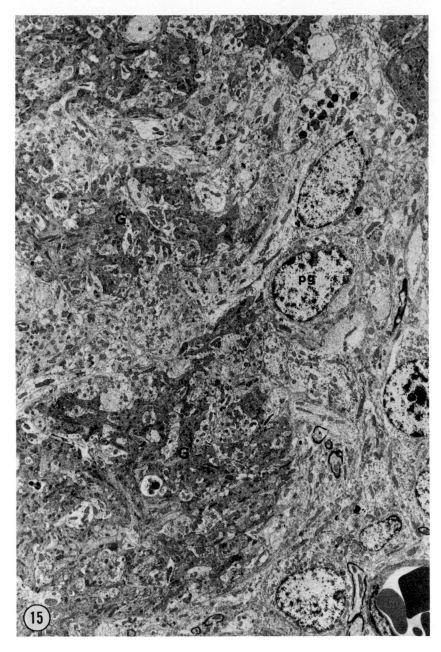

FIG. 15. Low power electron micrograph of the glomerular layer of the bulb in rat. The compact structure of the glomerulus (G) is obvious. Nuclei of periglomerular cells are indicated (pg). ×2,800.

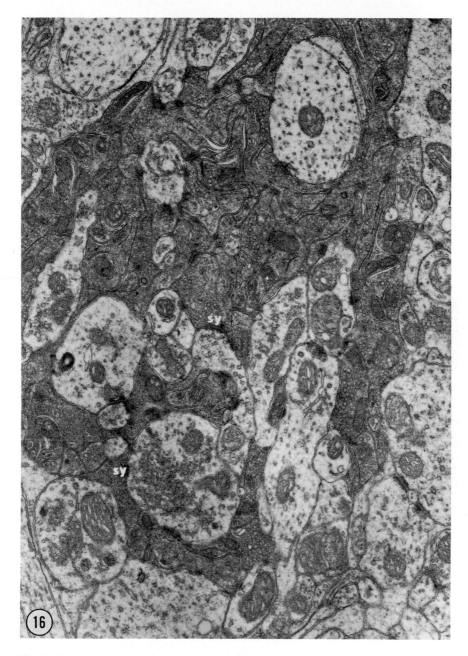

FIG. 16. Detail of a normal glomerulus in rat. The sensory axon terminals establish synaptic contacts (sy) with the dendritic profiles. X31,000.

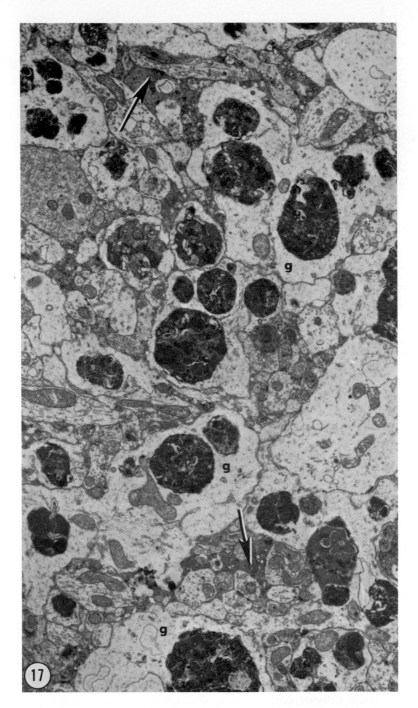

FIG. 17. Neuropile of the glomerulus of rat 44 hr after axotomy. Most terminals are engulfed in the glial processes which are expanded and occupy most of the area of the section. Some terminals, showing only an increased density of the cytoplasm, are still recognizable *(arrows).* This preparation was obtained from the rostroventral portion of the bulb (see text). X14,000.

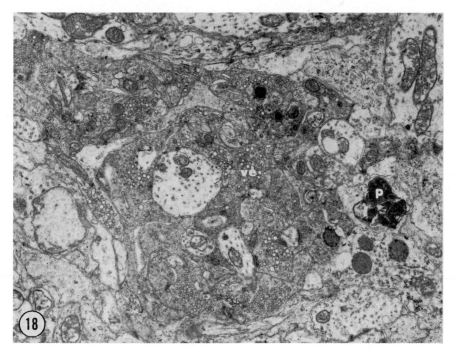

FIG. 18. Island of degeneration in a glomerulus located in the dorsocaudal portion of the bulb, from a rat sacrificed 76 hr after axotomy. The process of degeneration is characterized mostly by a swollen appearance of the vesicles (ve). One phagosome (p) is engulfed in a glial process. X19,000.

days after axotomy, the synaptic endings start to show the first signs of sufference, as exemplified by swollen vesicles and electron dense cytoplasm (Fig. 17).

The degeneration and reconstitution of the olfactory neurons and the regrowth of their axons into the olfactory bulb glomeruli have been further substantiated with biochemical techniques. After axotomy, the retrograde degeneration of the neurons is paralleled by a disappearance of the olfactory marker protein in the neuroepithelium and in the bulb. The morphological reconstitution of the neurons is followed by a reappearance of the marker protein in the neuroepithelium and subsequently in the olfactory bulb (30). With immunochemical techniques, using immunohistochemistry (57) the specific protein has been shown to be localized in the mature functional neurons and not in their precursor stem cells (45). These observations provide further documentation that indeed the neuron population has been reconstituted.

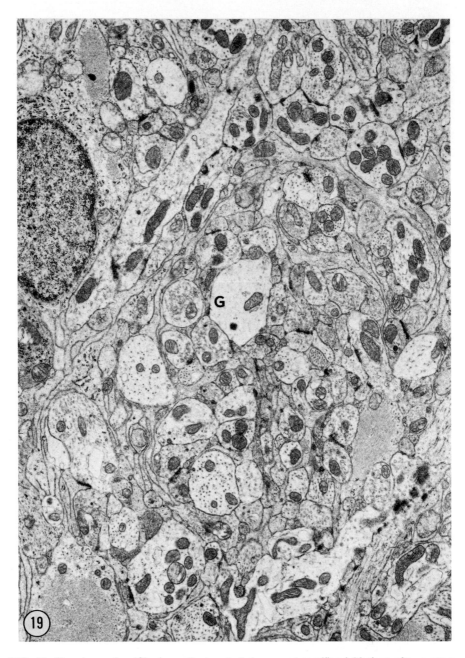

FIG. 19. The glomerulus (G) of an olfactory bulb from a rat sacrificed 20 days after axotomy shows absence of axon terminals. The glia, conspicuous during the first 10 days of degeneration (see Fig. 17), is not prominent at this time. The only synaptic contacts observed are established between dendrites. X16,500.

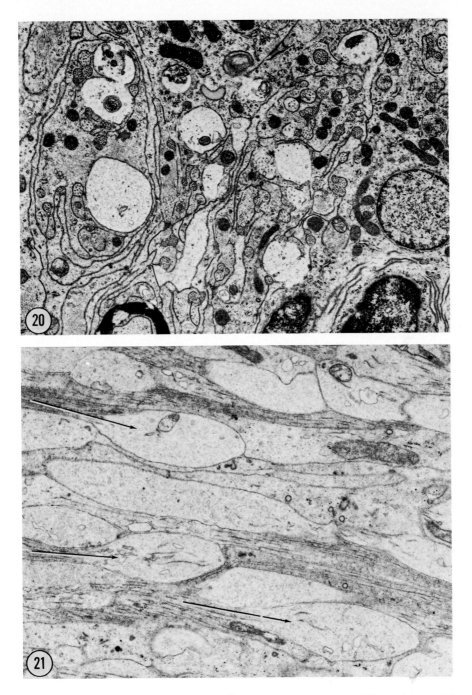

FIG. 20. Small axons of the reconstituted olfactory neurons reappear at the periphery of the glomerulus 20 days after surgery. They are sparse and singularly invaginated in the cytoplasm of the glial cells. X21,000.

FIG. 21. Same preparation as in Fig. 20 but in a portion of the external nerve layer where the regrowing olfactory axons are longitudinally sectioned. Some of them have been sectioned at the level of their growth cone *(arrows)*. X18,000.

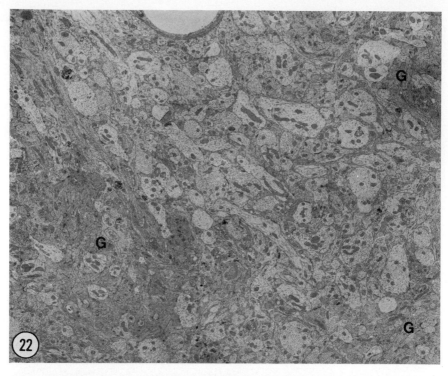

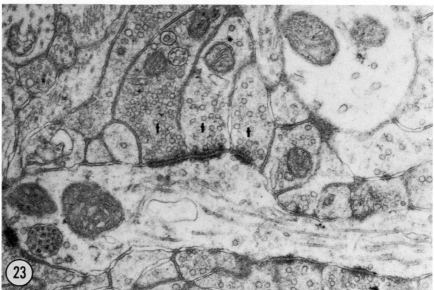

FIG. 22. Low power electron micrograph of a reinnervated olfactory bulb 33 days after denervation. The glomeruli (G) show the normal pattern of dense profiles (olfactory axons) and clear dendritic processes. X3,100.

FIG. 23. Detail of a reinnervated glomerulus 33 days after denervation showing the characteristic axon terminals (t) synapsing on a dendrite. X44,000.

CONCLUSIONS

In the nervous sytem of adult mammals, the primary olfactory neurons are the only known example of nerve cells which undergo turnover and are capable of regeneration after experimental injury. Furthermore, their axons provide a unique example of nerve fibers with the ability to regrow into the CNS and establish functional contacts (24,28).

That neurogenesis of microneurons may persist in the nervous system of mammals for some time after birth has been demonstrated in the olfactory bulb, hippocampus, and cerebellum (see ref. 4 for review). Recently Hinds and associates (33,35) have shown in rats that the granule cells of the olfactory bulb continue to increase in number well beyond maturity. These observations indicate that the nervous system, or at least parts of it, are not yet fully defined at birth and that some degree of plasticity may extend for a considerable time during the animal's life. However, the primary olfactory neurons are a unique model of a neuronal population that has well-defined and recognized lines of precursors and retains a constant number of cells via a dynamic process of death and rebirth. Our past and present studies indicate that this neurogenetic activity of the olfactory neuroepithelium is common to many vertebrates such as frogs, pigeons, gerbils, rats, and mice (23–28,30,44,48), and more recent work indicates that primates as well conform to this rule.

We do not understand the mechanisms that allow the olfactory matrix to maintain its neurogenetic activity (in contrast to the other portions of the nervous system). Equally unclear are the mechanisms that trigger the phenomena of differentiation and maturation of the stem cells. As yet, we do not have a working hypothesis to explain why the matrix remains into adult life, but we might suggest that the phenomenon of maturation of the stem cells may be triggered by the release of a "substance" provided by the decaying neurons. This hypothesis is consistent with the experimental observation that, when we determine the presence of massive destruction of the mature neurons, we simultaneously witness a rapid and tumultuous neurogenetic process, preceeded by active division of the stem cells.

Possibly the most puzzling property of the olfactory system is its ability to maintain an efficient sensory apparatus offering consistent performance in spite of the turnover of its primary neurons. The system has a simple morphological pattern; however, it is capable of an extremely sophisticated performance. There is considerable convergence of the primary neurons onto the mitral cells. For example, in the rabbit there are 50 million receptors converging onto 1,900 glomeruli, where the dendrites of approximately 45,000 mitral cells branch to receive the synaptic sensory input (3). Within the glomeruli the synaptic linkages are specific, and the patterns of connections repeat themselves with extreme regularity, albeit with species differences (52,53,56,59,60). Furthermore, electrophysiological and morphological observations reveal a distinct projection pattern from the olfactory sensory epithelium to the olfactory bulb (1,2,15–17,37–39).

If some degree of locus specificity is needed for the total performance of the organ and if different regions of the peripheral olfactory sheat project into specific regions of the bulb glomerular layer, then each neuron and each axon must have sufficient information to select the right glomerulus and the right site on the membrane of the postsynaptic element. Our experimental evidence shows that, following complete axotomy, the stream of newly growing axons reaches the bulb and occupies the rostroventral glomeruli first. As these are the "nearest" vacant loci, one could believe that connections are randomly formed. However, additional data are needed. But, we now believe that it is possible to explore how these new axons find their way to a target cell in the olfactory bulb, and to ask and answer the pertinent question of whether each new axon reoccupies a specific vacant site or contacts dendrites randomly in want of input. If the second hypothesis should be proven correct, then this may further imply that in the olfactory system the coding of information is implemented without a morphological-topographical substrate, in contrast to other sensory systems such as vision.

Whereas the parameters of the axonal regrowth demand investigation, our studies document that the CNS of adult mammals is not impervious to the penetration of axons and that functional recovery is possible. Here, we have a model where an input of homogeneous sensory fibers regrow to contact the second neurons (the mitral cells) that do not have the potential of accepting spurious elements and being distracted by the phenomena of collateral sprouting of neighboring elements after experimental deafferentiation. Actually, we may consider collateral sprouting as a "noise" phenomenon which does not allow the postsynaptic element to be receptive to the proper connections. Conversely, one could conceive that, in the maze of the CNS, fibers attempting to reach the proper target may be forbidden from doing so by the acceptance of their first attempted sprouting by nonspecific receptor elements in the neighborhood. We must also emphasize that the presence of scar tissue may play a limiting role in the regeneration of the CNS (29). In the course of our studies we have observed that newly generated axons invariably fail to reach the target when the surgical procedure has left a scar at the site of the lesion. But when the scar is essentially absent, regeneration is very robust.

We are pursuing the study of the olfactory system in an attempt to answer some of the questions mentioned above. For the first time we have at hand a disposable neuron that will continuously regenerate. This proves that regrowth of functional connections in the CNS of mammals can be achieved. Why not other places too?

ACKNOWLEDGMENT

This research was supported in part by a grant from the PHS NS 08943. The authors wish to thank Drs. R. R. Levine and D. W. Samanen for helpful criticism and for reading the manuscript and Mrs. H. M. Sloan for excellent technical assistance.

REFERENCES

1. Adrian, E. D. (1950): The electrical activity of the mammalian olfactory bulb. *Electroencephalog. Clin. Neurophysiol.,* 2:377–388.
2. Adrian, E. D. (1953): Sensory messages and sensation. The response of the olfactory organ to different smells. *Acta Physiol. Scand.,* 29:4–14.
3. Allison, A. C., and Warwick, R. T. (1949): Quantitative observations on the olfactory system of the rabbit. *Brain,* 72:186–197.
4. Altman, J. (1970): Postnatal neurogenesis and the problem of neural plasticity. In: *Developmental Neurobiology,* edited by W. A. Himwich, pp. 197–237. C C Thomas, Springfield, Ill.
5. Andres, K. H. (1965*a*): Der Feinbau des Bulbus olfactorius der Ratte unter besonderer Berücksichtigung der synaptischen Verbindindungen. *Z. Zellforsch. Mikroskop. Anat.,* 65:530–561.
6. Andres, K. H. (1965 *b*); Differenzierung und Regeneration von Sinnezellen in der Regio Olfactoria. *Naturwissenschaften,* 17:500.
7. Andres, K. H. (1966): Der Feinbau der Regio Olfactoria von Makrosmatikern. *Z. Zellforsch.,* 69:140–154.
8. Bedford, E. A. (1904): The early history of the olfactory nerve in Swine. *J. Comp. Neurol.,* 14:390–410.
9. Berger, B. (1971): Formes diverses de degenerescence des boutons synaptiques dans le glomerule olfactif de lapin apres lesion du nerf olfactif. *Brain Res.,* 33:218–222.
10. Berger, B. (1973): Degenerescence transynaptique dans le bulbe olfactif du lapin, apres desafferentiation peripherique. *Acta Neuropath.,* 24:128–152.
11. Bizzozero G. (1894): Growth and regeneration of the organism. *Brit. Med. J.,* 1:728–732.
12. Bizzozero, G. (1895): Accresimento e rigenerazione nell'organismo. *Arch. Sci. Med. It.,* 18:245–287.
13. Brookover, C., and Jackson, T. S. (1911): The olfactory nerve and nervus terminalis of Ameiurus. *J. Comp. Neurol.,* 21:237–259.
14. Cajal, S. R. (1911): *Histology du systeme nerveux de l'homme et des vertebres, Vol. II.* Maloine, Paris.
15. Clark, W. E. le gros (1951): The projection of the olfactory epithelium on the olfactory bulb in the rabbit. *J. Neurol. Neurosurg. Psychiatr,* 14:1–10.
16. Clark, W. E. le gros (1957): Inquiries into the anatomical basis of olfactory discrimination. *Proc. Roy. Soc. London,* Ser. B 146:299–319.
17. Costanzo, R. M., and Mozell, M. N. (1976): Electrophysiological evidence for a topographical projection of the nasal mucosa onto the olfactory bulb of the frog. *J. Gen. Physiol.,* 68:297–312.
18. Devor, M. (1976*a*); Fiber trajectories of olfactory bulb efferents in hamster. *J. Comp. Neurol.,* 166:31–48.
19. Devor, M. (1976*b*): Neuroplasticity in the rearrangement of olfactory tract fibers after neonatal transection in hamster. *J. Comp. Neurol.,* 166:49–72.
20. Dieulafe, L. (1906): Morphology and embryology of the nasal fossae of vertebrates. *Ann. Otol. Rhinol. and Laryngol.,* 15:560–567.
21. Estable-Puig, J. F., and deEstable, R. F. (1969): Acute ultrastructural changes in the rat olfactory glomeruli after peripheral deafferentiation. *Experimental Neurology,* 24:592–602.
22. Graziadei, P. P. C. (1971): The olfactory mucosa of vertebrates. In: *Handbook of Sensory Physiology, Vol. IV,* edited by L. M. Beidler. Springer-Verlag, New York.
23. Graziadei, P. P. C. (1973): Cell dynamics in the olfactory mucosa. *Tissue and Cell,* 5:113–131.
24. Graziadei, P. P. C. (1975): Neuronal plasticity in the vertebrate olfactory receptor organ. *Tenth Int. Cong. Anat. Tokyo,* p. 45.
25. Graziadei, P. P. C., and DeHan, R. S. (1973): Neuronal regeneration in frog olfactory system. *J. Cell Biol.,* 59:525–530.

26. Graziadei, P. P. C., and Metcalf, J. F. (1970): Autoradiographic studies of frog's olfactory mucosa. *Am. Zool.,* 10:559.
27. Graziadei, P. P. C., and Metcalf, J. F. (1971): Autoradiographic and ultrastructural observations on the frogs olfactory mucosa. *Z. Zell.,* 116:305–318.
28. Graziadei, P. P. C., and Monti Graziadei, G. A. (1977): Continuous nerve cell renewal in the olfactory system. In: *Handbook of Sensory Physiology, Vol. IX,* edited by M. Jacobson, Springer-Verlag, New York, Berlin, Heidelberg.
29. Guth, L. (1975): History of CNS regeneration research. *Experimental Neurology,* 48:3–15.
30. Harding, J., Graziadei, P. P. C., Monti Graziadei, G. A., and Margolis, F. L. (1977): Denervation in the primary olfactory pathway of mice. *Brain Res.,* 132:11–28.
31. Hinds, J. W. (1970): Reciprocal and serial dendro-dendritic synapses in the glomerular layer of the rat olfactory bulb. *Brain Research,* 17:530–534.
32. Hinds, J. W. (1972): Early neuron differentiation in the mouse olfactory bulb. I. Light microscopy. *J. Comp. neurol.,* 146:233–252.
33. Hinds, J. W., and McNelly, N. A. (1977a): Aging of the rat olfactory bulb: growth and atrophy of constituent layers and changes in size and number of mitral cells. *J. Comp. Neurol.,* 171:345–368.
34. Hirata, Y. (1964): Some observations of the fine structure of the synapses in the olfactory bulb of the mouse, with particular reference to the atypical synaptic configuration. *Arch. Histol. Okayama* (Saibo Kayu Byorigaku Zasshi), 24:293–302.
35. Kaplan, M. S., and Hinds, J. W. (1977b): Neurogenesis in the olfactory bulb and dentate gyrus in the adult rat: electron microscopic analysis of light radioautographs. *The Anat. Rec.,* 187:620.
36. Kolmer, W. (1927): Geruchsorgan. In: *Handbuck der Mikroskopische Anatomie des Menschen, Vol. III,* pp. 192–249. Springer, Berlin.
37. Land, L. J. (1973): Localized projection of olfactory nerves to rabbit olfactory bulb. *Brain Res.,* 63:153–166.
38. Land, L. J., Eager, R. P., and Shepherd, G. M. (1970): Olfactory nerve projections to the olfactory bulb in rat: demonstration by means of a simple ammoniacal silver degeneration method. *Brain Res.,* 23:250–254.
39. Land, L. J., and Shepherd, G. M. (1974): Autoradiographic analysis of olfactory receptor projections in the rabbit. *Brain Res.,* 70:506–510.
40. Leblond, C. P. (1964): Classification of cell populations on the basis of their proliferative behavior. *Nat. Cancer Monogr.,* 14:119.
41. Leblond, C. P., and Walker, B. E. (1956): Renewal of cell populations. *Physiol. Rev.,* 36:255–275.
42. Margolis, F. L. (1975): Biochemical markers of the primary olfactory pathway: A model neural system. In: *Advances in Neurochemistry Vol. I,* edited by B. W. Agranoff and M. H. Aprison, pp. 193–246. Plenum Press, New York and London.
43. Messier, B., and Leblond, C. P. (1960): Cell proliferation and migration as revealed by autoradiography after injection of Thymidine ^{3}H in male rats and mice. *Am. J. Anat.,* 131:247–285.
44. Metcalf, J. F. (1974): The olfactory epithelium: a model system for the study of neuronal differentiation and development in adult mammals. Ph.D. Thesis, Florida State University, Tallahassee, Florida.
45. Monti Graziadei, G. A., Margolis, F. L., Harding, J. W., and Graziadei, P. P. C. (1977): Immunochemistry of the olfactory marker protein. *J. Histochem. Cytochem.,* 25:1311–1316.
46. Moulton, D. G. (1975): Cell renewal in the olfactory epithelium of the mouse. In. *Olfaction and Taste,* edited by D. A. Denton and J. P. Coghlan, pp. 111–114 Academic Press, New York.
47. Okano, M., and Takagi, S. F. (1974): Secretion and electrogenesis of the supporting cells in the olfactory epithelium. *J. Physiol.,* 242:353–370.
48. Oley, N., DeHan, R. S., Tucker, D., Smith, J. C., and Graziadei, P. P. C. (1975): Recovery of structure and function following transection of the primary olfactory nerves in pigeons. *J. Comp. Physiol. Psychol.,* 88:477–495.
49. Pearson, A. A. (1941a): The development of the nervus terminalis in man. *J. Comp. Neurol.,* 75:39–66.
50. Pearson, A. A. (1941b): The development of the olfactory nerve in man. *J. Comp. Neurol.,* 75:199–217.

51. Pearson, A. A. (1942): The development of the olfactory nerve, the nervus terminalis and the vomeronasal nerve in man. *Ann. Otol. Rhinol. and Laryngol.,* 51:317–332.
52. Pinching, A. J., and Powell, T. P. S. (1971a): The neuron types of the glomerular layer of the olfactory bulb. *J. Cell Sci.,* 9:305–345.
53. Pinching, A. J., and Powell, T. P. S. (1971b): The neuropil of the glomeruli of the olfactory bulb. *J. Cell Sci.,* 9:347–377.
54. Pinching, A. J., and Powell, T. P. S. (1972): A study of terminal degeneration in the olfactory bulb of the rat. *J. Cell Sci.,* 10:585–619.
55. Rall, W., Shepherd, G. M., Reese, T. S., and Brightman, M. W. (1966): Dendrodendritic synaptic pathway for inhibition in the olfactory bulb. *Exp. Neurol.,* 14:44–56.
56. Shepherd, G. M. (1972): Synaptic organization of the mammalian olfactory bulb. *Physiol. Revs.,* 52:864–917.
57. Sternberger, L. A., Hardy, P. H., Jr., Cuculis, J. J., and Meyer, H. G. (1970): The unlabeled antibody enzyme method of immunochemistry. Preparation and properties of soluble antigen-antibody complex (horseradish peroxidase-Antihorseradish peroxidase) and its use in identification of spirochetes. *J. Histochem. Cytochem.,* 18:315–333.
58. Takagi, S. F. (1971): Degeneration and regeneration of the olfactory epithelium. In: *Handbook of Sensory Physiology, Vol. IV,* edited by L. M. Beidler, pp. 76–94. Springer Verlag, Berlin, Heidelberg, New York.
59. White, E. L., (1972): Synaptic organization in the olfactory glomerulus of the mouse. *Brain Res.,* 37:69–80.
60. White, E. L. (1973): Synaptic organization of the mammalian olfactory glomerulus: new findings including an intraspecific variation. *Brain Res.,* 60:299–313.

Neuronal Plasticity, edited by
Carl W. Cotman.
Raven Press, New York © 1978.

Role of the Nerve Cell Body in Axonal Regeneration

Bernice Grafstein and Irvine G. McQuarrie

Department of Physiology and Department of Surgery (Neurosurgery), Cornell University Medical College, New York, New York 10021

INTRODUCTION

Following axonal injury, the nerve cell body usually undergoes characteristic changes in structure. However, these morphological changes are only a superficial manifestation of major alterations in the metabolism and cytoplasmic dynamics of the neuron, alterations that may play a decisive role in determining whether successful regeneration of the axon can occur. The key to the relationship between the changes in the cell body and the replacement of the axon lies in the fact that the cell body is the major site of synthesis of proteins and other materials required for the growth of the axon, as well as its normal maintenance, and the delivery of materials by the cell body to the axon would therefore be expected to be an important factor in the regulation of axonal outgrowth.

In this review we propose to explore the nature of the support that the cell body provides for axonal regeneration, and conversely, the nature of the influences operating on the cell body that apparently enable it to respond to the special requirements of the regenerating axon. It is particularly important in an evaluation of this kind to delineate carefully the sequence of changes taking place in the cell body in relation to the time course of axonal regeneration. Unfortunately, there are relatively few studies in which a systematic approach of this kind has been undertaken, so we feel justified in giving special emphasis to our own extensive studies on the goldfish retinal ganglion cell. This neuron is phenomenally successful with respect to its capacity for axonal regeneration, almost invariably showing vigorous axonal outgrowth after the optic axons have been injured, which is especially remarkable in view of the fact that these axons constitute a tract of the central nervous system. Although the cell body of this neuron does not present what is usually considered to be a typical morphological response to axotomy, the underlying changes do not seem to be fundamentally different from those seen in other regenerating neurons, and it seems reasonable to assume that the basic mechanisms operating during regeneration are the same. Our understanding of the nature of these mechanisms and how they operate in any neuron is distressingly incomplete (52). Some of the many fundamental questions that still remain unanswered will be raised in our review, but the evidence that can be mustered in an effort to find the answers is still fragmentary and sometimes inconsistent, although a large literature exists, admirably reviewed in two papers by Lieberman (102,103). Our present formulation is therefore a tentative attempt to identify some general principles that may be emerging in this field, as a guide for further evaluation and experimentation.

One subject that comes up repeatedly for consideration is the phenomenon of axonal transport, which has been receiving increasing attention in recent years, as its essential role in determining neuronal structure and function has become more widely appreciated. This phenomenon stands at a central point in the process of axonal regeneration, not only because of its function in supplying materials for construction of the new axon, but also because of its potential role as a communication system between cell body and axon tip.

It is generally agreed that there are at least three forms of axonal transport—fast anterograde transport, fast retrograde transport, and slow anterograde transport. Some intermediate rate components may also exist, but these have not yet been well defined. The three main types can be distinguished from one another not only by differences in their rates but also by differences in the nature of the transported material and differences in mechanism (51,53). Fast anterograde transport (150–400 mm per day in mammals, 50–100 mm per day in fish and frogs) comprises mainly particulate material, including transmitter storage vesicles, plasma membrane precursor vesicles, elements of smooth endoplasmic reticulum, and some mitochondria. Retrograde transport (with a rate usually thought to be about half that of fast anterograde transport) appears to involve lysosomes or lysosome precursors in addition to some of the material delivered to the axon terminals by anterograde transport. Slow anterograde transport (1–5 mm per day in mammals, about 0.5 mm per day in fish) contains a large proportion of soluble proteins, and includes microtubule protein, neurofilament proteins, various soluble enzymes, and most of the mitochondria. A current view is that the slow component is generated by the movement of the cytoplasmic matrix of the axon, whereas the fast components involve the movement of organelles within this matrix. The possibility that the slow component might play a vital role in axonal growth and regeneration was already recognized by Weiss and Hiscoe (181) in their initial formulation of the concept of axonal transport. They emphasized the idea that this transport was responsible for the replenishment of the axon, both under normal conditions and during regeneration. Additional ways in which axonal transport may make an essential contribution to the reaction to axotomy will become evident in the course of this review.

NEURONAL CHANGES FOLLOWING AXOTOMY

Cell Body Changes

Morphological alteration of the cell body following axotomy was first described by Nissl in 1892 for the facial motor neurons of the rabbit (125). He found that by 24 hr after the operation, the "chromatinkörper" (i.e., chromatin bodies, now usually called "Nissl substance") of the neurons had begun to disintegrate, and that in the course of the next few days the cell bodies became completely chromatolytic, i.e., they lost the granular texture that is given by the Nissl substance upon staining with basic dyes. In addition, the cell bodies became swollen, and their nuclei migrated to the periphery. This combination of changes is now generally considered to represent the prototypical response to axotomy (28,102), although these features are not invariably seen, and in some cases in which they do occur, it is difficult to be certain that they do not in fact represent the early stages of cellular dissolution (e.g., 166). Nevertheless, these changes help us to identify some of the basic mechanisms being brought into play in response to axotomy: the change in staining pattern arises from an alteration in the arrangement and concentration of RNA-containing material in the cell, presumably leading to changes in protein synthesis, which will in turn have an important role in determining the success of axonal regeneration.

Changes in RNA

The chromatolysis, i.e., dispersion of the Nissl substance, that commonly occurs in axotomized neurons has been revealed by electron microscopy to be due to the disorganization of the structure of the rough endoplasmic reticulum (rER). Normally, the rER that constitutes the Nissl substance consists of concentrations of flattened elongate cisternae arranged in parallel arrays, the cisternae being lined on their outer surfaces with membrane-attached ribosomes and having numerous free polyribosomal elements lying among them (130,136). Upon axotomy, the regularity of the cisternal arrays is lost, the individual cisterns become shorter, and the total amount of ribosome-associated membranous material may be reduced (102). Concomitantly, the proportion of free polyribosomes increases, which accounts for the observation that the dispersion of the Nissl substance is often accompanied by an increase in diffuse cytoplasmic basophilia (102). In some cases this increase in basophilia is so intense that the cell body becomes frankly hyperchromic (124,167).

Another indication of changes in RNA metabolism that is often seen is nucleolar enlargement (102), which indicates an increased capacity for synthesis of ribosomal RNA (88,136). Also, the ultrastructure of the nucleolus may change in a way that suggests that normal reserves of ribosomal RNA within the nucleolus are being depleted (85,100).

Thus from these ultrastructural observations alone, it may be deduced that following axotomy the synthesis and turnover of ribosomal RNA are increased. This conclusion is supported by other kinds of data: the increased synthesis of RNA has been substantiated by the finding of an increased neuronal incorporation of RNA precursors (102), and an increase in the rate of RNA turnover has been revealed by an increased rate of disappearance of RNA after RNA synthesis was arrested by poisoning with actinomycin D (175). As a result of the above changes, the total cellular content of RNA usually increases (17,175). However, as a result of cell body enlargement, which may be due, in various cases, to an increase in either the cell body mass or its water content (102), the RNA concentration may remain constant or even decrease (17,36).

Like other neurons, the goldfish retinal ganglion cell undergoes rapid changes in RNA metabolism in response to axotomy, but some of the morphological manifestations are atypical (124): there is no chromatolysis, nucleolar enlargement is unusually dramatic, and the neurons become intensely hyperchromic as well as greatly enlarged. The underlying change, however, is a familiar one—RNA synthesis is increased. This is attested to by an increase in the incorporation of RNA precursors (121), a proliferation of free polyribosomes, and an increase in the amount of rER (which is normally scanty in these neurons) (122). There is also an increase in the incidence of single ribonucleoprotein particles, a condition that is usually associated with neuronal degeneration in mammals (102), but has also been seen in successfully regenerating neurons in the lizard and frog (131,137), and hence may be a characteristic feature of regeneration in lower vertebrates.

Changes in Protein

In view of the increased requirements for structural materials that may be assumed to accompany axonal replacement, an increase in protein synthesis would be expected following axotomy in neurons capable of regeneration. In general, this expectation appears to be borne out by numerous observations of increased incorporation of radioactive amino acids into proteins during axonal regeneration (18,38,58,119,124,146,172). Some objections can be raised to the method of evaluating protein synthesis from labeled amino acid incorporation, e.g., the increased incorporation might reflect a change in intraneuronal amino acid pools or easier access of the labeled material to the axotomized neuron (172). However, since the increased amino acid incorporation may be shortly followed by an increased protein content and increased cell size (17,18,124,146), it appears that net protein synthesis is indeed elevated.

Nevertheless, not all proteins produced by the neuron show an increased synthesis following axotomy. In sympathetic ganglia in which the postganglionic nerves have been cut, for example, changes in amino acid incorporation were detected for only about 10% of the 300 to 400 different proteins that could be recognized (62), and while most of those that did change showed an increase in incorporation, some showed a decrease. Thus decreased synthesis (or increased degradation) of some neuronal proteins can occur in response to axotomy. It is possible that in some neurons, this decrease would be so prominent that a net decrease in amino acid incorporation would result. This may be the explanation for the decreased incorporation that has been seen with axotomy in some neurons, such as the dorsal root ganglion cells and motor neurons of the rat (37,57). Even in these cases, however, there is evidence that the synthesis of some proteins may be increased, since there is an increase in the amount of some of the proteins exported from the cell body to the axon (56,99). It is not surprising, therefore, that in many instances the net changes in amino acid incorporation show a complex time course (e.g.,89,95).

One protein that evidently undergoes increased synthesis is tubulin, the protein constituent of microtubules. Heacock and Agranoff (67) found that the amount of tubulin extractable from the goldfish retina was increased as early as 5 days after section of the optic nerve, indicating an increase of tubulin synthesis in the axotomized retinal ganglion cells. An increase of tubulin in regenerating rat motor axons has also been described by Lasek and Hoffman (99).

A reduction in synthesis appears to be characteristic of proteins associated with synaptic transmitter metabolism. In hypoglossal neurons, which have acetyl-choline as their synaptic transmitter, acetylcholinesterase has been found to decrease beginning 2 to 3 days after axotomy (39,174), and at the same time muscarinic ACh receptors on these neurons begin to disappear (149); choline acetyltransferase is also decreased (44). In various aminergic neurons with cell bodies in either the central or peripheral nervous systems, enzymes involved in both transmitter synthesis and degradation exhibit decreased activity. These include dopamine-β-hydroxylase, tryosine hydroxylase, and monoamine oxidase (25,90,145). Characteristically, the levels of these enzymes in the cell body are elevated for 1 to 2 days after axotomy, then decline to less than 50% of normal over a period of 1 to 2 weeks. The decline has been shown to be due to a reduction in the amount of enzyme in the cell rather than merely a decrease in enzyme activity (49,145,148), but it is not yet clear whether a decrease in synthesis or an increase in breakdown occurs. The changes in enzyme levels are accompanied by corresponding changes in the amount of neurotransmitter (16,25,84).

Changes in Axonal Transport

Changes in protein synthesis would be expected to lead to corresponding changes in the delivery of materials to the axon. Evidence of changes in axonal transport with regeneration was first obtained by Grafstein and Murray (55) in the goldfish visual system, where the rate of slow transport was found to increase about 3-fold after section of the optic axons. An increase in the amount of protein carried by the slow transport has also been found (B. Grafstein, *unpublished results*). In the case of fast transport, measurements made shortly after regeneration was complete (as indicated by recovery of vision), showed that labeled protein was transported to the terminals of the regenerated axons at about twice the normal rate and that the amount was increased 3-fold (55). More recent experiments have shown that the amount of material began to increase within 24 hours after axotomy (54), and the rate a few days later (114). [Increased amounts of transported nucleotides and transfer RNA, as well as some polyamines, have also been reported in regenerating goldfish optic axons (75–77), but it is not clear whether these transported materials make a positive contribution to axonal regeneration, or whether their appearance in the axon is only an incidental accompaniment of cell body alterations.]

Changes in slow axonal transport following axotomy in mammalian nerves appear to be somewhat variable. In the hypoglossal nerve of the rabbit, Frizell and Sjöstrand (47) have shown that the slow transport of proteins labeled with ^{3}H-leucine had nearly doubled in rate by 7 to 9 days after a crush lesion, but had returned to close to normal by 23 to 31 days. It was not possible to determine whether the amount of transported labeled protein carried in the axon at any one moment was increased as well. In the vagus nerve, under comparable circumstances, both the rate and amount of slow transport were decreased. In the hypoglossal nerve of the guinea pig, Kreutzberg and Schubert (91) could not demonstrate a clear change in the rate of slow transport, but concluded that there was a "redistribution" of the transported material. Lasek and Hoffman (99) have proposed that in rat motor axons there is no change in the rate of slow transport, but an increase in the amount of some of the slowly transported material. They have shown that the slow component of transport carries microtubule protein in two different fractions, which they have called SCa and SCb. Normally, SCa, advancing at a rate of about 1.5 mm/day, is present in greater amount than SCb, which advances at a rate of 3 to 4 mm/day. In regenerating axons, the amount of SCb is increased, so that the overall rate of advance of the combined mass of material in the slow component appears to be increased, whereas in fact the rates of the two individual fractions are unaltered.

Changes in fast transport following axotomy in mammalian nerves appear to be confined to changes in the amount of transported material, with no change in rate. Thus an increase of about 20% in the amount of rapidly transported labeled proteins was detected at 3 to 5 days after transection of the hypoglossal nerve of guinea pig, and an increase of nearly 250% was seen by 28 to 30 days (91). In the rabbit hypoglossal, Frizell, Sjöstrand, and McLean (43,44,46) showed an increased amount of transported glycoproteins labeled with ^{3}H-fucose at 1 and 4 weeks after nerve crush. At 4 to 6 weeks, rapidly transported proteins labeled with ^{3}H-leucine also were increased in amount, but at 1 week the picture was more complex: the labeled proteins emerging from the cell body during the first 20 hr were decreased, while those emerging later were increased. In the vagus nerve the amount of labeled glycoproteins was consistently decreased (46). In cat sciatic nerve, Ochs's careful study (126) showed no change in either the rate or amount of transport in motor axons during regeneration, but in rat motor axons Griffin, Drachman, and Price (56) found an approximately 2-fold increase in the amount of labeled protein entering the axons, with no change in rate. These workers also showed that the rate of transport in the newly formed portion of the axons was the same as in the parent axons proximal to the lesion, but that the density of radioactivity in the sprouts reached five times the density in normal axons, indicating a preferential delivery of the transported material to the emerging sprouts.

Some of the material conveyed by anterograde transport normally reverses direction at the axon terminals and is returned to the cell body by retrograde transport. Retrograde transport during regeneration has been examined in hypoglossal nerve by Frizell et al.(43,45) and in sciatic nerve by Bisby and Bulger (9). Following axotomy, retrograde transport from the site of injury is established within about an hr (9), so that much of the material that would normally be distributed to the portion of the axon beyond the lesion is rapidly returned to the cell body. Although the amount of transported material prematurely returning in this way would increase as the amount of anterogradely transported material increases, there may be a disproportionate increase in the retrograde component of the transport (43).

Another fraction of retrograde transport involves materials taken up from the extracellular fluid by the axon terminals. The uptake of such materials during regeneration has been studied by applying an exogenous protein, horseradish peroxidase (HRP), to the site of the lesion. For a few hours after axotomy, the uptake of HRP was very much reduced, and then rose to levels somewhat above normal (64). In neurons of the avian visual system, which do not regenerate, the elevated level was found to be maintained for only 12 to 15 hours, and then fell below normal (64), but in goldfish optic axons the level appeared to be greatly elevated throughout the course of regeneration (J. Currie and M. Whitnall, *unpublished results*).

MECHANISMS INVOLVED IN ELICITING THE CELL BODY CHANGES

Since the cell body reaction obviously involves major changes in RNA metabolism, it is likely that a modification of gene activity is involved in the initiation of these changes. Some evidence exists to support this view. For example, Watson (173) has found an increased uptake of ^{3}H-thymidine in the perinucleolar region of some axotomized hypoglossal neurons, suggesting that DNA synthesis might be increased. Also, there may be increased nuclear binding of actinomycin-D, an inhibitor of RNA synthesis that appears to act by complexing with actively transcribing sites on DNA (179). The dispersion of the Nissl substance can be prevented by application of actinomycin-D to the cell body within a few hours after axotomy, leading to the suggestion that the Nissl substance changes might be mediated through enzyme synthesis induced by the production of new messenger RNA (167).

Some of the factors that are likely to lead to the process of gene activation have been critically analysed by Cragg (28). He has suggested that since the onset of cell body changes is later if the lesion is further from the cell body, a "signal" ascends the axon at a finite rate. Cragg calculated this rate to be 4 to 5 mm per day, based on observations by Watson (175) on the time of appearance of an increased nucleolar nucleic acid content in axotomized hypoglossal neurons. On the other hand, calculations made from the appearance of chromatolysis in rat dorsal root ganglion cells (94) indicate that the rate of ascent of the signal for this phenomenon would have to be some mm per *hour*. It is conceivable, however, that this signal might be different from the one involved in triggering the nucleolar changes described by Watson.

Cragg (28) has considered a number of mechanisms that might serve as possible signals for the initiation of the cell body reaction, and has concluded that more than one are likely to be operative. These mechanisms include: depolarization of the neuronal membrane; loss of action potentials; loss from the cell body of axonally transported constituents, such as transmitter-related materials or a substance that would act as a repressor of the genes regulating protein synthesis; loss of axoplasm and mitochondria; and loss of a trophic substance coming from the periphery. Few of these possibilities have been subjected to experimental testing as yet, and most of them still deserve serious consideration. Recent thinking, dominated by the increasing awareness of the importance of fast antero-grade and retrograde transport for regulating the status of the axon terminals, has focussed on the possible role of axonal transport in initiating the cell body changes.

One important consideration, for example, is that as a result of the rapid establishment of retrograde transport at the site of a lesion (see p. 161), materials that would normally be dissipated or modified at the axon terminals (or en route to or from the terminals) are prematurely returned to the cell body. An injury of the rat sciatic nerve in mid-thigh, for example, causes axonally trans-ported materials to be returned to the cell body 7 hr earlier than normal (9). The build-up of such materials in the cell body might then be the signal for a change in the pattern of protein synthesis. These materials would include a significant amount of transmitter-related enzymes and other constituents of syn-aptic vesicles, which are known to be conveyed to the axon terminals by fast anterograde transport (53). The observation that shortly after axotomy the level of transmitter-related materials in the cell body may show a transient increase and then a sharp decline (3,145) is consistent with the hypothesis that the excessive accumulation of these materials leads to a decrease in their synthesis.

A somewhat different role for axonal transport may be envisaged on the basis of recent observations (68,141) that some of the changes produced by axotomy in postganglionic sympathetic neurons can be reversed by nerve growth factor (NGF). This substance, which is normally supplied to the sympathetic neurons by their target cells, is taken up by the adrenergic nerve terminals and conveyed by retrograde transport to the cell body (159) where it acts to promote neuronal metabolism (5). Axotomy would therefore prevent the NGF from exerting its trophic effects. The view that some of the cell body changes in the sympathetic neurons are due to loss of NGF, which is congruent with one of the mechanisms considered by Cragg (28), is supported by the finding that changes reversed by NGF were also reversed when the regenerating axons reconnected with their target cells (see p. 174), i.e., when the supply of trophic material from the target cells would presumably have again become available.

Another relevant line of investigation has been opened by the observation that cell body changes resembling those elicited by axotomy can be produced by application to the axon drugs such as colchicine or the vinca alkaloids, which block axonal transport, presumably by disrupting microtubules (65,112). Even when these drugs do not interfere with electrical activity in the axon or cause overt axonal degeneration, they may nevertheless elicit, in various neurons, some of the changes usually associated with axotomy, including chromatolysis, nucleolar enlargement, decrease in neurotransmitter-synthesizing enzymes, re-traction of presynaptic terminals, and loss of synaptic transmission (83,90, 134,139,184,187). These findings indicate that at least some of the characteristic effects produced by axotomy are due to a block of axonal transport in the anterograde or retrograde direction. This would be consistent with either of the two mechanisms considered above, i.e., block of transport of a trophic factor originating at the terminals or the premature return to the cell body of materials normally conveyed to the axon terminals but now reflected from the site of transport block. In our own studies on the block of axonal transport by vinca alkaloids in the goldfish optic system, however, we have been impressed by the fact that although the retinal ganglion cell bodies could develop several features resembling the response to axotomy (e.g., increased nucleolar size, increased rate of slow transport), protein synthesis was not increased (W.R. White and B. Grafstein, *unpublished results*). This indicates that although block of axonal transport probably does contribute to the changes initiated by axotomy, it is not sufficient to initiate the whole array of changes. Apparently, some additional factors are operating.

One possibility originally raised by Cragg (28) and recently subjected to detailed consideration, is that axonal injury may permit the entry into the axon of some abnormal materials which would then be conveyed by retrograde axonal transport to the cell body. In line with this, Kristensson and Olsson (93) have shown that exogenous proteins, such as horseradish peroxidase, do enter the axon at the site of an injury and can reach the cell body within a few hours. This would be fast enough to account for the initiation of the cell body reaction.

Another possibility, proposed by Watson (176), is that the initial act of axonal sprouting is responsible for inducing the cell body changes. Membrane expansion during sprouting, for example, might be the operative factor. This suggestion was based on the observation that axonal sprouting induced by means other than axotomy was accompanied by cell body changes, including an increase in nucleolar nucleic acid, resembling those produced by axotomy. As will be seen below, this mechanism probably does not account for the initiation of chromatolysis. However, the possibility that axonal outgrowth can influence the cell body changes cannot be dismissed, and a considerable portion of this review will be devoted to examining the problem of the relationship between axonal outgrowth and the changes elicited by axotomy.

DOES AXONAL OUTGROWTH INFLUENCE THE CELL BODY CHANGES?

A number of different lines of evidence will be examined in relation to this question. One is the temporal relationship between axonal sprouting and the cell body changes—sprouting can be considered as a possible initiating factor for these changes only if it precedes them. A second is the nature of the cell body changes that are observed when sprouting is induced by means other than axotomy. A third relates to the question of whether the cell body changes are affected by the rate of axonal elongation. Finally, we shall consider the effects on the cell body of axonal reconnection.

Temporal Relationship Between Axonal Sprouting and Other Changes

Time of Initiation of Sprouting

There are some inherent problems in determining the time of initiation of sprouting. One difficulty is to identify the point on the axon at which the outgrowth begins, since axonal degeneration may extend for a variable distance back from the site of injury (143). The length of this zone of "traumatic degeneration" may vary with the nature of the injury, probably depending at least partly on the degree of local ischemia produced. Also, a considerable proportion of axon sprouts may arise in the form of collaterals from a point at some distance behind the nerve tip (120,143). Another problem is that immediately after an axon is cut, materials normally conveyed along the axon from the cell body by axonal transport may accumulate at the cut tip, to form a dilated but apparently stationary terminal end-bulb (82,143,186), which is sometimes difficult to distinguish from the terminal axonal dilatation, or growth cone, of an actively advancing axon (21,120,163).

In the goldfish optic tract, a study of the configuration of the tips of the cut axons (as seen in silver-stained sections by light microscopy) revealed that within 1 day after the cut the terminal bulbs were already well formed, but began to disappear by 3 days after the cut. At this time it was occasionally possible to detect thin axonal sprouts collecting into characteristic dense bundles near the edge of the cut, but such bundles were only rarely seen until 5 days after axotomy (50). These findings have now been confirmed by electron microscopic studies (N. Lanners and B. Grafstein, *unpublished results*). Recently, we have followed the progress of elongation of the optic axons after a crush of the optic nerve by measuring the outgrowth distance of the dense bundles of newly formed axons, and have estimated the time of initial sprouting (by backward extrapolation of the outgrowth values to zero distance) to be 4.3 days (Table 1) (114). Similar treatment of outgrowth measurements obtained from the rate of advance of the axons after radioactive labeling of the axonal proteins gave a value of 4.6 days (114). Thus all our data point to the conclusion that outgrowth in goldfish optic axons begins in a few axons as early as 3 days after axotomy but is not widespread until 4 to 5 days. The values obtained appear to be the same regardless of whether the optic tract was cut or the optic nerve was crushed.

In mammalian nerve, events would be expected to occur earlier because of the higher body temperature. In rat sciatic nerve, values for the initial delay before sprouting begins, calculated from outgrowth measurements obtained by various techniques (Table 1), are 1.3 days for adrenergic axons, 1.6 days for sensory axons, and 2.2 days for motor axons. The nature of the lesion appears to make a considerable difference, since values obtained after a cut and suture are clearly higher than those for a crush. Species differences are also important,

TABLE 1. *Axonal outgrowth characteristics*

Axons	Technique	Initial delay[a] (days)	Outgrowth rate (mm/day)	Lesion	Ref.
Goldfish optic	Silver-staining	4.3	0.34	Crush	(114)
Goldfish optic	Radioactive protein	4.6	0.42	Crush	(114)
Mouse sciatic	Silver-staining	4.0	0.15	Excision	(115)
Rat sciatic (motor)	Radioactive protein	3[b]	3.6[c]	Crush	(11)
Rat sciatic (motor)	Radioactive protein	3.2	3.0	Crush	(40)
Rat sciatic (fastest motor)	Radioactive protein	2.1	4.4	Crush	(40)
Rabbit sciatic (sensory)	Pinch test	7.3	3.5	Cut and suture	(60)
Rabbit sciatic (sensory)	Pinch test	5.2	4.4	Crush	(60)
Rat sciatic (sensory)	Pinch test	1.6	4.3	Crush	(117)
Rat sciatic (adrenergic)	^{3}H-norepi-nephrine uptake	1.3	3.9	Crush	(116)

[a] Calculated by backward extrapolation of outgrowth distance to zero.
[b] Calculated from values given by Black and Lasek (11).
[c] At 4 to 8 days.

since the value for sensory axons is significantly higher in the rabbit than in the rat (Table 1).

The above calculations of the initial delay of sprouting depend on measurements of axonal outgrowth from the site of the lesion. This delay would include not only the latent period before sprouting begins, but also the time required for the axons to traverse the zone of traumatic degeneration. Therefore, the actual latent period is somewhat less than the initial delay values indicate.

Detailed electron microscopic studies of regenerating sciatic nerve by Morris, Hudson, and Weddell (120) have provided consistent evidence of sprouting by 36 hr after axotomy. However, Zelena, Lubińska, and Gutmann (186) have claimed to see some sprouting already by 4 hr after nerve transection. The appearance of axonal sprouts within hours after peripheral nerve injury as detected by electronmicroscopy is, surprisingly, not inconsistent with the classical descriptions of Ramón y Cajal (143) whose phenomenal powers of observation presumably compensated for the limits of resolution imposed by the light microscope. His breakdown of the time required for axonal regeneration begins with the proposition that the initial 30 to 36 hours following a lesion is taken up by "the phase of dividing turgidity" in the axon tip prior to outgrowth (143, p. 227). He nevertheless has placed considerable emphasis (143, pp. 151,154) on the fact that in young animals collateral branching beginning at some distance from the axon tip may be evident in some axons by 6 hr after the injury and already quite profuse at 10 to 12 hours. It is obvious from his description, however, that this is not characteristic of the axonal population as a whole, and that in any case the time course in adult animals would be slower.

In our own electron microscopic studies in rat sciatic nerve (I.G. McQuarrie, *unpublished results*) we have seen some collateral sprout formation at nodes of Ranvier in myelinated axons by 9 hr after nerve crush; by 18 hr such sprouting was frequently seen but many of the sprouts showed signs of degeneration. It was not until 27 hr that there were numerous sprouts that were considered to be viable, as indicated by the presence of a smooth plasma membrane, an appreciable amount of neurofilaments and microtubules, and a normal population of longitudinally oriented mitochondria associated with the filaments and tubules.

The possibility suggested by our observations, that under normal conditions the early sprouts undergo degeneration or involution before the definitive phase of sprouting occurs, receives some support from the scanning electron micrographs of the ends of severed dorsal roots obtained by Duce, Reeves, and Keen (33). They showed that within a few hr after nerve injury, the tips of the severed axons began to emerge from the end of the root in the form of smooth bulbs, but that by 48 hr these bulbs had taken on a wrinkled appearance that suggested that degenerative changes were occurring. However, it is not clear whether the smooth bulbs can be considered to be growth cones, or whether they are terminal bulbs whose dissolution might be a prerequisite for sprouting, as appears to be the case in the goldfish optic nerve (see p. 165).

In summary, our tentative conclusion on the basis of the above evidence is that in mammalian nerve some sprouting may occur by 4 to 6 hr after axotomy, but it is quite rare before 12 hr, and definitive sprouting of the majority of the axons probably does not occur before 24 hr. It is possible that there is a wave of sprout degeneration following the initial outgrowth, but the fact that Cajal apparently did not observe this makes one cautious about advancing such a hypothesis, since it is hard to believe that such a phenomenon would have escaped his formidable eye.

Time of Initiation of Changes in RNA

Changes in the configuration or metabolism of RNA are generally regarded to be the earliest events detected thus far in the cell body's reaction to axotomy (52,102). In the goldfish retinal ganglion cells, for example, the earliest morphological change that we recognized was an increase in the proportion of cells containing nucleoli large enough to be detectable in the light microscope (124). This occurred between 2 and 3 days after axotomy, coincident with an increase in the incorporation of ^{3}H-uridine into RNA (121). The rER, which in these neurons is normally present as dissociated single cisterns was not obviously altered at this time. Proliferation of free polysomes became evident between 4 and 6 days after axotomy and proliferation of the rER began between 6 and 10 days (122).

In mammalian neurons, establishing the precise time at which the alteration in RNA begins is complicated by the fact that the distance of the lesion from the nerve cell body makes a significant difference to the latency of the cell body reaction (94,103). This is clearly seen, for example, in the hypoglossal nerve of the rat, where the beginning of an increase in nucleolar nucleic acid occurs about 5 to 6 hr later for each mm of increased distance from the cell body (28). The latency of the reaction may also be affected by the nature of the lesion. Thus Watson (175) observed that the nucleolar nucleic acid of hypoglossal neurons began to increase at 3 days after nerve ligation or nerve crush, but had already begun to increase by 2 days after the nerve was divided and avulsed. In spite of such variable factors, it is clear that in a variety of neurons (e.g., facial, hypoglossal, spinal motor) in a variety of species (mouse, hamster, rabbit, monkey), light-microscopically detectable dispersion of the Nissl substance may already be evident by 12 to 24 hr after the lesion (17,24,48,100, 125,168,169). Dorsal root ganglion cells in the rat showed chromatolysis in 50% of the neuronal population at 30 hr after crush of the sciatic nerve 20 mm from the ganglia; in the mouse the response developed more slowly (94). The earliest reaction reported has been in rat postganglionic sympathetic neurons with axons cut only 1 to 2 mm from the ganglion, where chromatolysis was already seen in 25% of the neurons as early as 6 hr after axotomy (111).

Indicators of increased RNA synthesis usually appear somewhat later than the first signs of chromatolysis. In rabbit hypoglossal neurons, incorporation of ^{14}C-orotic acid into RNA showed no change at 24 hr after axotomy (18), though chromatolysis was already evident (18). Nucleolar enlargement in mouse facial neurons only became evident at 48 hr (168), and changes in nucleolar basophilia in hamster facial neurons were not observed until 3 days (100). In mouse hypoglossal neurons an increase in the rate of transfer of RNA from nucleus to cytoplasm was not evident until 48 hr (172). In rat hypoglossal neurons nucleolar nucleic acid usually began to increase at 2 to 3 days and cell body nucleic acid at 3 to 4 days (175). Thus far there have been only a few reports of earlier changes (aside from chromatolysis): mouse hypoglossal neurons showed an increase in the incorporation of ^{3}H-uridine into RNA by 12 hr after axotomy (61); rat hypoglossal neurons injured close to the cell body showed an increase in nucleolar nucleic acid content within 24 hr (175).

Even before the first signs of chromatolysis or other RNA changes appear, however, the neurons may have undergone a significant alteration. This is evident from the fact that actinomycin-D could prevent the development of chromatolysis in mouse facial neurons if it was given by 9 hr after axotomy, whereas at 12 hr it no longer had a blocking effect, even though chromatolysis was not yet evident (167). This indicates that at 9 to 12 hours the neurons undergo some change that is critical for the subsequent development of chromatolysis.

The difficulties of trying to correlate the scattered data on the time of initiation of the cell body reaction with the equally diverse data on the time of axonal sprouting are obvious. The general impression that arises, however, is that the cell body changes begin before there is any significant degree of axonal outgrowth. This impression is clearly confirmed by two cases in which both the cell body reaction and axonal sprouting have been carefully observed: in goldfish retinal ganglion cells the RNA changes began between 2 and 3 days, when sprouting was rarely seen, if at all (50,121,124); in sympathetic postganglionic neurons, chromatolysis had already developed in about 25% of the neurons by 6 hr, but sprouting was not evident until 24 to 38 hr (109,111). It is difficult, therefore, to accept the proposal (176) that the initial act of sprouting is responsible for inducing the RNA changes.

Time of Initiation of Changes in Protein Metabolism

It would be reasonable to expect that changes in protein synthesis should appear somewhat later than the changes in RNA. In mammals, the existing data are inadequate to resolve this point. Mostly, they only serve to show that increased amino acid incorporation into hypoglossal and spinal motor neurons could be seen by 24 to 48 hr after axotomy (18,27,41,89,172). In one case (172), an increase in ^{3}H-lysine incorporation into protein in mouse hypoglossal neurons was seen at 48 hr together with an increase in ^{3}H-uridine incorporation into RNA, but the precise timing of these two events was not explored. For rabbit dorsal root ganglion cells, one study showed that an increase in protein synthesis began between 2 and 7 days after axotomy (119), whereas in another study chromatolysis was already obvious at 30 hr (94). In goldfish retinal ganglion cells, on the other hand, a sequential relationship was readily apparent: increased incorporation of ^{3}H-leucine was seen by 4 days after axotomy, 1 day later than the earliest detectable RNA changes (121,124).

It is interesting that both the mammalian and goldfish data suggest that increased protein synthesis occurred at about the time that axonal sprouting began. The possibility that the increased synthesis may play a positive role in the initiation of sprouting will be considered in detail below (p. 175).

Time of Initiation of Changes in Axonal Transport

It is inevitable that the changes in protein synthesis should result in changes in axonal transport. Even before protein synthesis is altered, however, there are some marked disturbances in the circulation of proteins within the neuron. As has been discussed above, the amount of transmitter-related materials in the cell body initially increases after axotomy, presumably as a result of the premature return of transported materials from the site of the lesion. Such increases have been seen, for example, by 48 hr after axotomy in locus ceruleus neurons (145), but this change undoubtedly begins much earlier; in postgangli-onic sympathetic neurons, it has been seen at 12 hr (90). With the usual rates of retrograde transport (158) one would expect the disturbance to begin to make itself felt in the cell body within a few hr after axotomy, depending, of course, on the distance of the lesion from the cell body. For example, proteins conveyed by retrograde transport from a sciatic nerve lesion in the mid thigh of mice or rats could reach the cell bodies in 6 to 18 hr (9,94).

In goldfish retinal ganglion cells an early event following axotomy may be an increase in the amount of fast-transported protein delivered to the axon. Within 18 to 24 hr after optic tract section we have seen an increase in the amount of transported protein-bound radioactivity appearing in the optic axons at 2 to 6 hr after application of a labeled amino acid to the retinal ganglion cells (54). This change, which occurred before any alteration in RNA synthesis or protein synthesis was evident, may represent an increase in the proportion of newly synthesized protein diverted to the axon relative to the proportion retained in the cell body. At later times, the amount delivered to the axon continued to increase, presumably due, at least in part, to increasing protein synthesis. At 4 to 5 days after axotomy of the goldfish optic axons, when axonal outgrowth was starting and protein synthesis had just begun to increase, there was also an abrupt increase in the amount of axonally transported labeled phos-pholipid appearing in the axons after application of either labeled glycerol or labeled choline to the retinal ganglion cell bodies (43) (B. Grafstein and R. A. Alpert, *unpublished results*). In addition, the rate of accumulation of the labeled phospholipid in the tips of the axons was increased, which may be interpreted as either an increase in the rate of axonal transport or the preferential deposition of transported material in the emerging sprouts.

An increase in the amount of material carried by slow transport in the goldfish optic axons appeared to develop at some time between 3 and 6 days after axotomy. (B. Grafstein, *unpublished results*), probably reflecting the increased protein synthesis beginning at that time, whereas the rate of slow transport began to increase at 6 to 8 days after axotomy (55), a time of rapid axonal elongation.

In summary, it is evident from the above description that the sequence of changes in axonal transport following axotomy is quite complex. The transport pattern is altered by premature return of materials reflected at the site of the lesion, by alterations in the synthesis of various transported materials, and prob-ably also by the emergence of the axonal sprouts. In addition, there may be a change in the proportion of material diverted to the axon even before the overall level of protein synthesis is altered.

Effects on the Cell Body of Sprouting Initiated Without Axotomy

Axonal sprouting may be induced in a number of ways that do not involve axotomy. For example, degeneration of nearby nerves induces collateral sprout-ing in both peripheral and central axons (35,104,107,123,142). Sprouting of motor nerve terminals may also be induced by injection of botulinum toxin (165,176), a drug which blocks ACh release from the terminals (23), presumably by preventing the recycling of synaptic vesicles in the terminals (15,81), possibly by inhibiting entry of Ca^{++} (106).

Watson (176–178) has shown that sprouting induced by either of these means is accompanied by cell body changes that to some extent resemble those produced by axotomy. For example, 70 days after the hypoglossal nerve had been implanted into a foreign muscle (sternomastoid muscle), sprouting of the hypoglossal axons could be induced by cutting the original nerve to the muscle (spinal accessory nerve). At 5 days after the nerve had been cut, nucleolar dry mass, nucleolar nucleic acid content, and cell body nucleic acid content all began to increase, reaching a peak at about 10 days, and declining over the next 10 to 20 days. If the hypoglossal nerve had been implanted into the median nerve, similar changes occurred in the hypoglossal neurons when sprouting of the hypoglossal axons was induced by cutting the median nerve. Almost identical changes were produced when sprouting was induced in normal hypoglossal axons by injection of botulinum toxin into the tongue. The hypothesis that these changes may be evoked in each case by axonal sprouting would depend on the demonstration that the cell body changes were preceded by sprouting. However, this relationship has not yet been satisfactorily established. Sprouting was reported to have been evident by 6 days after either spinal accessory nerve section or botulinum toxin injection, but it would require more detailed studies, possibly involving electron microscopy, to determine when the sprouting had actually begun.

Although the above changes in the hypoglossal neurons differed from those produced by distal axotomy only in that the latter began about a day earlier, it is important to note that sprouting elicited without axotomy may be associated with an increase, instead of a decrease, in transmitter-related materials. Thus, in hypoglossal neurons poisoned with botulinum toxin the cholinesterase activity was increased (176), whereas it was decreased following axotomy (174). In substantia nigra neurons undergoing collateral sprouting within the olfactory tubercle in response to removal of the olfactory bulb, there was a transient increase of tyrosine hydroxylase activity, but no decline such as was characteristically seen following axotomy (49). Nucleic acid changes in dorsal root ganglion cells undergoing collateral sprouting may be more intense than the corresponding changes in response to axotomy (178).

Cell Body Changes Associated with Axonal Elongation

Aside from the question of whether the beginning of axonal sprouting is responsible for the initiation of cell body changes (see p. 169), it is difficult to escape the impression that what happens in the cell body is soon affected by whether or not successful axonal outgrowth occurs. This impression is probably mainly derived from experiments in which different kinds of lesions, either permitting or preventing outgrowth, result in a different effect on the cell body.

In some cases, the differences in cell body function appear so late that they must be correlated with whether or not the severed axons have succeeded in reestablishing their terminal connections (see p. 173). In other cases, however, the difference in the cell body reaction is already evident before reconnection could possibly have occurred. For example, in the experiments of Karlström and Dahlström (84), who studied the accumulation of noradrenaline in the sympathetic axons of cut, ligated, or crushed sciatic nerves, the amount of noradrenaline accumulating proximal to the lesion initially declined with the same time course in all three cases, but it may be discerned that by 7 days after the lesion there was a greater accumulation in the crushed nerves than in those subjected to the other types of lesions. Although axonal sprouts were observed after each type of lesion, the sprouts in the crushed nerves readily penetrated into the nerve beyond the crush, beginning at 3 days, whereas the sprouts in the other nerves were found mainly in the scar tissue around the lesion site. In another case, Torvik and Skjörten (168) found that after injury of the facial nerve in mice, the dissolution of the rER proceeded with the same time course regardless of whether the nerve had been cut or crushed, but by 8 days the Nissl substance had begun to reappear in the facial neurons if the nerves had been crushed, and did not reappear if they had been cut; reconnection of the crushed axons was observed at 10 to 11 days. There are also other reports of the rapid recovery of the Nissl substance in successfully regenerating neurons while their axons are still undergoing rapid elongation: monkey spinal motor neurons showed return of the Nissl substance at 2 weeks after sciatic nerve crush although reconnection was unlikely to have occurred by that time (14); rabbit facial neurons, which reconnect at 2 weeks after nerve crush, showed recovery of the Nissl substance beginning at 5 days (169). In goldfish retinal ganglion cells, which do not undergo chromatolysis, the phenomenon analogous to recovery of the Nissl substance may be the proliferation of the rER, which began at 6 to 10 days after optic tract section (122), a week or more before any signs of reconnection appeared (55) (B. Grafstein, *unpublished results*).

These observations may be interpreted as suggesting that rapid axonal elongation may somehow encourage an increased production of rER. It is possible to imagine that some feature of the process of elongation itself, e.g., expansion of the membrane (176), increased polymerization of microtubules (99), or increased diversion of axonally transported materials into the elongating segment, might be the trigger for the appropriate cell body mechanisms. Another possibility is that the actively growing axon tip, which shows vigorous endocytosis (22,74,135), is taking up trophic substances from the extracellular fluid. The fact that NGF, which can be identified as a trophic substance in some neurons, may be produced by cells which the growing axon tip would come in contact with, e.g., fibroblasts and glia (171), lends some credibility to this hypothesis. A third alternative is that the exaggerated endocystosis at the axon tip may result in an excessive discharge of materials produced by the rER, and thus provoke a compensatory increase in the rER.

Although the view that the rER may be influenced by an appropriate feedback mechanism from the growing axon is a reasonable and attractive one, the data are also consistent with the opposite view, namely that it is the proliferation of the rER, presumably proceeding according to a cell body program determined by the nature of the original axon injury, that makes sustained elongation possible. There is little evidence at present that would help decide which of these views is correct.

In a preliminary attempt to explore the question of whether axonal outgrowth can influence cell body mechanisms, we looked for changes in slow axonal transport after axonal outgrowth had been blocked by application of colchicine to the tips of growing goldfish optic axons (50). We found that the amount of labeled protein available for slow transport was elevated above normal, just as it was in neurons in which outgrowth was proceeding normally. This indication that the increased synthesis of at least some proteins may be seen independently of whether or not axonal outgrowth is occurring, provides some tentative support in favor of the view that once the changes in protein synthesis are initiated, they are not influenced by feedback from the axon tip.

Changes Associated with Reconnection of the Regenerating Axons

Some of the metabolic changes initiated by axotomy are likely to reach their peak at about the time that the regenerating axons begin to reconnect with their target cells. For example, in Watson's (175) study of rat hypoglossal neurons, nucleolar nucleic acid content reached a peak at 5 to 10 days after nerve injury, and nerve fibers were seen to reinnervate the geniohyoid muscle at 6 to 10 days (29,175). In goldfish retinal ganglion cells, where the average time for recovery of vision following optic tract section was 21 days (55), incorporation of ^{3}H-leucine into the retinal ganglion cells was found to be maximal at this time (124). We have observed that the amount of axonally transported ^{3}H-fucose-containing glycoprotein in the regenerating goldfish optic axons also reached its maximum at this time (B. Grafstein and R. Alpert, *unpublished results*). Such findings appear to suggest that the reconnection of the axons might serve as a signal for the subsidence of the cell body changes. However, the correspondence is not always so close: Watson's data (175) show that when the hypoglossal nerve was injured farther from the cell body, the nucleolar nucleic acid content not only began to increase later, but also reached its peak later, even though the regenerating axons did not have as far to go. Moreover, Watson demonstrated that when the regenerating nerve was prevented from making terminal connections, the nucleolar and cell body nucleic acid content began to decline at the same time as normal (175). In view of these observations we must assume that the dissipation of the cell body changes does not depend on reconnection with target cells, but follows a time course that is set when axonal injury occurs. To at least some extent, this time course, and also the latency and intensity of the changes provoked, are determined by how near the injury is to the cell body (175).

On the other hand, there are clearly certain effects on the cell body that are linked to successful reconnection. The final size attained by the cell body, for example, shows at least a partial dependence on whether or not connections have been reestablished, so that axotomized neurons that remain disconnected from their target cells characteristically remain reduced in size, and the nucleic acid content of both the nucleolus and cell body may fall to levels below normal (175); also these cells are more likely to degenerate completely (103,140). Therefore, reconnection is presumably able to attenuate the downhill course of cellular metabolism that sets in after the changes produced by axotomy have reached their peak. In addition to this preventive role, reconnection may have a positively beneficial effect. This may be seen, for example, in the increased level of amino acid incorporation occurring in regenerating rat spinal neurons at the time of reconnection (37). In some cases, there may be a phase of neuronal hypertrophy at the time of reconnection (17,132).

Another feature of axotomized cells that develops upon disconnection of the axon and recovers with reconnection is removal of boutons from the cell surface (161,162), which results in the disruption of synaptic function (110,138). Since these changes appear to be the result of a decrease in the production of postsynaptic receptor proteins (149), it is probable that the production of these receptor proteins shows corresponding effects. Moreover, disconnection and reconnection of the axon, rather than axonal injury itself, is also the basis for the reaction of glial cells in the vicinity of the axotomized cell bodies, since the glial reactions are apparently secondary to the bouton changes (reviewed by Watson, 180). Thus (a) division of the microglia is specifically associated with retraction of the boutons (no division occurs if the axon is divided a second time, provided that the axon has not yet been allowed to reestablish its connections); (b) metabolic changes of the astroglia occur both when boutons are removed from the cell body and when they are restored; (c) metabolic activity of myelin-forming oligodendrocytes is increased only when boutons are reapplied to the neuron, presumably in relation to myelination of the terminal portion of the presynaptic axon.

It has been proposed that the changes in the axotomized neuron related to disconnection of the axon from its end-organ result from the loss of a trophic influence exercised by the peripheral target cells on the neuron (140). In the sympathetic system, for example, the trophic factor operating between neurons and their target cells may be NGF, since application of NGF to axotomized sympathetic neurons leads to reestablishment of normal functional relations with the presynaptic elements (141) and an increased probability of neuronal survival (68). It is conceivable that within the cells of the nervous system and peripheral target tissues there is a whole array of trophic factors, having effects similar to those that NGF specifically exerts on sympathetic neurons, responsible for the long-term maintenance of the neurons that terminate on them.

Does Axonal Outgrowth Influence the Cell Body Changes?

Most of the evidence indicates that axonal outgrowth probably has little, if any, influence on the cell body changes following axotomy. Axonal sprouting is apparently not responsible for the initiation of the cell body changes, since these changes begin before sprouting occurs. Also, reconnection of the axon is apparently not responsible for the subsidence of the changes, since the changes subside even if reconnection is prevented. Cell body features that are affected by axonal reconnection, e.g., cell body size, basal levels of RNA and protein synthesis, and attachment of presynaptic terminals, may be responding to a trophic factor originating in the target cells, rather than cessation of axonal outgrowth. Nevertheless, the possibility that axonal outgrowth may have some effect on the cell body has not been ruled out, e.g.,when rapid elongation is occurring prior to reconnection of the axon or when sprouting has been initiated by means other than axotomy.

DOES THE CELL BODY HAVE AN ACTIVE ROLE IN REGULATING AXONAL OUTGROWTH?

In evaluating how the cell body might regulate axonal outgrowth, we shall consider what mechanisms may be involved in the initiation of outgrowth, and what factors may affect the rate of elongation. Separate attention will be given to the action of NGF in promoting the outgrowth of neurites from neurons or related cells, as an example of the manner in which peripheral factors may act on both the axon tip and the cell body. Finally, we shall consider the implications of the fact that axonal outgrowth is altered in neurons that have undergone a prior injury, a phenomenon that we believe points to the importance of the cell body in regulating axonal outgrowth.

Mechanisms Involved in Initiation of Sprouting

Axonal sprouting can be initiated in a number of ways in addition to axotomy. Two examples, sprouting evoked by degeneration of nearby nerves and sprouting evoked in motor axons by intramuscular injection of botulinum toxin, have been considered above (p. 170). Sprouting also occurs in axons in which action potential activity has been blocked by tetrodotoxin (20) and in the undamaged axon branches of neurons in which some of the branches have been previously removed (133,152). In these various cases, a number of different mechanisms might be operating to cause axonal sprouting. For example, it has been suggested that a sprout-inducing chemical might be released from degenerating tissue (71) or from denervated or inactive muscles (20). Another possibility is that nerve terminals normally release a factor that prevents sprouting, so that when some nerves are damaged, sprouting of nearby nerves is no longer inhibited (30).

An ingenious hypothesis recently proposed by Lasek and Hoffman (99), which might serve to unify at least some of the concepts of how sprouting is initiated under various conditions, envisages a central role for Ca^{++} in the regulation of axonal sprouting. These workers propose that axonal sprouting is normally prevented by the continual disassembly of neurofilaments and microtubules in the axon terminal. An increased concentration of Ca^{++} in the terminal might alter the equilibrium between polymerized microtubules and free tubulin, and might also activate an endogenous axoplasmic protease which cleaves the polypeptide backbone of neurofilaments. In conditions of low internal Ca^{++}, the disassembly mechanism would be inactivated, the neurofilaments and microtubules would therefore continue to advance, and axonal elongation would occur. This mechanism can be readily reconciled with the initiation of sprouting in conditions that block activity of the nerve terminal, e.g., intramuscular injection of botulinum toxin or application of tetrodotoxin to the nerve, when there would be a reduction in the entry of Ca^{++} into the nerve terminal that normally occurs as a prelude to transmitter release.

In addition to such mechanisms involving the microtubules, other factors probably regulate the initiation of axonal sprouting. Following axotomy, most axonal sprouts do not form at the axon tip but at points farther proximal, i.e., the nodes of Ranvier in the case of myelinated axons (120, 143, 156), and it is possible that the initial event at these sites may be an incease in the fluidity of the plasma membrane. An increase in plasma membrane fluidity associated with cell growth and division has been seen in cultured fibroblasts (26,66), and appears to involve specific changes in the composition of plasma membrane lipids.

The relationship between the various kinds of peripheral events leading to axon sprouting in the absence of axotomy and events in the cell body has not been well explored. As has been discussed above (p. 171), the evidence that sprouting precedes the cell body changes is weak in the few cases in which such a correlation has been sought. On the contrary, the possibility that the stimulus leading to sprouting may be operating via an initial effect on the cell body receives some support from the observation that with injection of botulinum toxin into the tongue an increase in the dry mass of the hypoglossal cell bodies was already evident at 2 to 3 days after the injection, i.e., well in advance of sprouting (175).

Factors Affecting the Rate of Axonal Outgrowth

Axonal elongation involves the deposition of materials at, or close to, the emerging axon tip, rather than along the shaft of the axon or at the cell body (19,21). The rate of elongation is believed to depend primarily on conditions at the axon tip, particularly the strength of adhesion of the tip to the surface on which it is growing (157). The relative autonomy of the axon tip in determining its rate of elongation is apparent from observations on nerve cells in tissue culture, in which axonal outgrowth was seen to continue for at least several hr after protein synthesis in the cell body had been blocked by cycloheximide (154) or after the axon had been physically separated from the cell body (155, 183). However, these observations were made under conditions in which outgrowth was already under way, and the axons might already have been more abundantly stocked with materials necessary for elongation, compared to axons preparing to sprout for the first time. In the absence of a large reserve of such materials, a greater dependence on support from the cell body might be manifest.

Can materials synthesized in the periaxonal glial cells contribute to axonal elongation? Invertebrate axons obtain a significant part of their protein requirements from periaxonal glial cells, both in normal nerves (12,97,98) and in axotomized nerves (150). However, vertebrate axons are somewhat less well supplied by local means. Normally, less than 20% of the different types of nerve polypeptides are synthesized locally (42,160), and the number remains low following axotomy (164). For vertebrate axons, therefore, it seems clear that most axonal proteins, including those essential for sprout elongation, are transported from the nerve cell body.

Can the level of protein synthesis in the cell body influence the rate of axonal elongation? As we have seen above (p. 169), there is a close correspondence between the time at which protein synthesis increases following axotomy and the initiation of axonal sprouting. However, the critical experiments to determine whether the increase in protein synthesis is necessary for sprouting have not yet been performed. We have found that when cell body protein synthesis is inhibited by cycloheximide, axonal elongation following a crush of the goldfish optic nerve is reduced by about 50% (114). This result suggests that when protein synthesis is very low it may become a limiting factor for axonal outgrowth.

Action of NGF in Promoting Neurite Outgrowth

In postganglionic sympathetic neurons and immature dorsal root ganglion cells, axonal outgrowth can be accelerated by NGF treatment (10,101). This effect of NGF can be attributed at least partly to an enhancement of protein synthesis by the nerve cell body. For example, the NGF treatment caused increased cell body incorporation of RNA and protein precursors (4). Also, examination of the cells by light microscopy showed neuronal enlargement, increased cytoplasmic basophilia, and enlarged nucleoli, whereas electron microscopy revealed increased amounts of rER, free polyribosomes, Golgi membranes, neurofilaments, and neurotubules (5). In a neuron-related cell line *in vitro*, NGF caused changes in protein synthesis before the onset of neurite outgrowth, including increased synthesis of a few proteins and decreased synthesis of one other (113). Both the alteration in polypeptide synthesis and the formation of neurites could be prevented by inhibiting RNA synthesis at the time of the NGF treatment, suggesting that the protein synthesis changes may be necessary for neurite outgrowth.

The actions of NGF on the cell body are presumably made possible by the fact that the NGF is carried to the cell body by retrograde transport from the axon terminals (159). In addition, however, it appears that NGF may promote axonal outgrowth by a direct effect on the neuronal surface membrane. Studies on sympathetic ganglion cells *in vitro* suggest that the two different mechanisms may regulate different aspects of neurite outgrowth: whereas the rate of elongation of the axons may be determined by NGF transported to the cell body, the number of neurites produced may be determined by NGF bound to the surface membrane (70). The latter effect is independent of protein synthesis in the cell body and may result from a change in the adhesion of the neuronal membrane to cell surfaces and tissue culture substrata (153). It probably involves a different part of the NGF molecule than that responsible for the cell body effects (118).

Alteration of Axonal Outgrowth as the Result of a Prior Injury: the Conditioning Lesion

Axonal outgrowth may be accelerated in neurons that have undergone a prior axonal injury (Table 2). This was demonstrated by measuring the rate of outgrowth of axons following a crush of the sciatic nerve. If this "testing" lesion had been preceded by a nerve injury, i.e., a "conditioning" lesion, some time earlier, the rate of outgrowth was faster than in animals in which only a sham operation had been performed instead of the conditioning lesion. For example, the rate of advance of the fastest-growing sensory axons, as determined by the response to direct mechanical stimulation of the nerve (i.e., the "pinch test" of Young and Medawar, 185), was 4.9 mm/day in animals in which a

TABLE 2. *Effects of conditioning lesions on initial delay and outgrowth rate of axons[a]*

Axons	Outgrowth measurement technique	Initial delay (days)		Outgrowth rate (mm/day)		Ref.
		Sham operation	Conditioning lesion	Sham operation	Conditioning lesion	
Mouse sciatic	Axon counts (silver-stained)	4.0	3.5	0.15	0.19	(115)
Rat sciatic (sensory)	Pinch test	1.4	1.2	4.0	4.9	(117)
Rat sciatic (motor)	Radioactive labeling	—	—	2.4[b]	3.2[b]	(I.G., McQuarrie, unpublished results)
Rat sciatic (adrenergic)	Norepinephrine uptake	1.3	0.6	3.9	1.9	(116)
Goldfish optic	Axon counts (silver-stained)	4.3	2.5	0.34	0.74	(114)
Goldfish optic	Radioactive labeling	4.6	—	0.42	0.7	(114)

[a] Conditioning lesion or sham operation followed 2 weeks later by testing lesion.
[b] Average rate for the interval 0–8 days, i.e., effects on initial delay, as opposed to outgrowth rate, not distinguished.

conditioning lesion, section of the tibial nerve, had been performed 2 weeks earlier, whereas the rate was 4.0 mm/day in sham-operated animals (117). Thus the outgrowth rate was 25% faster as a result of the conditioning lesion. We have obtained similar results in experiments in which the outgrowth of the sciatic axons following nerve excision was measured by axon counts from silver-stained histological sections (115), or in which the outgrowth of motor axons following a crush was determined from the rate of advance of radioactively labeled protein in the tips of axons (I. G. McQuarrie, *unpublished results*). In the experiments involving pinch testing or silver staining, the conditioning lesion produced only a slight decrease in the delay before the initiation of sprouting (Table 2). However, the average number of branches produced by a single severed axon was increased from 1.5 to 1.7, and the time course of formation of branches was accelerated (I. G. McQuarrie, *unpublished results*).

In goldfish optic axons, the effects of the conditioning lesion were even more dramatic: the rate of axonal outgrowth following a crush of the optic nerve was normally 0.34 mm/day, but was increased to 0.74 mm/day if the axons had been subjected to a conditioning lesion 2 weeks earlier (114). In addition, the delay before axonal outgrowth began was reduced from about 4.5 days to 2.5 days. A dramatic decrease in the time required for initiation of neurite outgrowth has also been observed in explants of either goldfish or *Xenopus* retina as a result of crushing the optic nerve 1 to 2 weeks before explantation (2,96): the goldfish explants often showed outgrowth within hours if the optic nerve had been subjected to the conditioning lesion, whereas normally 2 to 4 days passed before outgrowth was usually seen.

The above results show that the effects of a conditioning lesion can lead to an increased rate of outgrowth, and, in at least some neurons, an earlier initiation of outgrowth. The mechanism by which these effects are produced is not known. The hypothesis initially proposed by Ducker et al. (34) is that since protein synthesis is increased after the conditioning lesion, an enhanced supply of materials to support outgrowth is already available at the time of the second lesion. Our own findings are in accord with this view, since we have found that the effect is seen even if the testing lesion is separated by 10 to 50 mm from the conditioning lesion (116,117), and even if the nerve stump distal to the site of the testing lesion is excised (2,96,115). Therefore the effect does not depend on local changes at the site of the conditioning lesion or changes along the path of the growing axons, such as Schwann cell proliferation.

The evidence that the cell body is involved in the conditioning lesion effect is suggestive, though incomplete. It has long been known that the cell body reaction can be intensified by a series of axotomies made at intervals of 1 to 2 weeks (73,127,147). In goldfish retinal ganglion cells we have found that if a second axotomy is performed 20 days after the first, i.e., before the effects of the first have completely subsided, the increase in cell size is greater the second time (124). More recent studies have shown that with a 2-week interval between lesions, the amount of axonally transported protein entering the goldfish optic axons was greatly increased following the second lesion. Thus, the amount of labeled protein in the fast component of axonal transport at 24 hr after a crush of the optic nerve was increased about 11-fold in axons that had been subjected to a conditioning lesion, and the amount in the slow component of transport showed a corresponding 6-fold increase (114). By 8 days after the crush, however, axonal transport in the axons that had been subjected to the conditioning lesion was no different than in those that had not. Therefore, the enhancement of axonal outgrowth resulting from a conditioning lesion may be attributable to the delivery of abundant amounts of protein to the growing axon tip within the first week after the second lesion. Nevertheless, it is not out of the question that some other kind of mechanism, such as a change in membrane properties over the whole neuron, may contribute to the effect of the conditioning lesion.

An interesting finding which may eventually prove to be a clue to the nature of the conditioning lesion effect is that it does not always result in the enhancement of outgrowth, and that the effect on elongation need not be congruent with the effect on the initiation of outgrowth. In adrenergic neurons in rat sciatic nerve, we found that as a result of the conditioning lesion the rate of elongation was reduced from 3.9 mm/day to 1.9 mm/day (116). However, the average number of branches produced during regeneration of these axons was 1.7 in both the animals that had been subjected to a conditioning lesion and those that had not, indicating that this aspect of regeneration had not been impaired. The initiation of outgrowth appeared to be accelerated, since the initial delay, determined by backward extrapolation of the outgrowth curve, was reduced from 31 hr to 14 hr. The difference between the conditioning lesion effect in adrenergic axons and sensory axons of the same nerve is especially striking in view of the fact that, in the absence of a conditioning lesion, the rates of regeneration in the two kinds of axons are virtually identical, i.e., about 4 mm/day. The cell body reaction of the adrenergic neurons is not obviously different from that of other neurons, except that adrenergic neurons appear to develop more intense lysosomal activity (31,72,111).

Enhancement of axonal regeneration by a prior lesion has been seen in a number of other situations. In rabbit peroneal nerve, the time for functional recovery from a crush lesion was reduced by 10% in animals whose nerves had been subjected to a more distal lesion 16 to 42 days before the crush (59). In chimpanzee peripheral nerve, in which axonal outgrowth is normally not yet observed by 14 days after transection (87), outgrowth occurred "almost immediately" if 3 weeks were allowed to pass after the transection and then the nerve stumps were trimmed (thereby removing the first crop of sprouts) and sutured together (34). Wells (182) found that the rate of outgrowth of regenerating axons in the rat sciatic nerve was significantly greater when a conditioning lesion had been made 2 weeks prior to the testing lesion, compared to the rate obtained if the conditioning and testing lesions were made at the same time. Hall-Craggs and Brand (63) have demonstrated improved reinnervation of transplanted rat muscles if the nerves destined to innervate the transplants had been crushed 2 weeks before transplantation. Scheff, Benardo, and Cotman (151) have found that sprouting of axons in the dentate gyrus of the hippocampus following removal of the ipsilateral entorhinal cortex was enhanced if a small lesion had been made in the entorhinal cortex 4 or more days earlier. In this case, the initiation of outgrowth was accelerated, so that the degree of outgrowth was greater at 2 days in the animals subjected to the conditioning lesion than at 4 days in the previously unlesioned animals; also the final amount of axonal outgrowth achieved was greater in the animals that had received the conditioning lesion.

Recently, Kao et al. (78–80) reported regeneration of spinal cord axons under conditions that we believe evoke the conditioning-lesion effect. After the spinal cord in dogs had been subjected to an experimental injury they waited 1 week, then removed the necrotic cord tissue at the site of the injury and replaced this tissue with multiple grafts taken from a peripheral nerve. Penetration of the spinal axons into the nerve grafts could be observed microscopically, and (in 3 of 4 animals) conduction of electrical activity between the limbs and the cerebral cortex was shown to occur. Two of the animals could stand and 1 could also walk, presumably as a consequence of the successful regeneration of the spinal axons. Kao et al. attribute the success of this procedure to the removal, during the nerve grafting, of the portion of the spinal axons that had undergone traumatic degeneration following the initial injury. We believe, however, that it is likely that in the grafting operation many of the spinal axons were injured for a second time, and that following this second injury, their outgrowth was more vigorous than it would have been after the initial insult alone.

The above findings emphasize the potential importance of the conditioning-lesion effect in relation to recovery from injury, not only in peripheral nerves but also in the CNS. Determining the mechanism involved in the enhancement of outgrowth by the conditioning lesion is therefore of considerable interest, particularly as it might be applicable in attempts to enhance recovery from nervous system damage under clinical conditions.

Does the Cell Body have an Active Role in Regulating Outgrowth?

The evidence appears to be very strong in support of the view that the cell body has a critical influence on axonal outgrowth. On the one hand, block of protein synthesis in the cell body interferes with outgrowth; on the other hand, outgrowth may be enhanced in conditions in which the synthesis of materials in the cell body, and hence the supply of axonally transported materials from the cell body, is elevated. Even when sprouting is initiated without axotomy, under conditions in which the sprout-inducing factor appears to have access initially to the axon terminals, it appears that in at least some instances the axonal outgrowth is consequent upon an alteration of the cell body. It is possible that the contribution of the cell body may primarily influence the rate of axonal elongation, whereas mechanisms directed toward alteration of the neuronal surface membrane may be responsible for determining whether axonal sprouting will occur at all.

ROLE OF THE NERVE CELL BODY IN AXONAL REGENERATION: A SYNTHESIS

Current theories of protein synthesis and axonal transport can provide a framework for connecting together some of the events occurring in the cell body in response to axotomy. Our starting point is the fact that in neurons, as in other cells, protein synthesis occurs mainly on polyribosomes that are either free in the cytoplasm or attached to membranes of the endoplasmic reticulum, whereas single free ribosomes are believed to be relatively inactive in protein synthesis (129). The free polyribosomes are generally thought to be responsible for the production of cytoplasmic proteins, whereas the membrane-bound ribosomes of the rER are responsible for the production of cellular membranes and secretion products (69,128,144). Extending this dichotomy, we may approximately identify the products of free polyribosomes with the materials involved in the slow component of axonal transport and the products originating in the rER with the materials carried in the fast component (32,137). The products of the free polyribosomes would include the constituent proteins of the microtubules, neurofilaments and soluble phase of the axoplasm; the products of the rER would include not only materials involved in synaptic transmitter metabolism and function, but also those participating in the formation of certain structural elements, such as the plasma membrane and smooth endoplasmic reticulum (32,53). It is likely, therefore, that the materials required for replacement of the axon, quite apart from the recovery of transmitter function, would be derived to at least some extent from the rER, as well as from the free polyribosomes.

The balance of protein synthesis between free polyribosomes and membrane-bound ribosomes is determined by the various kinds of messenger RNA (mRNA) that are active in the cell at a given moment. The mRNA, which specifies the kind of protein to be produced, also specifies whether or not the synthesis must proceed with the ribosomes attached to the membranes of the endoplasmic reticulum (13). The attachment of the ribosomes to the membrane appears to involve two kinds of linkages: one is a linkage that depends on the presence of a nascent polypeptide; the other is a linkage sensitive to the intracellular concentration of inorganic ions (1,170). Sometimes the conditions that lead to disruption of the salt-sensitive linkage may also cause damage to the ribosomes, so they are unable to participate again in protein synthesis (1). Normally, however, ribosomes that detach from the endoplasmic membranes at the conclusion of protein synthesis are available for reentry into either the free or membrane-bound polyribosomal pools (105).

These general principles provide us with a basis for some speculations on a few of the long-standing problems about the characteristics of the reaction of the nerve cell body to axotomy (52) and serve as a point of departure in integrating some of the specific issues that have been dealt with in the present review.

Mechanism of Chromatolysis

It appears to us to be likely that the loss of membrane-bound ribosomes during chromatolysis is due to (a) a decreased production or increased turnover of mRNAs coding for proteins synthesized on the rER, and (b) a nonspecific inhibition of polyribosome attachment resulting from an alteration in intracelluar milieu, including inorganic ion balance. Thus, chromatolysis may involve both a physiological alteration of mRNA metabolism and a pathological disruption of ribosomal RNA function which, in some cases, may make the ribosomes incompetent for further protein synthesis. The mechanisms for initiating these two kinds of changes are not yet known, but it is likely that the changes in mRNA are related to the pile-up in the cell body of materials returning prematurely from the site of the lesion, and possibly also to the disruption in the supply of trophic factors from the periphery. On the other hand, the nonspecific inhibition of ribosome attachment may be caused by the accumulation of exogenous materials in the cell body, which might result from the retrograde transport of such materials from the site of the lesion or their direct penetration into the cell body consequent to membrane permeability changes and other effects of trauma (52). It is obvious that the intensity of the changes produced by mechanisms of this kind would be increased with lesions closer to the cell body. The variability in the degree of chromatolysis seen in various cells and with various kinds of injuries is presumably due to differences in the balance among the various factors contributing to chromatolysis.

To the extent that chromatolysis may involve a nonspecific inhibition of ribosome attachment, the synthesis of all proteins originating from the rER would be inhibited; moreover, to the extent that the competence of the detached ribosomes may be impaired, the synthesis of proteins on free polyribosomes would probably suffer as well, and a larger proportion of ribosomal material would appear in the form of single free ribosomes. This may be the basis for the appearance of single ribosomes in CNS neurons that do not regenerate (6,8). This phenomenon should not be confused, however, with the appearance of single ribosomes in regenerating neurons in lower vertebrates (122,131,137), which probably represents the formation of new ribosomal material in excess of that required for immediate association with the available mRNA.

Changes in mRNA contributing to chromatolysis are likely to entail more selective alterations in protein synthesis than those described above. The observed decrease in transmitter-related materials, for example, is probably a result of mRNA changes. In some neurons the decrease in transmitter-related materials may occur in the absence of overt chromatolysis (148), presumably indicating that the total amount of protein synthesis on membrane-bound ribosomes has not changed significantly. Thus the production of transmitter-related materials in these cells may normally represent only a minor proportion of the output from the rER. Alternatively, the decreased production of transmitter-related materials may be balanced by an increase in the production of other kinds of proteins by the rER, but there is as yet no evidence for this hypothesis.

RNA and Protein Synthesis Changes Subsequent to Chromatolysis

Shortly after the initiation of chromatolysis, RNA synthesis may increase, as indicated by an increase in the nucleic acid content of the nucleolus, an increase in the amount of ribosomal material in the cytoplasm, or an increase in the incorporation of RNA precursors. Absence of increased RNA synthesis in response to axotomy, or even a decrease in synthesis, appears to be characteristic of neurons that fail to regenerate, such as neurons lying wholly within the CNS and immature neurons (7,86). LaVelle and his coworkers (86,100) have suggested that neurons lacking a potential for increased RNA synthesis may be recognized by their lack of an "intranucleolar body," a structure that apparently indicates the presence of a storage reserve of ribosomal subunits. This has led to the view that neurons already engaged in a maximal turnover of nucleic acid cannot further increase their metabolism in response to axotomy and are therefore likely to show only deleterious effects from axotomy (86).

In neurons in which RNA synthesis increases following axotomy, the augmented ribosomal mass is at first directed predominantly into the formation of free polyribosomes (122,137). Thus an axotomized neuron may come to resemble an immature neuron in having its protein synthesis based mainly on free polyribosomes. The suggestion that the change in the axotomized neuron represents a "regressive" shift to an earlier state of development (58) appears not to be justified, however, since only a minority of the numerous proteins characteristic of the mature neuron are affected by axotomy (62).

Subsequent to the increase in free polyribosomes, there is an increase in rER, which may be seen in successfully regenerating neurons even before reconnection occurs. In neurons that have previously undergone chromatolysis, this change would lead to reappearance of the Nissl substance, but, since an increase in rER can also occur in the absence of chromatolysis, the increase should perhaps be regarded as a positive reaction to axotomy rather than a return to the preaxotomized condition. In any case, the increase in rER, as the basis for an increased supply of structural membranes, may be essential for successful outgrowth, and in some cases may also be essential for survival of the axotomized cell. For example, immature neurons, which are likely to die following axotomy, will survive longer if the axotomy occurs after they have acquired a substantial amount of rER (108).

Contribution of Axonally Transported Materials to Axonal Outgrowth

In studies of protein synthesis in the cell body following axotomy, no attempt has been made thus far to differentiate between changes in the production of proteins on the rER and on free polyribosomes. However, such changes might be deduced from corresponding changes in the amount of material that would become available for the fast component of axonal transport and the slow component, respectively. In principle, either a change in the capacity of the transport channel, or a change in the rate (velocity) of transport could occur. In the case of fast protein transport, changes in rate have thus far been observed only in the goldfish retinal ganglion cell. The amount of protein transported, on the other hand, was seen to be either increased or decreased in various cases, according to the type of neuron involved, the type of protein, and the time after axotomy. We presume that these differences reflect a different balance in the synthesis of various fractions of fast transport. Since transmitter-related materials decrease in amount soon after axotomy, an increased fast component presumably represents an increased supply of structural elements. The importance of these elements for axonal outgrowth is underlined by the fact that fast-transported protein is preferentially deposited in the newly formed portion of the axons (56).

The slow component of axonal transport, which carries cytoplasmic proteins, may show a change in rate as well as in amount during regeneration. However, in at least one case, the observation of an increased rate could be explained by an increase in the amount of one fraction of the slow component, advancing slightly faster than the rest. In this case, the rate of elongation of the axons was found to be equal to the rate of advance of the fraction that had been augmented (99). The close correspondence between the rate of slow transport and the rate of elongation was originally remarked upon by Weiss and Hiscoe (181), who were led to suggest that the movement of the column of axonal cytoplasm by slow transport was actually responsible for elongation. In a number of instances, however, the rate of slow transport is actually about twice as fast as the rate of elongation (47,55,114). Precisely how slow axonal transport contributes to axonal elongation is therefore not clear, and the problem cannot be adequately dealt with until more is known about the mechanism of slow transport and the dynamics of deposition of the transported material in the axon proximal to the lesion, as well as in the newly formed segment. For example, the observation that regenerating axons may become greatly thinned out above the level of the lesion (92) probably has an important bearing, but how it fits into the picture has not yet been established. Nevertheless, our general view at present is that both slow and fast transport provide the axon with a reserve of materials essential for growth, upon which the axon tip can draw as it advances, and that in some circumstances the amount of these materials and the rate at which they are delivered might be growth-limiting factors. It appears likely that the effects of a conditioning lesion on axonal outgrowth are attributable to changes in this supply of materials, which are in turn determined by changes in the synthetic activity of the cell body. However, it is possible that there is also a change in the properties of the neuronal surface membrane.

Initiation of Increased RNA and Protein Synthesis

There is unfortunately no clear answer to the critical question of what the stimulus may be that leads to an increased supply of materials necessary for axonal regeneration, i.e., the stimulus that triggers increased RNA and protein synthesis. This stimulus appears to be distinct from the events responsible for chromatolysis, since some neurons, such as goldfish retinal ganglion cells, show the increase in synthesis without chromatolysis (121,122,124), and conversely, chromatolysis is not always followed by increased synthesis (7). One attractive possibility, that the stimulus for increased synthesis is generated by axonal outgrowth, unfortunately has very little evidence to support it. At the present time, therefore, it seems most probable that the sequence of events leading to the increased synthesis develops according to a fixed program in the cell body, initiated by the axonal injury, but subject to little if any feedback from the subsequent events at the axon tip that may lead to axonal outgrowth. The characteristics of the cell body program would presumably be determined by the genetic endowment of the neuron, but might be modified to some extent by the nature of the injury. In successfully regenerating neurons, axonal injury may have a dual action [for which the dual action of NGF in promoting neurite outgrowth (p. 177) might be considered to be the model]: on the one hand, the injury may elicit changes in the neuronal membrane leading to the initiation of axonal sprouting; and on the other hand, the injury may act by an independent mechanism to trigger increased RNA and protein synthesis in the cell body, thus increasing the supply of material to support axonal elongation. Drawing a further analogy between the effects of the injury and the action of NGF in promoting outgrowth, we may tentatively suggest that the trigger mechanism might involve the retrograde axonal transport of some factor from the site of the injury.

We must emphasize that the view that the cell body program is not affected by feedback from the growing axon is only intended to apply to the initial stages of the cell body's reaction to axotomy. The possibility still exists that at a slightly later stage rapid axonal elongation may have some effect on the cell body, particularly in promoting the production of rER. Furthermore, there is no question that as reconnection of the axon occurs, trophic factors emanating from the target cells may not only prevent the full development of the involutional changes dictated by the declining phase of the cell body program, but may also make a positive contribution to the process of recovery.

SUMMARY

In this review an attempt has been made to explore the nature and significance of the changes that occur in the nerve cell body in response to axotomy, with particular emphasis on the possible role of these changes in axonal regeneration, and on the possible mechanisms involved in the production of these changes. This speculative treatment is of necessity based on evidence that is still fragmentary and sometimes inconsistent; it must therefore be viewed as a tentative guide for further evaluation and experimentation, rather than a definitive statement of strongly-held opinions.

Within hours after an axon has been injured, visible changes may occur in the nerve cell body, in the form of chromatolysis or dispersion of the Nissl substance. At the electron microscopic level, this is seen to be due to disorganization of the rough endoplasmic reticulum (rER), often accompanied by an increase in the proportion of free polyribosomes. These events may involve two mechanisms: 1, a physiological reduction in the amount of messenger RNA (mRNA) coding for proteins synthesized on the rER; and 2, a pathological disturbance of the intracellular milieu (particularly the balance of inorganic ions), leading to defective attachment of ribosomes to membranes and possibly also to damage of the ribosomes. The changes in mRNA, which may be responsible for the subsequent decrease in the neuronal content of materials associated with synaptic transmission, may be initiated by the pile-up in the cell body of axonally transported materials prematurely returning from the site of the lesion, or by disruption of the supply of trophic factors from the periphery. The pathological changes, which may lead to an overall decrease in protein synthesis and an increase in the proportion of free single ribosomes, may result from the presence in the cell body of exogenous materials, possibly conveyed to the cell body by retrograde axonal transport from the site of the lesion, or penetrating into the cell body directly from the extracellular space.

Even in the absence of chromatolysis, signs of increased RNA synthesis may be seen (except in neurons incapable of regeneration), beginning at about 1 to 3 days after axotomy. The augmented ribosomal mass is at first directed primarily into the production of free polyribosomes, which leads to a certain resemblance between the axotomized neuron and an immature one. Subsequently, there is an increase in rER, which often becomes evident even before axonal reconnection occurs. This increase, as the basis for an increased supply of structural membranes, is probably an essential factor in successful outgrowth.

The increase in RNA synthesis is shortly followed by an increase in the synthesis of certain neuronal proteins, including tubulin. These changes, together with the earlier changes in protein synthesis associated with chromatolysis, may be reflected in alterations in the supply of materials reaching the axon by axonal transport. Both the fast and slow components of axonal transport contribute to axonal outgrowth by providing a pool of materials essential for growth, materials that the axon tip can utilize as it advances. Although the rate of axonal outgrowth may be determined to some extent by conditions at the axon tip, e.g., the strength of adhesion between the tip and the surface over which it advances, or the internal Ca^{++} concentration, the amount of the materials delivered to the axon tip and the rate at which they are delivered can become major factors in the regulation of axonal outgrowth. The supply of these materials may be increased somewhat by the diversion of an increased proportion of cell body products to axonal transport. For the most part, however, the supply of transported materials during regeneration (and hence the rate of axonal outgrowth) is regulated by the level of synthesis in the cell body. Whereas the contribution of the cell body may primarily influence the rate of axonal elongation, it is possible that mechanisms directed toward alteration of the neuronal surface membrane are responsible for determining whether axonal sprouting will occur at all.

The hypothesis that the cell body, by determining the supply of materials to the growing axon, has a critical influence on axonal outgrowth is consistent with the observation that block of protein synthesis in the cell body interferes with outgrowth. Conversely, outgrowth may be enhanced by conditions in which the synthesis and delivery of axonally transported materials are increased. Changes of this kind are probably responsible for the "conditioning lesion effect," which is manifested in the fact that the rate of axonal outgrowth following the second of two successive axotomies is different from the rate following a single axotomy; in this case, the supply of axonally transported material at the time of the second axotomy is different from normal as a result of the cell body's response to the first axotomy.

The stimulus for the increased RNA and protein synthesis in axotomized neurons is probably distinct from the mechanisms leading to chromatolysis, since the increased synthesis may appear in the absence of chromatolysis, and vice versa. Available evidence also provides little support for the possibility that increased synthesis is triggered by the initiation of axonal outgrowth. A feasible hypothesis is that the trigger mechanism might involve the retrograde transport of some factor from the site of the injury.

ACKNOWLEDGMENTS

This article was written with the support of USPHS grant NS-09015 to Dr. Grafstein from NINCDS and a Fellowship to Dr. McQuarrie from the Schepp Foundation. Dr. McQuarrie is currently an Andrew W. Mellon Teacher-Scientist.

REFERENCES

1. Adelman, M. R., Sabatini, D. D., and Blobel, G. (1973): Ribosome-membrane interaction. Nondestructive disassembly of rat liver rough microsomes into ribosomal and membranous components. *J. Cell Biol.,* 56:206–229.
2. Agranoff, B. W., Field, P., and Gaze, R. M. (1976): Neurite outgrowth from explanted *Xenopus* retina: an effect of prior optic section. *Brain Res.,* 113:225–234.
3. Andén, N. -E., Dahlström, A., Fuxe, K., Larsson, K., Olson, L., and Ungerstedt, O. (1966): Ascending monoamine neurons to the telencephalon and diencephalon. *Acta Physiol. Scand.,* 67:313–326.
4. Angeletti, P. U., Gandini-Attardi, D., Toschi, G., Salvi, M. L., and Levi-Montalcini, R. (1965): Metabolic aspects of the effect of nerve growth factor on sympathetic and sensory ganglia: protein and ribonucleic acid synthesis. *Biochim. Biophys. Acta,* 95:111–120.
5. Angeletti, P. U., Levi-Montalcini, R., and Caramia, F. (1971): Ultrastructural changes in sympathetic neurons of newborn and adult mice treated with nerve growth factor. *J. Ultrastruct. Res.,* 36:24–36.
6. Barron, K. D., Dentinger, M. P., Nelson, L. R., and Mincy, J. E. (1975): Ultrastructure of axonal reaction in red nucleus of cat. *J. Neuropathol. Exp. Neurol.,* 34:222–248.
7. Barron, K. D., Dentinger, M. P., Nelson, L. R., and Scheibly, M. E. (1976): Incorporation of tritiated leucine by axotomized rubral neurons. *Brain Res.,* 116:251–266.

8. Barron, K. D., Means, E. D., and Larson, E. (1973): Ultrastructure of retrograde degeneration in thalamus of rat. I. Neuronal somata and dendrites. *J. Neuropathol. Exp. Neurol.,* 32:218–244.
9. Bisby, M. A., and Bulger, V. T. (1977): Reversal of axonal transport at a nerve crush. *J. Neurochem.,* 29:313–320.
10. Bjerre, B., and Rosengren, E. (1974): Effects of nerve growth factor and its antiserum on axonal regeneration of short adrenergic neurons in the male mouse. *Cell Tissue Res.,* 150:299–322.
11. Black, M. M., and Lasek, R. J. (1976): The use of axonal transport to measure axonal regeneration in rat ventral motor neurons. *Anat. Rec.,* 184:360–361.
12. Black, M. M., and Lasek, R. J. (1977): The presence of transfer RNA in the axoplasm of the squid giant axon. *J. Neurobiol.,* 8:229–237.
13. Blobel, G., and Dobberstein, B. (1975): Transfer of proteins across membranes. I. Presence of proteolytically processed and unprocessed nascent immunoglobulin light chains on membrane-bound ribosomes of murine myeloma. *J. Cell Biol.,* 67:835–851.
14. Bodian, D., and Mellors, R. C. (1945): The regenerative cycle of motoneurons, with special reference to phosphatase activity. *J. Exp. Med.,* 81:469–487.
15. Boroff, D. A., del Castillo, J., Evoy, W. H., and Steinhardt, R. A. (1974): Observations on the action of type A botulinum toxin on frog neuromuscular junctions. *J. Physiol. (Lond.),* 240:227–253.
16. Boyle, F. C., and Gillespie, J. S. (1970): Accumulation and loss of noradrenaline central to a constriction on adrenergic nerves. *Eur. J. Pharmacol.,* 12:77–84.
17. Brattgård, S. -O., Edström, J. -E., and Hydén, H. (1957): The chemical changes in regenerating neurons. *J. Neurochem.,* 1:316–325.
18. Brattgård, S. -O., Hydén, H., and Sjöstrand, J. (1958): Incorporation of orotic acid-^{14}C and lysine-^{14}C in regenerating single nerve cells. *Nature,* 182:801–802.
19. Bray, D. (1973): Model for membrane movements in the neural growth cone. *Nature,* 244:93–96.
20. Brown, M. C., and Ironton, R. (1977): Motor neurone sprouting induced by prolonged tetrodotoxin block of nerve action potentials. *Nature,* 265:459–461.
21. Bunge, M. B. (1973): Fine structure of nerve fibers and growth cones of isolated sympathetic neurons in culture. *J. Cell Biol.,* 56:713–735.
22. Bunge, M. B. (1977): Initial endocytosis of peroxidase or ferritin by growth cones of cultured nerve cells. *J. Neurocytol.,* 6:407–439.
23. Burgen, A. S. V., Dickens, F., and Zatman, L. J. (1949): The action of botulinum toxin on the neuromuscular junction. *J. Physiol. (Lond.),* 109:10–24.
24. Cammermeyer, J. (1963): Differential response of two neuron types to facial nerve transection in young and old rabbits. *J. Neuropathol. Exp. Neurol.,* 22:594–616.
25. Cheah, T. B., and Geffen, L. B. (1973): Effects of axonal injury on norepinephrine, tyrosine hydroxylase and monoamine oxidase levels in sympathetic ganglia. *J. Neurobiol.,* 4:443–452.
26. Colard, J. G., deWildt, A., Oomen-Meulemans, E. P. M., Smeekens, J., Emmelot, P., and Inbar, M. (1977): Increase in fluidity of membrane lipids in lymphocytes, fibroblasts and liver cells stimulated for growth. *FEBS Lett.,* 77:173–178.
27. Cova, J. L., and Barron, K. D. (1977): Uptake of leucine ^{3}H by axotomized cervical motoneurons. *Anat. Rec.,* 187:558.
28. Cragg, B. G. (1970): What is the signal for chromatolysis? *Brain Res.,* 23:1–21.
29. Cull, R. E. (1974): Role of nerve-muscle contact in maintaining synaptic connections. *Exp. Brain Res.,* 20:307–310.
30. Diamond, J., Cooper, E., Turner, C., and Macintyre, L. (1976): Trophic regulation of nerve sprouting. *Science,* 193:371–377.
31. Dixon, J. S. (1967): Phagocytic lysosomes in chromatolytic neurons. *Nature,* 215:657–658.
32. Droz, B. (1975): Synthetic machinery and axoplasmic transport: maintenance of neuronal connectivity. In: *The Nervous System, Vol. I: The Basic Neurosciences,* edited by D. B. Tower, pp. 111–127. Raven Press, New York.
33. Duce, I. R., Reeves, J. F., and Keen, P. (1976): A scanning electron microscope study of the development of free axonal sprouts at the cut ends of dorsal spinal nerve roots in the rat. *Cell Tissue Res.,* 170:507–513.
34. Ducker, T. B., Kempe, L. G., and Hayes, G. J. (1969): The metabolic background for peripheral nerve surgery. *J. Neurosurg.,* 30:270–280.

35. Edds, Jr., M. W. (1953): Collateral nerve regeneration. *Quart. Rev. Biol.,* 28:260–276.
36. Edström, J. E. (1959): RNA changes in the motoneurons of the frog during axon regeneration. *J. Neurochem.,* 5:43–49.
37. Engh, C. A., Schofield, B. H., Doty, S. B., and Robinson, R. A. (1971): Perikaryal synthetic function following reversible and irreversible peripheral axon injuries as shown by radioautography. *J. Comp. Neurol.,* 142:465–480.
38. Fischer, J., Lodin, Z., and Kolousek, J. (1958): A histoautoradiographic study of the effect on section of the facial nerve in the uptake of methionine-^{35}S by the cells of the facial nucleus. *Nature,* 181:341–342.
39. Flumerfelt, B. A., Lewis, P. R. (1975): Cholinesterase activity in the hypoglossal nucleus of the rat and the changes produced by axotomy: a light and electron microscopic study. *J. Anat.,* 119:309–332.
40. Forman, D. S., and Berenberg, R. A. (1977): Regeneration in the rat sciatic nerve studied by labeling the motor fibers with axonally transported radioactive proteins. *Neurosci. Abstr.,* 3:425.
41. Francoeur, J., and Olszewski, J. (1968): Axonal reaction and axoplasmic flow as studied by radioautography. *Neurology,* 18:178–184.
42. Frankel, R. D., and Koenig, E. (1977): Identification of major indigenous protein components in mammalian axons and locally synthesized axonal protein in hypoglossal nerve. *Exp. Neurol.,* 57:282–295.
43. Frizell, M., McLean, W. G., and Sjöstrand, J. (1976): Retrograde axonal transport of rapidly migrating labelled proteins and glycoproteins in regenerating peripheral nerves. *J. Neurochem.,* 27:191–196.
44. Frizell, M., and Sjöstrand, J. (1974): Transport of proteins, glycoproteins, and cholinergic enzymes in regenerating hypoglossal neurons. *J. Neurochem.,* 22:845–850.
45. Frizell, M., and Sjöstrand, J. (1974): Retrograde axonal transport of rapidly migrating proteins in the vagus and hypoglossal nerves of the rabbit. *J. Neurochem.,* 23:651–658.
46. Frizell, M., and Sjöstrand, J. (1974): The axonal transport of [3H] fucose labelled glycoproteins in normal and regenerating peripheral nerves. *Brain Res.,* 78:109–123.
47. Frizell, M., and Sjöstrand, J. (1974): The axonal transport of slowly migrating [3H]leucine labelled proteins and the regeneration rate in regenerating hypoglossal and vagus nerves of the rabbit. *Brain Res.,* 81:267–284.
48. Gersh, I., and Bodian, D. (1943): Some chemical mechanisms in chromatolysis. *J. Cell. Comp. Physiol.,* 21:253–274.
49. Gilad, G. (1977): Biochemical and immunocytochemical studies of the axon reaction and collateral sprouting in dopaminergic neurons of rat brain. Ph.D. Thesis. Cornell University Graduate School of Medical Sciences.
50. Grafstein, B. (1971): Role of slow axonal transport in nerve regeneration. *Acta Neuropath., (Berl.), Suppl. V:*144–152.
51. Grafstein, B. (1975): Principles of anterograde axonal transport in relation to studies of neuronal connectivity. In: *The Use of Axonal Transport for Studies of Neuronal Connectivity,* edited by W. M. Cowan and M. Cuénod, pp. 47–67. Elsevier, Amsterdam.
52. Grafstein, B. (1975): The nerve cell body response to axotomy. *Exp. Neurol.,* 48 (No. 3, pt. 2):32–51.
53. Grafstein, B. (1977): Axonal transport: the intracellular traffic of the neuron. In: *Cellular Biology of Neurons, Part I, Handbook of Physiology, Section 1: The Nervous System, Vol. I,* edited by Eric R. Kandel, pp. 691–717. Amer. Physiol. Soc., Bethesda.
54. Grafstein, B., and Alpert, R. (1976): Early changes in the metabolism of goldfish retinal ganglion cells following axotomy. *Neurosci. Abst.,* 2:46.
55. Grafstein, B., and Murray, M. (1969): Transport of protein in goldfish optic nerve during regeneration. *Exp. Neurol.,* 25:494–508.
56. Griffin, J. W., Drachman, D. B., and Price, D. L. (1976): Rapid axonal transport in motor nerve regeneration. *J. Neurobiol.,* 7:355–370.
57. Griffin, J. W., Price, D. L., and Drachman, D. B. (1977): Impaired axonal regeneration in acrylamide intoxication. *J. Neurobiol.,* 8:355–370.
58. Griffith, A., and LaVelle, A. (1971): Developmental protein changes in normal and chromatolytic facial nerve nuclear regions. *Exp. Neurol.,* 33:360–371.
59. Gutmann, E. (1942): Factors affecting recovery of motor function after nerve lesions. *J. Neurol. Neurosurg. Psychiatr.,* 5:81–95.

60. Gutmann, E., Guttmann, L., Medawar, P. B., and Young, J. Z.: (1942): The rate of regeneration of nerve. *J. Exp. Biol.,* 19:14–44.
61. Haddad, A., Iucif, S., and Cruz, A. R. (1969): Synthesis of RNA in neurons of the hypoglossal nerve nucleus after section of the axon in mice. *J. Neurochem.,* 16:865–868.
62. Hall, M. E., Wilson, D. L., and Stone, G. C. (1977): Changes in protein metabolism following axonotomy: a two-dimensional analysis. *Neurosci. Abst.,* 3:426.
63. Hall-Craggs, E. C. B., and Brand, P. (1977): Effect of previous nerve injury on the regeneration of free autogenous muscle grafts. *Exp. Neurol.,* 57:275–281.
64. Halperin, J. J., and LaVail, J. H. (1975): A study of the dynamics of retrograde transport and accumulation of horseradish peroxidase in injured neurons. *Brain Res.,* 100:253–269.
65. Hammond, G. R., and Smith, R. S. (1977): Inhibition of the rapid movement of optically detectable axonal particles by colchicine and vinblastine. *Brain Res.,* 128:227–242.
66. Hatten, M. E., Horwitz, A. F., and Burger, M. M. (1977): The influence of membrane lipids on the proliferation of transformed and untransformed cell lines. *Exp. Cell Res.,* 107:31–34.
67. Heacock, A. M., and Agranoff, B. W. (1976): Enhanced labeling of a retinal protein during regeneration of optic nerve in goldfish. *Proc. Natl. Acad. Sci., USA* 73:828–832.
68. Hendry, I. A. (1975): The response of adrenergic neurons to axotomy and nerve growth factor. *Brain Res.,* 94:87–98.
69. Hicks, S. J., Drysdale, J. W., and Munro, H. N. (1969): Preferential synthesis of ferritin and albumin by different populations of liver polysomes. *Science,* 164:584–585.
70. Hill, C. E., and Hendry, I. A. (1976): Differences in sensitivity to nerve growth factor of axon formation and tyrosine hydroxylase induction in cultured sympathetic neurons. *Neuroscience,* 1:489–496.
71. Hoffman, H. (1950): Local re-innervation in partially denervated muscle: a histo-physiological study. *Aust. J. Exp. Biol. Med. Sci.,* 28:383–397.
72. Holtzmann, E., Novikoff, A. B., and Villaverde, H. (1967): Lysosomes and GERL in normal and chromatolytic neurons of the rat ganglion nodosum. *J. Cell Biol.,* 33:419–435.
73. Howe, H. A., and Bodian, D. (1941): Refractoriness of nerve cells to poliomyelitis virus after interruption of their axons. *Johns Hopkins Hosp. Bull.,* 69:92–103.
74. Hughes, A. F. (1953): The growth of embryonic neurites. A study on cultures of chick neural tissue. *J. Anat.,* 87:150–162.
75. Ingoglia, N. A., Sturman, J. A., and Eisner, R. A. (1977): Axonal transport of putrescine, spermidine and spermine in normal and regenerating goldfish optic nerves. *Brain Res.,* 130:433–445.
76. Ingoglia, N. A., and Tuliszewski, R. (1976): Transfer RNA may be axonally transported during regeneration of goldfish optic nerves. *Brain Res.,* 112:371–382.
77. Ingoglia, N. A., Weis, P., and Mycek, J. (1975): Axonal transport of RNA during regeneration of the optic nerves of goldfish. *J. Neurobiol.,* 6:549–564.
78. Kao, C. C., Chang, L. W., and Bloodworth, J. M. B., Jr. (1977): Axonal regeneration across transected mammalian spinal cords: an electron microscopic study of delayed microsurgical nerve grafting. *Exp. Neurol.,* 54:591–615.
79. Kao, C. C., Chang, L. W., and Bloodworth, J. M. B., Jr. (1977): The mechanism of spinal cord cavitation following spinal cord transection. Part 3: Delayed grafting with and without spinal cord retransection. *J. Neurosurg.,* 46:757–766.
80. Kao, C. C., Faricllo, R. G., Quaglieri, C. E., Messert, B., and Bloodworth, J. M. B., Jr. (1977): Functional recovery of contused spinal cords repaired by delayed nerve grafting. *Proc. Am. Assoc. Neurol. Surg.,* Ann. Meeting, Toronto, Canada, pp. 1–6.
81. Kao, I., Drachman, D. B., and Price, D. L. (1976): Botulinum toxin: mechanism of presynaptic blockade. *Science,* 193:1256–1258.
82. Kapeller, K., and Mayor, D. (1967): The accumulation of noradrenaline in constricted sympathetic nerves as studied by fluorescence and electron microscopy. *Proc. R. Soc. Lond. (Biol.),* 166:282–292.
83. Karlsson, J. -O., Hansson, H. -A., and Sjöstrand, J. (1971): Effect of colchicine on axonal transport and morphology of retinal ganglion cells. *Z. Zellforsch.,* 115:265–283.
84. Karlström, L., and Dahlström, A. (1973): The effect of different types of axonal trauma on the synthesis and transport of amine storage granules in rat sciatic nerve. *J. Neurobiol.,* 4:191–200.
85. Kinderman, N. B., and LaVelle, A. (1976): Ultrastructural changes in the developing nucleolus following axotomy. *Brain Res.,* 108:237–248.

86. Kinderman, N. B., and LaVelle, A. (1977): Uridine incorporation by axotomized facial neurons. *Anat. Rec.,* 187:624.
87. Kline, D. G., Hayes, G. J., and Morse, A. S. (1964): A comparative study of the response of species to peripheral nerve injuries. *J. Neurosurg.,* 21:968–979.
88. Knowland, J., and Miller, L. (1970): Reduction of ribosomal RNA synthesis and ribosomal RNA genes in a mutant of *Xenopus laevis* which organizes only a partial nucleolus. I. Ribosomal RNA synthesis in embryos of different nucleolar types. *J. Mol. Biol.,* 53:321–328.
89. Ko, Y. (1971): Neuronal and glial reaction after peripheral nerve section in rats. *Yonago Acta Med.,* 3:197–207.
90. Kopin, I. J., and Silberstein, S. D. (1972): Axons of sympathetic neurons: transport of enzymes *in vivo* and properties of axonal sprouts *in vitro. Pharmacol. Rev.,* 24:245–254.
91. Kreutzberg, G. W., and Schubert, P. (1971): Changes in axonal flow during regeneration of mammalian motor nerves. *Acta Neuropath.* (Berl.) Suppl. V:70–75.
92. Kreutzberg, G. W., and Schubert, P. (1971): Volume changes in the axon during regeneration. *Acta Neuropath. (Berl.),* 17:220–226.
93. Kristensson, K., and Olsson, Y. (1974). Retrograde transport of horseradish peroxidase in transected axons. I. Time relationships between transport and induction of chromatolysis. *Brain Res.,* 79:101–109.
94. Kristensson, K., and Olsson, Y. (1975): Retrograde transport of horseradish peroxidase in transected axons. II. Relations between rate of transfer from the site of injury to the perikaryon and the onset of chromatolysis. *J. Neurocytol.,* 4:653–661.
95. Kung, S. H. (1971): Incorporation of tritiated precursors in the cytoplasm of normal and chromatolytic sensory neurons as shown by autoradiography. *Brain Res.,* 25:656–660.
96. Landreth, G. E., and Agranoff, B. W. (1977): Explant culture of adult goldfish retina: effect of prior optic nerve crush. *Brain Res.,* 118:299–303.
97. Lasek, R. J., Dabrowski, C., and Nordlander, R. (1973): Analysis of axoplasmic RNA from invertebrate giant axons. *Nature (New Biol.),* 244:162–165.
98. Lasek, R. J., Gainer, H., and Przybylski, R. J. (1974): Transfer of newly-synthesized proteins from Schwann cells to the squid giant axon. *Proc. Natl. Acad. Sci., USA,* 71:1188–1198.
99. Lasek, R. J., and Hoffman, P. N. (1976): The neuronal cytoskeleton, axonal transport and axonal growth. In: *Cell Motility, Book C., Microtubules and Related Proteins.,* edited by R. Goldman, T. Pollard, and J. Rosenbaum. pp. 1021–1051. Cold Spring Harbor Laboratory, Cold Spring Harbor.
100. LaVelle, A., and LaVelle, F. W. (1975): Changes in an intranucleolar body in hamster facial neurons following axotomy. *Exp. Neurol.,* 49:569–579.
101. Levi-Montalcini, R., and Angeletti, P. U. (1968): Nerve growth factor. *Physiol. Rev.,* 48:534–569.
102. Lieberman, A. R. (1971): The axon reaction: a review of the principal features of perikaryal responses to axon injury. *Int. Rev. Neurobiol.,* 14:49–124.
103. Lieberman, A. R. (1974): Some factors affecting retrograde neuronal responses to axonal lesions. In: *Essays on the Nervous System,* edited by R. Bellairs and E. G. Gray, pp. 71–105. Clarendon Press, Oxford
104. Liu, C. -N., and Chambers, W. W. (1958): Intraspinal sprouting of dorsal root axons. *Arch. Neurol. Psychiatr.,* 79:46–61.
105. Lucas-Lennard, J., and Lipmann, F. (1971): Protein biosynthesis. *Ann. Rev. Biochem.* 40:409–448.
106. Lundh, H., Cull-Candy, S. G., Leander, S., and Thesleff, S. (1976): Restoration of transmitter release in botulinum-poisoned skeletal muscle. *Brain Res.,* 110:194–198.
107. Lynch, G., Deadwyler, S., and Cotman, C. (1973): Postlesion axonal growth produces permanent functional connections. *Science,* 180:1364–1366.
108. Matthews, M. A., Narayanan, C. H., Narayanan, Y., and St. Onge, M. F. (1977): Neuronal maturation and synaptogenesis in the rat ventrobasal complex: alignment with developmental changes in rate and severity of axon reaction. *J. Comp. Neurol.,* 173:745–772.
109. Matthews, M. R. (1973): An ultrastructural study of axonal changes following constriction of postganglionic branches of the superior cervical ganglion in the rat. *Philos. Trans. R. Soc. Lond. (Biol.),* 264:479–508.
110. Matthews, M. R., and Nelson, V. H. (1975): Detachment of structurally intact nerve endings from chromatolytic neurones of rat superior cervical ganglion during the depression of synaptic transmission induced by postganglionic axotomy. *J. Physiol. (Lond.),* 245:91–136.

111. Matthews, M. R., and Raisman, G. (1972): A light and electron microscopic study of the cellular response to axonal injury in the superior cervical ganglion of the rat. *Proc. R. Soc. Lond. (Biol.)*, 181:43–79.

112. McClure, W. O. (1972): Effect of drugs upon axoplasmic transport. *Adv. Pharmacol. Chemother.*, 10:185–220.

113. McGuire, J. C., and Greene, L. A. (1977): NGF alters specific protein synthesis in rat PC12 cells. *Neurosci. Abst.*, 3:526.

114. McQuarrie, I. G. (1977): Axonal regeneration in the goldfish optic system: the role of the nerve cell body. Ph.D. Thesis, Cornell University Graduate School of Medical Sciences.

115. McQuarrie, I. G., and Grafstein, B. (1973): Axon outgrowth enhanced by a previous nerve injury. *Arch. Neurol.*, 29:53–55.

116. McQuarrie, I. G., Grafstein, B., Dreyfus, C. F., and Gershon, M. D. (1978): Regeneration of adrenergic axons in rat sciatic nerve: effect of a conditioning lesion. *Brain Res.*, 141:21–34.

117. McQuarrie, I. G., Grafstein, B., and Gershon, M. D. (1977): Axonal regeneration in the rat sciatic nerve: effect of a conditioning lesion and of dbcAMP. *Brain Res.*, 132:443–453.

118. Merrell, R., Pulliam, M. W., Randono, L., Boyd, L. F., Bradshaw, R. A., and Glaser, L. (1975): Temporal changes in tectal cell surface specificity induced by nerve growth factor. *Proc. Natl. Acad. Sci. USA*, 72:4270–4274.

119. Miani, N., Rizzoli, A., and Bucciante, G. (1961): Metabolic and chemical changes in regenerating neurons. II. *In vitro* rate of incorporation of amino acids into proteins of the nerve cell perikaryon of the C. 8 spinal ganglion of rabbit. *J. Neurochem.*, 7:161–173.

120. Morris, J. H., Hudson, A. F., and Weddell, G. (1972): A study of degeneration and regeneration in the divided rat sciatic nerve based on electron microscopy. II. The development of the "regenerating unit." *Z. Zellforsch.*, 124:103–130.

121. Murray, M. (1973): ^{3}H-uridine incorporation by regenerating retinal ganglion cells of goldfish. *Exp. Neurol.*, 39:489–497.

122. Murray, M., and Forman, D. S. (1971): Fine structural changes in goldfish retinal ganglion cells during axonal regeneration. *Brain Res.*, 32:287–298.

123. Murray, M., and Goldberger, M. E. (1974): Restitution of function and collateral sprouting in the cat spinal cord: the partially hemisected animal. *J. Comp. Neurol.*, 158:19–36.

124. Murray, M., and Grafstein, B. (1969): Changes in the morphology and amino acid incorporation of regenerating goldfish optic neurons. *Exp. Neurol.*, 23:544–560.

125. Nissl, F. (1892): Ueber die Veränderungen der Ganglienzellen am Facialiskern des Kaninchens nach Ausreissung der Nerven. *Allg. Z. Psychiatr.*, 48:197–198.

126. Ochs, S. (1976): Fast axoplasmic transport in the fibres of chromatolyzed neurones. *J. Physiol. (Lond.)*, 255:249–261.

127. Oliver, Jr., J. E., Bradley, W. E., and Fletcher, T. F. (1969): Identification of preganglionic parasympathetic neurons in the sacral spinal cord of the cat. *J. Comp. Neurol.*, 137:321–328.

128. Palade, G. (1975): Intracellular aspects of the process of protein synthesis. *Science*, 189:347–358.

129. Palay, S. L., Billings-Gagliardi, S., and Chan-Palay, V. (1974): Neuronal perikarya with dispersed, single ribosomes in the visual cortex of *Macaca mulatta*. *J. Cell Biol.*, 63:1074–1089.

130. Palay, S. L., and Palade, G. E. (1955): The fine structure of neurons. *J. Biophys. Biochem. Cytol.*, 1:68–88.

131. Pannese, E. (1963): Investigations on the ultrastructural changes of the spinal ganglion neurons in the course of axon regeneration and cell hypertrophy. I. Changes during axon regeneration. *Z. Zellforsch.*, 60:711–740.

132. Pannese, E. (1963): Investigations on the ultrastructural changes of the spinal ganglion neurons in the course of axon regeneration and cell hypertrophy. II. Changes during cell hypertrophy and comparison between the ultrastructure of nerve cells of the same type under different functional conditions. *Z. Zellforsch.*, 61:561–586.

133. Pickel, V. M., Segal, M., and Bloom, F. E. (1974): Axonal proliferation following lesions of cerebellar peduncles. A combined fluorescence microscopic and radioautographic study. *J. Comp. Neurol.*, 155:43–59.

134. Pilar, G., and Landmesser, L. (1972): Axotomy mimicked by localized colchicine application. *Science*, 177:1116–1118.

135. Pomerat, C. M., Hendelman, W. J., Raiborn, C. W., Jr., and Massey, J. F. (1967): Dynamic

activities of nervous tissue in vitro. In: *The Neuron,* edited by Hydén, H., pp. 119–178. Elsevier, Amsterdam.

136. Porter, K. R., and Bonneville, M. A. (1973): *Fine Structure of Cells and Tissues, 4th edition,* pp. 196. Lea and Febiger, Philadelphia.

137. Price, D. L., and Porter, K. R. (1972): The response of ventral horn neurons to axonal transection. *J. Cell Biol.,* 53:24–37.

138. Purves, D. (1975): Functional and structural changes in mammalian sympathetic neurones following interruption of their axons. *J. Physiol. (Lond.),* 252:429–463.

139. Purves, D. (1976): Functional and structural changes in mammalian sympathetic neurones following colchicine application to post-ganglionic nerves. *J. Physiol. (Lond.),* 259:159–175.

140. Purves, D. (1976): Long-term regulation in the vertebrate peripheral nervous system. *Int. Rev. Physiol.,* 10:125–178.

141. Purves, D., and Njå, A. (1976): Effect of nerve growth factor in synaptic depression after axotomy. *Nature,* 260:535–536.

142. Raisman, G. (1969): Neuronal plasticity in the septal nuclei of the adult rat. *Brain Res.,* 14:25–48.

143. Ramón y Cajal, S. (1928): *Degeneration and Regeneration of the Nervous System, Vol. I,* translated by R. M. May. Oxford Univ. Press, Cambridge.

144. Redman, C. M. (1969): Biosynthesis of serum proteins and ferritin by free and attached ribosomes of rat liver. *J. Biol. Chem.,* 244:4308–4315.

145. Reis, D. J., and Ross, R. A. (1973): Dynamic changes in brain dopamine-β-hydroxylase activity during anterograde and retrograde reactions to injury of central noradrenergic neurons. *Brain Res.,* 57:307–326.

146. Rhodes, A., Ford, D., and Rhines, R. (1964): Comparative uptake of DL-lysine-H^3 by normal and regenerative hypoglossal nerve cells in euthyroid, hypothyroid and hyperthyroid male rats. *Exp. Neurol.,* 10:251–263.

147. Romanes, G. J. (1951): The motor cell columns of the lumbrosacral spinal cord of the cat. *J. Comp. Neurol.,* 94:313–364.

148. Ross, R. A., Joh, T. H., and Reis, D. J. (1975): Reversible changes in the accumulation and activities of tyrosine hydroxylase and dopamine-β-hydroxylase in neurons of nucleus locus coeruleus during the retrograde reaction. *Brain Res.,* 92:57–72.

149. Rotter, A., Birdsall, N. J. M., Burgen, A. S. V., Field, P. M., and Raisman, G. (1977): Axotomy causes loss of muscarinic receptors and loss of synaptic contacts in the hypoglossal nucleus. *Nature,* 266:734–735.

150. Sarne, Y., Neale, E. A., and Gainer, H. (1976): Protein metabolism in transected peripheral nerves of the crayfish. *Brain. Res.,* 110:73–90.

151. Scheff, S., Benardo, L., and Cotman, C. (1977): Progressive brain damage accelerates axonal sprouting in the adult rat. *Science,* 197:795–797.

152. Schneider, G. E. (1973): Early lesions of superior colliculus: factors affecting the formation of abnormal retinal projections. *Brain Behav. Evol.,* 8:73–109.

153. Schubert D., and Whitlock, C. (1977): Alteration of cellular adhesion by nerve growth factor. *Proc. Natl. Acad. Sci., USA,* 74:4055–4058.

154. Seeds, N. W., Gilman, A. G., Amano, T., and Nirenberg, M. W. (1970): Regulation of axon formation by clonal lines of a neural tumor. *Proc. Natl. Acad. Sci., USA,* 66:160–167.

155. Shaw, G., and Bray, D. (1977): Movement and extension of isolated growth cones. *Exp. Cell. Res.,* 104:55–62.

156. Shawe, G. D. H. (1954): On the number of branches formed by regenerating nerve fibers. *Br. J. Surg.,* 42:474–488.

157. Sidman, R. L., and Wessells, N. K. (1975): Control of direction of growth during the elongation of neurites. *Exp. Neurol.,* 48 (No. 3, pt. 2):237–251.

158. Stoeckel, K., Schwab, M., and Thoenen, H. (1977): Role of gangliosides in the uptake and retrograde axonal transport of cholera and tetanus toxin as compared to nerve growth factor and wheat germ agglutinin. *Brain Res.,* 132:273–285.

159. Stoeckel, K., and Thoenen, H. (1975): Retrograde axonal transport of nerve growth factor: specificity and biological importance. *Brain Res.,* 85:337–341.

160. Stone, G. C., Wilson, D. L., and Hall. M. E. (1977): Two-dimensional mapping of proteins in rapid axoplasmic transport. *Neurosci. Abst.,* 3:32.

161. Sumner, B. E. H. (1975): A quantitative analysis of the response of presynaptic boutons to postsynaptic motor neuron axotomy. *Exp. Neurol.,* 46:605–615.

162. Sumner, B. E. H. (1976): Quantitative ultrastructural observations on the inhibited recovery of the hypoglossal nucleus from the axotomy response when regeneration of the hypoglossal nerve is prevented. *Exp. Brain Res.,* 26:141–150.

163. Tennyson, V. M. (1970): The fine structure of the axon and growth cone of the dorsal root neuroblast of the rabbit embryo. *J. Cell. Biol.,* 44:62–79.

164. Tobias, G. S., and Koenig, E. (1975): Influence of nerve cell body and neurolemma cell on local axonal protein synthesis following neurotomy. *Exp. Neurol.,* 49:235–245.

165. Tonge, D. A. (1977): Effect of implantation of an extra nerve on the recovery of neuromuscular transmission from botulinum toxin. *J. Physiol. (Lond.),* 265:809–820.

166. Torvik, A. (1972): Phagocytosis of nerve cells during retrograde degeneration. An electron microscopic study. *J. Neuropathol. Exp. Neurol.,* 31:132–146.

167. Torvik, A., and Heding, A. (1969): Effect of actinomycin D on retrograde nerve cell reaction. Further observations. *Acta Neuropathol. (Berl.),* 14:62–71.

168. Torvik, A., and Skjörten, F. (1971): Electron microscope observations on nerve cell regeneration and degeneration after axon lesions. I. Changes in the nerve cell cytoplasm. *Acta Neuropathol. (Berl.),* 17:248–264.

169. Torvik, A., and Söreide, A. J. (1972): Nerve cell regeneration after axon lesions in newborn rabbits. *J. Neuropathol. Exp. Neurol.,* 31:683–695.

170. Unwin, P. N. T. (1977): Three-dimensional model of membrane-bound ribosomes obtained by electron microscopy. *Nature,* 269:118–122.

171. Varon, S. (1975): Nerve growth factor and its mode of action. *Exp. Neurol.,* 48 (No. 3, pt. 2):75–92

172. Watson, W. E. (1965): An autoradiographic study of the incorporation of nucleic-acid precursors by neurones and glia during nerve regeneration. *J. Physiol. (Lond.),* 180:741–753.

173. Watson, W. E. (1965): DNA synthesis in injured neurons of adult mice. *J. Neurochem.,* 12:907–908.

174. Watson, W. E. (1966): Quantitative observations upon acetylcholine hydrolase activity of nerve cells after axotomy. *J. Neurochem.,* 13:1549–1550.

175. Watson, W. E. (1968): Observations on the nucleolar and total cell body nucleic acid of injured nerve cells. *J. Physiol., (Lond.),* 196:655–676.

176. Watson, W. E. (1969): The response of motor neurones to intramuscular injection of botulinum toxin. *J. Physiol. (Lond.),* 202:611–630.

177. Watson, W. E. (1970): Some metabolic responses of axotomized neurones to contact between their axons and denervated muscle. *J. Physiol. (Lond.),* 210:321–344.

178. Watson, W. E. (1973): Some responses of dorsal root ganglia to axotomy. *J. Physiol. (Lond.),* 231:41P–42P.

179. Watson, W. E. (1974): The binding of actinomycin D to the nuclei of axotomised neurones. *Brain Res.,* 65:317–322.

180. Watson, W. E. (1974): Cellular responses to axotomy and to related procedures. *Brit. Med. Bull.,* 30:112–115.

181. Weiss, P., and Hiscoe, H. B. (1948): Experiments on the mechanism of nerve growth. *J. Exp. Zool.,* 107:315–395.

182. Wells, M. R. (1977): [³H]lysine incorporation into rat spinal cord and brain after simultaneous transection and crush or transection followed by crush of sciatic nerve. *Anat. Rec.,* 187:745.

183. Wessells, N. K., Spooner, B. S., Ash, J. F., Bradley, M. O., Luduena, M. A., Taylor, E. L., Wrenn, J. T., and Yamada, K. M. (1971): Microfilaments in cellular and developmental processes. *Science,* 171:135–143.

184. White, W. R., and Grafstein, B. (1973): Changes in goldfish retinal ganglion cells following intraocular injection of vincristine. *Abst. Soc. Neurosci,* 4th Ann. Meeting, 274.

185. Young, J. Z., and Medawar, P. B. (1940): Fibrin suture of peripheral nerves. Measurement of the rate of regeneration. *Lancet,* 2:126–128.

186. Zelena, J., Lubińska, L., and Gutmann, E. (1968): Accumulation of organelles at the ends of interrupted axons. *Z. Zellforsch.,* 91:200–219.

187. Zimmerman, E., Karsh, D., and Humbertson, A., Jr. (1971): Initiating factors in perineuronal cell hyperplasia associated with chromatolytic neurons. *Z. Zellforsch.,* 114:73–82.

Neuronal Plasticity, edited by
Carl W. Cotman.
Raven Press, New York © 1978.

Reaction of Central Catecholaminergic Neurons to Injury: Model Systems for Studying the Neurobiology of Central Regeneration and Sprouting

Donald J. Reis, Robert A. Ross, Gad Gilad and Tong Hyub Joh

*Laboratory of Neurobiology, Department of Neurology, Cornell University Medical College,
New York, New York 10021*

INTRODUCTION

The reaction to injury of the neurons of the central nervous system (CNS) which synthesize, store, and release the catecholamine neurotransmitters dopamine (DA) and norepinephrine (NE) have been examined since the discovery of these chemically specific systems in brain over a decade ago. At first, axonal lesions were only utilized as a tool for mapping the intracerebral distribution of these systems within the brain (2,3,19,59,69,71,92,103). Thus the projections of the catecholamine systems were delineated by observing histochemically or biochemically the disappearance of transmitter or biosynthetic enzymes in terminal regions following lesions of the axons or cell bodies. The distribution of cell bodies, on the other hand, was mapped by observing the enhancement of fluorescence in the perikaryon and proximal axons subsequent to axonal damage.

More recently, the central NE and DA systems have been increasingly utilized as models for studies of the general processes by which nerve cells respond to injury (30,84,86,87,91). The value of these systems, particularly the NE ones, as models for analysis of the reaction of intrinsic neurons of the CNS to injury are several.

First, the anatomy of these systems is reasonably well defined. The cell bodies are collected in relatively discrete nuclear areas, the trajectories of the axons are established, and their terminal areas have been mapped (36,57,78,103). Such information therefore makes it possible to place lesions at various sites along the axon and to selectively separate and examine the morphological and biochemical changes in the cell bodies, axon terminals, axonal pathways, uninjured collaterals, and even, in some instances, the dendrites.

Second, the transmitter produced by these neurons is known and can be visualized by histofluorescence or measured biochemically (16,72). Metabolites are also identifiable. The ease of measurement of transmitter and/or metabolites has permitted not only the examination of change in the steady state level of the neurotransmitters but also analysis of dynamic changes in transmitter synthesis and release in various parts of the neuron as a consequence of injury (44,107).

Third, the enzymes which specifically subserve the biosynthesis of the catecholamine neurotransmitters are well characterized, and can be assayed in tissue homogenates. These enzymes include the specific enzymes tyrosine hydroxylase (TH), which catalyzes the rate-limiting step in the biosynthesis of DA and NE, and dopamine-β-hydroxylase (DBH), the enzyme catalyzing the conversion of DA to NE in the NE neurons, and the relatively nonspecific enzyme 1-amino acid decarboxylase (DDC) (Fig. 1). Of great importance is the fact that

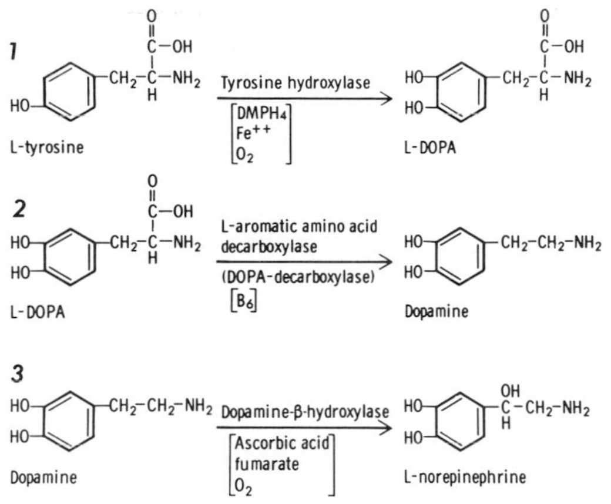

FIG. 1 Biosynthetic pathway of catecholamines.

these enzymes have been purified and antibodies produced to them (29,37,41). Antibodies have permitted the use of immunochemical techniques for determination of the amounts of enzyme protein (41,58,87,91), the relative rates of their synthesis in CNS neurons (43), and their immunocytochemical localization, both by light and electron microscopy (76,77). Since the enzymes TH and DBH represent identifiable proteins which, in brain, are exclusively neuronal and selectively contained in a clearly defined population (27,36,75), they can serve as powerful biochemical probes in the examination of the effects of axonal injury on neuronal function.

A fourth advantage is that the catecholamine neurons in CNS undergo both regenerative and collateral sprouting (9,10,45,66,78,79,82,100). They thereby represent a useful central counterpart to peripheral systems in which regenerative sprouting occurs, particularly with respect to relating the events at the damaged axon tip to those within the cell body.

Fifth, the central NE system has a biochemical counterpart in the sympathetic ganglion cell of the peripheral nervous system. It is thus possible to directly compare the effects of injury of a central neuronal system to that of a peripheral system of comparable biochemical constitution.

Finally, the importance of the central catecholamine systems in the expression of a number of behaviors (4,18,35,94), as substrates for the mediation of the action of a variety of psychotrophic drugs (12,52), and as a possible substrate for diseases such as Parkinsonism, schizophrenia, and depressive illnesses (38,-65,97,106) makes comprehension of their biology of relevance to psychiatry and medicine.

In this chapter we will review selective studies on the reaction of central catecholamine systems to injury, largely focusing on changes in the activities and amounts of the biosynthetic enzymes. As indicated above, these biosynthetic enzymes can be viewed not only as catalysts, but also as neuron-selective macro-molecules of brain. Moreover, the availability of antibodies to these enzymes has permitted a degree of analysis which has not been possible by examining enzyme activity alone.

REACTION OF CENTRAL NORADRENERGIC NEURONS TO INJURY IN ADULT ANIMALS

Noradrenergic Model System: The Nucleus Locus Ceruleus

The central NE system of rat has been extensively mapped by histofluorescence methods combined with biochemical and axonal transport techniques (78,92,-103). In general, the system consists of a group of nerve cell bodies distributed in relatively discrete nuclear groups designated A1 to A7 (19) which reside in the pons and medulla oblongata. The neuronal group singled out for the greatest scrutiny has been that of the nucleus locus ceruleus (A6 group) whose cell bodies are in a small, paired pontine nucleus. The utility of the locus ceruleus as an experimental model is that all of its neurons are noradrenergic and its axonal projections are widespread.

The nucleus locus ceruleus in rat contains approximately 1,400 nerve cells on each side (2,20,91). It sends highly collateralized axons through well-defined trajectories to innervate the upper brainstem (including hypothalamus), telencephalon, cerebellum, and probably portions of the lower brainstem and spinal cord (59,69,71,78,92). Most, but not all, of the innervation is ipsilateral. Indirect anatomical and biochemical evidence favors the view that branches from at least some of the neurons in the locus ceruleus innervate territories as widely separated as cerebellum, hippocampus, and spinal cord (69,71).

The ascending axons from neurons of the locus ceruleus form the so-called dorsal noradrenergic bundle (54,103). In the midbrain, this pathway joins with a more ventrally distributed bundle of NE fibers ascending from other brainstem nuclei. The projections from the locus ceruleus ascend through the median forebrain bundle sending collaterals into hypothalamus and proceed to form the major innervation of the forebrain. Because of its precisely defined location and biochemical homogeneity, the locus ceruleus has served as an ideal model system for studying the effects of axonal damage on its biochemically identified neuronal population.

In most studies of the response of these nerve cells to injury, damage to the NE neurons has been produced by electrolytic lesions placed stereotaxically at different sites in its trajectory, or by the administration, either stereotaxically or intraventricularly, of the selective neurotoxic agents 6-hydroxy-dopamine (6-OHDA) or 6-hydroxydopa (6-OH-DOPA) (20,86). An example of the experimental model is the one utilized by ourselves (86,91) and illustrated in Fig. 2. This figure demonstrates an idealized locus ceruleus neuron with axons ascending in the dorsal bundle, sending off collateral branches to hypothalamus, and inner-

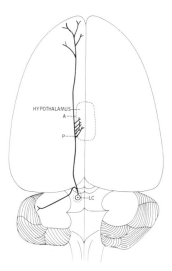

FIG. 2. Schematic horizontal view of rat brain portraying a representative neuron in the locus ceruleus (LC), its ascending projections through frontal cortex, and collateral branches to hypothalamus and cerebellum. lum. Lesions placed in the medial forebrain bundle posteriorly in the lateral hypothalamus (P) and will interrupt the axon before most hypothalamic collaterals leave the parent axon. A lesion placed anteriorly (A) will lie distal to emergence of collaterals. (From ref. 86.)

vating the frontal cortex. A collateral branch is illustrated arising from the main axon trunk to innervate the cerebellum. Lesions of the ascending axon are produced electrolytically at various sites along its trajectory, usually in the posterolateral hypothalamus in the median forebrain bundle and proximal to the hypothalamic collaterals. However, lesions can be placed further distally in the anterior hypothalamus, thereby preserving the hypothalamic collateral field. The possibility for flexibility in the placement of lesions with respect to proximity to the cell body provides a means for examining in central NE neurons the effects of the distance from cell body on the response of the NE neurons to injury.

Animals are killed at various days after placement of lesions. For biochemical analysis the brain is removed and dissected. In our own studies in degenerating terminals, the frontal cortex is removed for analysis of the *anterograde reaction;* for analysis of the *retrograde reaction* the locus ceruleus is removed by microdissection; for analysis of *changes in uninjured collateral* the cerebellum is isolated. For histology animals are killed by perfusion through the heart and regions of terminals, collaterals, or cell bodies appropriately sectioned and examined.

Anterograde Reaction of Central Noradrenergic Neurons

Lesions of the cell bodies, axons, or axon terminals of central NE neurons produced by electrolytic coagulation, mechanical transection of the axon, or by administration of 6-OHDA or 6-OH-DOPA elicits a characteristic pattern of biochemical and morphological changes in the degenerating axon and nerve terminal. Biochemically, in the terminal fields, there is a permanent reduction in the content of the neurotransmitter (25,67), in the capacity of the terminals to take up and store neurotransmitter via the high affinity uptake system (54,107), and in the catalytic activities of the biosynthetic enzymes TH, DBH, and DDC (85–87) (Fig. 3). The reduction of the activities of TH and DBH are almost complete and, as demonstrated immunochemically (Fig. 4) or immunocytochemically, is entirely due to loss of enzyme protein (87).

In contrast to the changes of TH and DBH, DDC activity is reduced only partially (87) (Fig. 3). This partial reduction is probably due to the fact that the enzyme is contained within other tissues in the terminal fields (e.g., serotonergic fibers and capillary endothelium) which themselves would not necessarily be damaged by the lesion. The biochemical changes are associated morphologically with evidence of degeneration of axon terminals presumed to be NE by the presence of dense core vesicles (82,83,87).

The reduction in the neurotransmitter and its biosynthetic enzymes during the anterograde reaction is undoubtedly a consequence of the separation of the axon from the perikaryon, the major source of newly synthesized macromolecules. Thus, the reduction in the amount of enzyme (and as a consequence the content of neurotransmitter) is due to both degradation of enzyme protein and an absence of replenishment.

The time course for the disappearance of TH, DBH, and NE in degenerating NE axons is remarkably slow, taking 14 days to reach a minimal value. This slow disappearance of the contents of the terminals stands in contrast to the much more rapid rate at which the same transmitter and its enzymes disappear in the peripheral sympathetic neuron (3,46,62,81,98) and in central DA systems (60,84), usually 24 to 48 hr. The prolonged time for the anterograde response in central NE terminals probably reflects an intrinsic property of the system; it is exactly the same in all terminal fields irrespective of whether the lesions

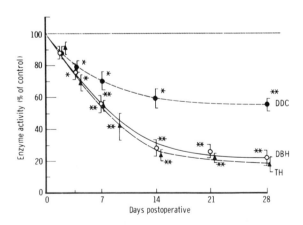

FIG. 3. Time course of changes in the activities of TH, DDC, and DBH in the ipsilateral frontal cortex following unilateral lesion of the posterolateral hypothalamus. Each point represents ± SEM of 6–20 animals and is expressed as percent of the mean of 6 unoperated controls. * $p < 0.01$; ** $p < 0.001$.

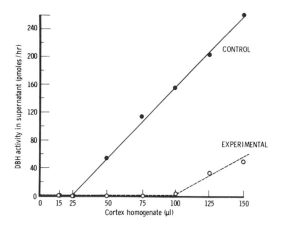

FIG. 4. Immunoprecipitation by a specific antibody to DBH of enzyme protein in homogenates of cerebral cortex from lesioned and control animals. In this experiment increasing amounts of a homogenate of frontal cortex (enzyme) ipsilateral to a 40-day-old hypothalamic lesion or from control animals were added to a constant amount of a specific antibody to DBH. The amount of enzyme in the lowest dilution of cortex is precipitated by available antibody and hence no enzyme activity is detectable in the supernatant. As more tissue homogenate is added, the antibody is saturated, and enzyme activity appears in the supernatant. The point at which enzyme activity first appears in the supernatant is called the equivalence point and represents the amount of enzyme (in microliters of homogenate) required to saturate the antibody. In this experiment it may be seen that the equivalence point for enzyme in the lesioned (experimental) cortex is shifted to the right of control. Four times as much tissue from the lesioned cortex is required to reach the equivalence point. Each curve was derived from pooled frontal cortex from 6–8 rats. Enzyme activity in samples measured individually from the lesioned animals was approximately 25% of control. Thus the reduction of enzyme activity in the cerebral cortex as a consequence of hypothalamic lesions is entirely attributable to a loss of specific enzyme protein and not to any increase in enzyme inhibitors.

destroy axon terminals, transect the axon in midpassage, or destroy the cell body (92).

The mechanism accounting for the slow time course of degeneration of central NE neurons and its biological significance remain obscure. Whether the difference in the rate of degeneration between the central NE systems and that of the peripheral sympathetic and central DA systems is due to a prolonged preservation of isolated NE terminals and their contents in astroglia (an interpretation we favor), differences of the molecular form of the enzymes (42), or even due to the prolonged preservation in the axon of some trophic factor is unknown.

Retrograde Response

Biochemical Changes

Damage of axons of NE neurons in the CNS results in a characteristic pattern of change in the biochemistry of the parent neurons in the locus ceruleus (86,-87,91) (Fig. 5). At present the most marked changes have been observed in

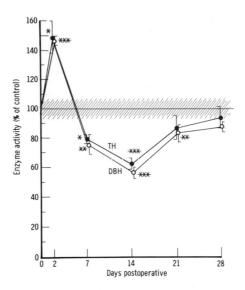

FIG. 5. Time course of changes in TH and DBH activity in the locus ceruleus at various days following axonal transection produced by electrolytic lesions of the medial forebrain bundle in the lateral hypothalamus of the rat. (Adapted from ref. 91.)

the activities and amounts of the specific biosynthetic enzymes TH and DBH. These changes occur in three distinct phases and will be described in some detail below.

Phase of Pile Up (Days 1–3)

The first response to lesions of ascending branches of central NE neurons in adult rats is a phase of "pile up." This consists of an increase in the amount of neurotransmitter (as defined by histofluorescence) which begins in the axonal stump proximal to the lesion and rapidly piles up to fill the cell body (19). Associated is a marked enhancement in the activities of TH and DBH, within the cell body, probably representing an increased accumulation of enzyme protein (86,91) (Fig. 5). The increase in fluorescence is seen within the first 24 to 48 hr, but a more careful timing of the enzyme changes indicates that it begins with a slightly longer latency: it is first seen approximately 24 hr after the lesion and reaches a maximum by 48 hr where it remains elevated for several days and then declines. This "pile up" phase of central NE neurons is comparable to that observed in peripheral sympathetic ganglia following postganglionic transection (19).

The magnitude of the augmentation in enzyme and transmitter in central NE neurons appears roughly proportional to the proximity of the lesion to the cell body: the more proximal the lesion, the greater the magnitude of the response and the more prolonged its duration. Thus following lesions of the

NE axon at distal sites in the anterior hypothalamus, little or no pile up is seen. Lesions of the posterolateral hypothalamus result in a spike of enzyme activity 48 to 72 hr later, whereas lesions of the dorsal bundle in the midbrain and close to the cell bodies result in an elevation of enzyme activity which could last a longer period (86) (Pickel, Joh, and Reis, *unpublished observations*).

At present, no studies have examined concurrently the changes of enzyme and transmitter in the locus ceruleus following a single lesion. However, it is of interest that lesions of the posterolateral hypothalamus have resulted in increased fluorescence in locus ceruleus neurons which appear to persist for over 1 week, and thereby into a time when enzyme activity has become reduced (see below). This finding suggests that after an initial increase of both enzyme and transmitter, a dissociation may occur, the transmitter persisting while enzyme diminishes. The persistence of transmitter in the face of reduction in the activity of biosynthetic enzymes could represent augmented storage, diminished release, and/or reduced degradation of the neurotransmitter in the affected cell body.

The simplest explanation of pile up is, as the name implies, mechanical. This interpretation would assume that under steady-state conditions the nerve cell body is producing sufficient enzyme to maintain relatively constant levels of neurotransmitter within the terminal fields. Following axonal transection, there is a loss of cytoplasm in which to disperse these macromolecules. Hence, they accumulate behind the lesion until the cell readjusts its program of enzyme biosynthesis to accommodate to the reduction in cytoplasmic volume. The increased concentration of enzyme/unit of cytoplasm during the pile up phase, of course, would result in an elevated quantity of the neurotransmitter. Hence, the elevated quantities of neurotransmitter which follow transection could be secondary to the enhanced accumulation of biosynthetic enzymes.

An alternative explanation of pile up is that lesions result in an alteration in the activity of the biosynthetic enzymes producing a catalytically more potent molecule, i.e., an activated one resulting thereby in greater quantities of neurotransmitter. Present evidence does not support this view.

Phase of Reduced Accumulation of Neurotransmitter Enzymes (Days 4–21)

The phase of pile up of neurotransmitter-synthesizing enzymes in locus ceruleus cells after hypothalamic lesions is followed by a relatively rapid decline in the activity of TH and DBH in the cell bodies (91). The time course of the decline is much more rapid than the loss of enzymes in the anterograde reaction. The time course and magnitude of these retrograde changes in TH and DBH activities are remarkably similar (Fig. 5) and not associated with changes in the activities of DDC or monoamine oxidase (MAO) (Fig. 6). The activities of TH fall to about 60% of control from approximately days 7 to 14 (87).

Reduction in the activities of TH and DBH can be demonstrated by immunotitration to be entirely a consequence of reduced accumulation of enzyme protein

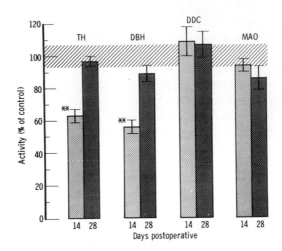

FIG. 6. Changes in the activities of TH, DBH, DDC, and MAO in the ipsilateral locus ceruleus at 14 *(light stipple)* and 28 days *(dark stipple)* following an electrolytic lesion of the hypothalamus. Activity is expressed as percent of mean activity of unlesioned controls ± SEM. *N*, 6–12. * * *p* < 0.001. (From ref. 86.)

(Fig. 7). The reduction in accumulation of these enzymes can be due to reduced synthesis, increased degradation or export, or a combination of these processes. By pulse labeling **DBH** in locus ceruleus neurons *in vivo* with ³H-amino acids perfused into the fourth ventricle and then by isolating DBH protein from the locus ceruleus by immunochemical techniques, it is possible to estimate changes in the relative rate of synthesis of the enzyme during the retrograde reaction. Such studies have demonstrated that the reduced accumulation of DBH, occurring 12 days after a lesion, can be attributed almost entirely to a relative reduction in the rate of synthesis of enzyme protein (31). Presumably a comparable mechanism accounts for the change in accumulation of TH.

The mechanism which triggers the reduction of synthesis of neurotransmitter synthesizing enzyme in the retrograde reaction is not known. One possibility would relate it to the preceding phase of pile up. It can be envisioned that as a result of pile up more biosynthetic enzymes are available in the cell body producing more NE. As a consequence there is an increase in end-product inhibition of the biosynthesis not only in the neurotransmitter but also of the relative rate of synthesis of enzyme protein. As neurotransmitter is gradually metabolized and lost, the negative feedback signal is diminished, enzyme synthesis resumes, and full activity is recovered.

Phase of Recovery

Two to three weeks following axonal lesions the activity of the biosynthetic enzymes resulting from the central lesions is returned to normal (Fig. 5). Recovery appears to be due to the recovery of the complement of enzymes in

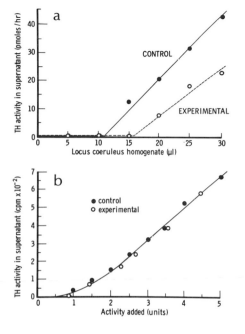

FIG. 7. Immunoprecipitation of TH in the locus ceruleus 14 days following hypothalamic lesions. Immunotitration in **A** as described in Fig. 4. In **B** the curve represents an experiment in which homogenates from lesioned and control animals are prepared so that equal volumes have equal activity. The overlapping curves indicate that differences in enzyme activity are due to differences in enzyme protein. Note that the reduced enzyme activity during the retrograde response is entirely attributable to reduction of enzyme protein. (Adapted from ref. 91.)

each of the injured nerve cells and not a consequence of death of some neurons with compensatory exaggeration of enzyme content in those that remain: careful morphometric analysis of the number of locus ceruleus neurons at various times following lesions has failed to demonstrate any loss as a consequence of retrograde cell death (Table 1).

Biochemical Changes in Remote Collaterals

The highly ramified structure of central NE neurons of the locus ceruleus has cast light on an interesting aspect of the reaction of nerve cells to injury,

TABLE 1. *Effect of hypothalamic lesion on nucleus ceruleus size and cell number*[a]

	N	Length (μm)	Cell number
Control	6	665 ± 48	1,449 ± 67
Experimental	6	712 ± 43[b]	1,409 ± 35[b]

[a]The nucleus locus ceruleus from both sides of the brainstem of 3 unoperated rats (control) and from the side ipsilateral to a unilateral lesion of the posterolateral hypothalamus placed 14 days earlier in 6 rats (experimental) were prepared for quantitative morphometry. Serial sections through each nucleus were examined and the total number of cells and the total length of the nucleus locus ceruleus determined. There were no significant changes in either the size or cell number of the locus ceruleus following the lesion. In control animals, the number of cells and the total length of the locus ceruleus were the same on the left and right sides of the brain. N, number of loci cerulei counted.
[b]Not significant.

namely that changes in the cell body initiated by damage to one axonal branch can initiate changes in remote collaterals. The earliest demonstration of this reaction in remote collaterals was shown biochemically; it was observed that transection of ascending branches of NE fibers produced by lesions in the postero-lateral hypothalamus not only results in a reversible reduction of DBH activity in the injured cell body of the locus ceruleus (86), but in addition, produces a depression of DBH activity in the ipsilateral cerebellum parallel in time course and intensity to the response within the locus ceruleus neurons themselves (Fig. 8).

The most reasonable interpretation of the phenomenon is that the initiation of reduced accumulation of enzyme in the cell bodies by axonal injury results in diminished availability of enzyme molecules for distribution and transport into the uninjured collaterals.

There also appears to be a morphological corollary of the response in uninjured collaterals. When cerebellar branches of central NE neurons are damaged, there appears to be transient sprouting in the remote, uninjured collaterals extending into the hippocampus (79).

Evidence that the Responses are Retrograde

In the foregoing discussion we have made the assumption that the chain of events initiated in central NE neurons of the locus ceruleus produced by axonal damage represents a retrograde reaction in the parent cell body and not a transynaptic effect due to interruption of fibers descending to synapse on these cells. We have discussed in detail elsewhere (86) the justification for our conclusion.

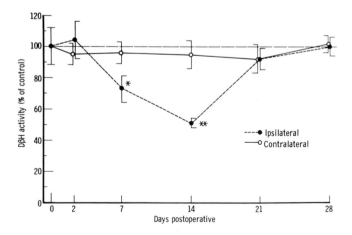

FIG. 8. Time course of changes in DBH activity in cerebellar hemisphere of rat following unilateral lesion of posterolateral hypothalamus. Enzyme activity is expressed as a per cent of mean activity in at least 6 matched, unoperated controls. Each point represents mean ± SEM of 6–12 animals. Ipsilateral cerebellum is represented by solid circles (●———●), contralateral cerebellum by open circles (○———○). * $p < .05$; ** $p < .001$. (From ref. 86.)

The arguments include the fact that the retrograde response differs from transynaptic neuronal reactions in central peripheral neurons by virtue of: (a) pile up; (b) a decrease in the activity of neurotransmitter enzyme measured in days; (c) a parallelism of the time course of enzyme changes in the central neuron to those seen in peripheral sympathetic ganglia and to the timing of the other associated concomitants of the retrograde reaction in peripheral systems; (d) the reversibility of the response; (e) the dependency of the response on the proximity of the lesion to the cell body; and (f) the paucity of evidence the lesions which we have made in the hypothalamus will interrupt projections to the locus ceruleus.

However, the observations that hypothalamic lesions will result in some reduction in the number of synapses onto locus ceruleus neurons (a finding in concordance with the well-established principle of synaptic retraction during retrograde cell changes) (104), raises the question as to whether or not some of the retrograde reaction may be indeed secondary to a reduction of input to these neurons. It is well established that the amount and activity of neurotransmitter-synthesizing enzymes within the NE neurons of the locus ceruleus may be regulated transynaptically. The administration of reserpine (88), or cholinergic agonists (53), may indeed modify the activity of the enzymes in the neuron. Conceivably, therefore, some of the changes of enzyme activity could be initiated, or modulated, by alterations of cell neuronal activity in turn resulting from synaptic retraction. However, our observation that even during the retrograde response NE neurons are capable of inducing an induction of TH response to reserpine (Ross and Reis, *unpublished observations*) suggests that some synaptic mechanisms are still in effect.

Morphological Concomitants of the Response

Cell Body

The classical morphological perikaryal response to axotomy comprises the chromatolytic reaction (17,33,55,56,104). By light microscopy, chromatolysis consists of swelling of the cell, enlargement of the nucleolus, eccentricity of the nucleus, and a dissolution of the Nissl substance (5,33,55,68). By electron microscopy there is a loss of the rough endoplasmic reticulum and retraction of synapses (105). These responses have been well characterized in peripheral NE neurons (14,23,40,63,64). The intensity of the chromatolytic response in peripheral neurons depends on a number of factors, including the specific neural system injured, the species of animal, the age of the animal, and the proximity of the lesion to the cell body (28,51,56). The younger the animal and the more proximal the lesion to the perikaryon, the more intense the response.

There is at present relatively little in the way of systematic data with respect to the morphological changes of central NE neurons to axonal injury. By fluorescence histochemistry some nucleolar swelling and eccentricity has been observed in the NE neurons of the A1 group (which innervate the spinal cord) following lesions of the cervical cord at C8 (19) and in neurons of the locus ceruleus in younger animals following cerebellar lesions (71).

Lesions of the posterior hypothalamus in adult rats which produce profound changes in enzyme activity in cell bodies do not result in any signs of chromatolysis within locus ceruleus neurons by light microscopy. By electron microscopy, however, some changes can be observed.

A detailed analysis (Field et al., *unpublished results*) of ultrastructural changes in locus ceruleus neurons at different days following lesions of the posterior hypothalamus is indicated in Table 2. During the phase of pile up, there is an increase in the number of dense core vesicles and autophagic vesicles, observations similar to those seen in peripheral sympathetic neurons during retrograde responses (23,64). There is also a small reduction in the stacked endoplasmic reticulum. The changes in the endoplasmic reticulum persisted until full biochemical recovery after day 21. However the changes in the autophagic vacuoles and dense core vesicles were reversed by day 14. Another finding of interest is evidence of the reduction in the number of synapses, an event which is characteristic of retrograde reaction in other neuronal systems (63,104,105).

It is evident therefore that the changes in the amount of neurotransmitter-synthesizing enzymes in central NE neurons in response to axonal damage can occur without classic signs of chromatolysis as demonstrated by light microscopy. However they are accompanied by subtle changes in the ultrastructure of the neurons similar qualitatively to, but substantially attenuated from, classical retrograde changes.

Terminals

Lesions of the axons of the locus ceruleus neurons within the hypothalamus result, as already described, in a reversible reduction in the activity and amount

TABLE 2. *Ultrastructural changes in locus ceruleus cell bodies during the retrograde reaction*

Structure	Control	Time following hypothalamic lesion			
		2–3d	5–12d	14–21d	41d
Stacked ER	0.91 ± 0.19	0.30 ± 0.07^a	0.38 ± 0.14^a	0.53 ± 0.07^a	0.75 ± 0.35
Dense cored vesicles	0.14 ± 0.10	0.64 ± 0.14^b	0.11 ± 0.08	0.17 ± 0.10	—
Autophagic vacuoles	0.09 ± 0.06	0.26 ± 0.05^b	0.29 ± 0.08^b	0.03 ± 0.02	0.06 ± 0.01
Multivesicular bodies	0.73 ± 0.29	0.86 ± 0.12	0.67 ± 0.15	0.59 ± 0.10	0.50 ± 0.12
Dense bodies	5.6 ± 0.8	6.4 ± 0.5	5.6 ± 0.9	5.8 ± 0.9	5.7 ± 0.9
Synapses	1.77 ± 0.27	1.06 ± 0.15^a	1.10 ± 0.18^a	1.49 ± 0.30	—

[a] $p < .01$.
[b] $p < .001$, Mann-Whitney U-test.
N, 18–74 cells/group.

of neurotransmitter-synthesizing enzymes in the remote collaterals within the cerebellum (86). In addition to the biochemical effects, morphological changes in remote collaterals may also occur in adult animals. Pickel et al. (79) have demonstrated that lesions of the cerebellar projections of locus ceruleus neurons produced by damage to the cerebellar peduncles will be followed by 30 days in an increase in the number of adrenergic terminals within the hippocampus. The increase in the number of terminals can be demonstrated by histofluorescence and by an increased density of radioactive particles seen within the hippocampus, following injection of the isotope into the locus ceruleus. Since projections which might traverse the cerebellar peduncles to innervate the hippocampus are unknown, the most reasonable interpretation is that the changes occur in the ascending uninjured collaterals of locus ceruleus neurons. The nature of the hyperinnervation of the hippocampus must remain at present a mystery. It is not known whether such terminals form synapses. Since many monoamine neurons have terminal interactions which do not necessarily involve the formation of structural synapses (21,74,75,102), it is conceivable that this innervation may act through field mechanisms.

The hyperinnervation and proliferation of axon terminals in the hippocampus following cerebellar lesions may be a counterpart to the extensive proliferation in the brainstem of young animals following destruction by 6-OHDA or 6-OH-DOPA of the terminal fields (44,47,70) (discussed below) and representing the persistence, in the adult, of a propensity highly developed in the neonate. Similar proliferative biochemical changes in remote collaterals of central NE neurons also may follow vascular lesions of the brain (89).

Relationship to Regenerative Sprouting

It has often been proposed that in the peripheral nervous system the cellular events of chromatolysis are intimately related to the development of regenerative sprouting from the lesioned axon (33,55,87). One of the arguments for this relationship is based on the temporal relationship between the appearance of sprouts, usually within 2 to 5 days, following a lesion and the onset of marked chromatolysis. It is now well established that the NE system, like other monoamine systems in the brain, can undergo regenerative sprouting from lesioned axonal tips. Such regeneration can be elicited by electrolytic lesions or by administration of the drug 6-OHDA (10,44,45). Fine regenerative sprouts can be seen by 5 to 15 days following the lesion. With mechanical or electrolytic damage to the axon, these sprouts, which are exuberant, appear to remain indefinitely. However, when produced by 6-OHDA, the sprouts appear to form, but after many weeks gradually regress, a condition likened to abortive sprouting and suggesting the possibility that the neurotoxin may have an additional effect on the nerve cell body.

The close association of the production of new axoplasm at a time (from 5–15 days) when there is reduced biosynthesis and accumulation of neurotransmitter-synthesizing enzymes has suggested that one aspect of the retrograde reaction may be a shifting of priorities of protein biosynthesis away from the production of macromolecules required for neurotransmission in favor of those required for reconstitution of cellular membrane (14,33,87,91).

Role of Nerve Growth Factor

Nerve growth factor (NGF), a protein which stimulates growth and differentiation of sympathetic neurons in the periphery, has only recently been analyzed with respect to its potential role in the regeneration of central neurons following nerve injury. Imaginative studies by Bjerre, Bjorklund and Stenevi (7,8) have examined and attempted to manipulate the growth of NE fibers into iris explants in the brain by the administration of NGF or an antibody to it (7,8). They demonstrated that when NGF was injected into the lateral ventricle at the time of iris implantation and examined some days later, there was an augmentation of the new growth of NE fibers into the implanted iris and it was most effective when given at the time of transplantation. This study, while suggesting a pharmacological action of NGF, did not itself address the question as to whether NGF normally plays a role. That it might was suggested by the converse experiment in which antiserum to NGF was administered either into the brain or by pre-incubation of the iris prior to implantation. Such treatment substantially inhibited the regeneration of fibers into the tissue. The authors concluded that the action of NGF was directed towards the A6 locus ceruleus system, since it did not appear to have comparable effects on fibers projecting through the ventral bundle and arising from other NE groups in the lower brainstem. The role of NGF in promoting recovery of function after lesions of central systems is controversial. Readers are referred to the excellent review by Freed for further discussion of the role of NGF in CNS (26).

Reaction in Young Animals

It has long been known that the retrograde response in young animals differs from that of adults. Not only is the retrograde reaction more intense, but it is more likely to result in retrograde cell death (11,48–50,90). In recent years examination of the biochemical and morphological effects of lesions of central NE neurons in neonatal animals has demonstrated that they exhibit responses differing substantially from those of the adult. The most extensive studies have been those of Jonsson and Sachs (44,95,96) in which damage to terminals of central NE neurons was produced by the administration of 6-OHDA to neonatal rats. In these animals the damage is restricted primarily to the NE terminals innervating forebrain and spinal cord, whereas the cell bodies themselves are undamaged. Such injury produces (as do surgical lesions in the developing animal) a permanent loss of NE fibers in the forebrain (25,61,71). However, following such lesions there is the relatively rapid increase in the amount of NE, and in the activities of TH and DBH in the brainstem, associated with a marked enhancement of the number of fluorescent NE fibers in this region. The source of this abundant overgrowth appears to arise from locus ceruleus neurons (39,-47,71,73,99,101). The exaggerated sprouting in this model is age-dependent; it is not seen in adults following administration of 6-OHDA systemically or into the brain itself (71,96).

The capacity for NE neurons to hyperinnervate the brainstem is reminiscent of the effects of NGF on peripheral sympathetic neurons. This overabundance in the regenerative capacity of these neurons has been interpreted as being similar to the pruning effect described by Devor and Schneider (22) in other neuronal systems in the brain and may represent a principle that neurons are programmed to express a terminal field of defined proportions and, that if one branch of a neuron is not permitted to develop as a consequence of a lesion there is, during the phase of development, compensatory overgrowth from the other.

REACTION OF DOPAMINERGIC NEURONS TO INJURY

The system of neurons in the CNS which synthesize, store, and release the neurotransmitter DA are of two principal types. The first consists of long, ascending systems with neurons and cell bodies and is designated as the A8 to A10 group (located within the midbrain) (19,57,103). Their axons project in specific trajectories to their terminal field. These systems consist of the nigrostriatal, mesolimbic, and mesocortical systems. It is these ascending systems to which the greatest attention has been directed over the past decade, particularly in view of their presumed importance in mediating a variety of motivated and motor behaviors, their role as substrates for the action of a number of psychoactive drugs, and their postulated role in diseases of brain, including Parkinsonism and schizophrenia (38,65). The existence of other long DA systems, including a descending one, has been proposed on the basis of the presence of DA within the spinal cord (6). The second major type of DA neurons are those of short trajectory, located in hypothalamus and a few other sites such as olfactory bulb and retina (24,34).

Studies on the reaction of central DA neurons to injury have primarily utilized the nigrostriatal or the mesolimbic system. The strategy of such studies is comparable to that used in analyzing the reaction of NE neurons to injury. The model for the system which we have used for our studies is demonstrated in Fig. 9. Lesions can be placed close to the cell bodies of nigrostriatal (A9) or mesolimbic (A10) neurons or in their terminal fields in striatum (caudate) or olfactory tubercle (OT). At various days after the lesion, animals are killed and brains dissected for biochemical analysis or prepared for histological examination. The reaction of central DA neurons to injury, in broad outline, are, with few exceptions, comparable to those of their central NE counterparts.

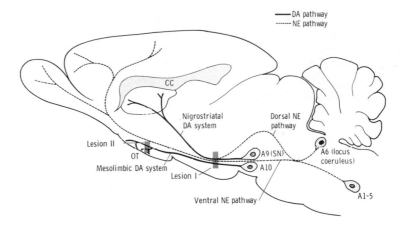

FIG. 9. A schematic parasagital view of the rat brain illustrating the experimental model. The projections of the mesolimbic and nigrostriatal dopaminergic (DA) systems are illustrated as well as the principal ascending noradrenergic (NE) systems. Lesion I interrupts DA axons close to their midbrain cell bodies and also the ascending NE pathways in the posterior lateral hypothalamus. Lesion II within the olfactory tubercle (OT) injuries mesolimbic axons distal from their A10 cell bodies. (From ref. 30.)

Anterograde Reaction

Lesions of the cell bodies, axons, or terminals of central DA neurons produced by electrolytic coagulation, mechanical damage, or 6-OHDA result in biochemical and morphological changes in degenerating axons qualitatively similar to those of the NE system (1,32,37,60,103). Immediately following the lesions of the DA axons, either of the nigrostriatal or mesolimbic systems, there is a brief surge of TH activity, possibly as a consequence of release of this enzyme from presynaptic inhibition (13,93). Thereafter, there is a rapid decline of enzyme activity of both TH and DDC (60,84). The nadir in TH activity is reached by 2 to 3 days after the lesion and remains permanently depressed (Fig. 10). The rate of decline of TH and DDC is comparable in central DA neurons to that of peripheral sympathetic axons and, as indicated above, differs substantially

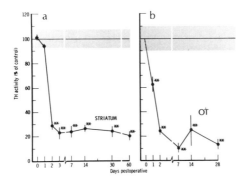

FIG. 10. Time course of the changes in TH activity in the striatum **A** and olfactory tubercle **B** following electrolytic lesions of the ipsilateral medial forebrain bundle. Note the irreversible reduction in enzyme activity. Enzyme activity is expressed as the percent of unoperated controls. Each point represents the mean ± SEM of 5–7 animals. **$p < 0.001$.

from the much slower rate of degeneration in the central NE system (see Fig. 3). The loss of TH activity during the anterograde reaction can be demonstrated by immunocytochemistry or immunochemical titration to be due to a loss of enzyme protein (Figs. 11, 12). Morphologically, the biochemical changes are accompanied by evidence of rapid disappearance within the striatum of axons containing dense core vesicles (37,103).

Retrograde Reaction

The retrograde reaction on central DA neurons differs in one important respect from those of the central NE system: the nature of the response is entirely dependent on the proximity of the lesion to the cell body (see below).

Pile Up

As with central NE neurons, lesions of the axons of central DA neurons of the nigrostriatal or mesolimbic system, in hypothalamus, and hence close to the cell bodies, result in an initial marked elevation of TH activity (Fig. 13) and DA fluorescence within the parent cell bodies within 24 to 48 hours following the lesion (2,84,103). Distal lesions, placed in terminal fields, do not result in pile up biochemically (Fig. 13), indicating therefore that the magnitude of the pile up is directly related to the proximity of the lesion to the cell body. The augmented enzyme activity is a consequence of increased amounts of enzyme protein, and this alone could account for the increased accumulation of the neurotransmitter in the cell body (84).

Phase of Reduced Enzyme Accumulation

Following the initial period of pile up produced by hypothalamic lesions, there is a rapid fall in the activity and amount of TH in the area of the substantia

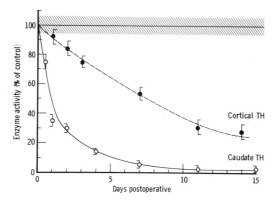

FIG. 11. Time course of fall in TH activity in ipsilateral caudate nucleus and frontal cortex following unilateral lesion of medial forebrain bundle in posterolateral hypothalamus.

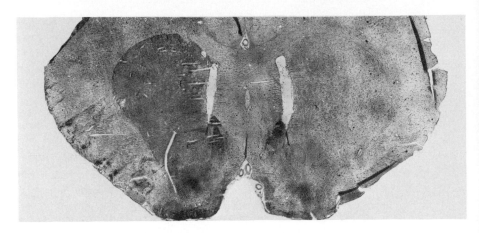

FIG. 12. Cross section of rat midbrain 26 days after unilateral *(left)* lesion of the medial forebrain stained by the PAP method for TH. Note the loss of specific staining in the striatum, nucleus accumbens, and olfactory tubercle on the lesioned side (at *right*). ×7.

nigra or of the A10 neurons innervating the olfactory tubercle (60,84). Enzyme activity reaches minimal values of about 40% of control approximately 5 days following the lesion. The reduction of enzyme activity can be demonstrated by immunocytochemistry or immunochemical titration to be due to a reduced accumulation of enzyme proteins and thus is comparable to the response in central NE neurons (30,84).

The outcome of this period of reduced enzyme accumulation is highly dependent upon the proximity of the lesion to the parent cell body. Lesions reasonably close to the neuronal cell body, such as those placed in the lateral hypothalamus, result in a failure of enzyme activity to recover (Fig. 13). This is a consequence of retrograde cell death which such lesions produce in the DA system (2,80,84).

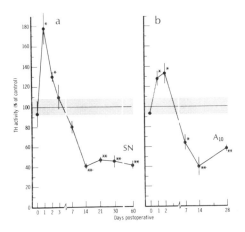

FIG. 13. Time course of changes in TH activity in the substantia nigra (SN) **A** and A10 dopamine nucleus **B** ipsilateral to a unilateral electrolytic lesion of the medial forebrain bundle near parent cell body. Note the irreversible changes in TH activity. $*p < .01$; $**p < .001$.

Phase of Recovery

The recovery of enzyme activity in neurons of the DA system from axonal lesions only occurs if the lesions placed in the terminal fields damage only a portion thereof. Thus, lesions of moderate size placed in the striatum or in the olfactory tubercle result after approximately days 12 to 14 in a recovery of enzyme activity to control levels (Fig. 14). Examination of the substantia nigra or the midbrain tegmentum does not demonstrate any loss of TH-containing neurons, and hence recovery is probably due to the reaccumulation of enzyme in those cells reacting to injury.

Comparison of the Perikaryal Response to Axotomy with that Occurring During Collateral Sprouting in DA Neurons

It is now well established that catecholamine neurons of both DA and NE systems have the capacity to undergo collateral sprouting (66). The stimulus appears to be degeneration of fibers which are not catecholaminergic within an area containing catecholamine terminals. As the noncatecholamine fibers disappear, the remaining catecholamine fibers sprout in an apparent effort to reoccupy abandoned synaptic sites and thereby enlarge their terminal fields. The cellular events associated with collateral sprouting have not been characterized.

Gilad and Reis (30) studied the changes in TH activity initiated in the mesolimbic neurons of the A10 group innervating the olfactory tubercle. Sprouting was elicited by removal of the ipsilateral olfactory bulb whose mitral cells heavily innervate intrinsic neurons of the olfactory tubercle which, in turn, are innervated by DA neurons of the A10 group. Within 1 week following olfactory bulb ablation there was evidence of collateral sprouting of DA fibers in the tubercle: there was an increase in the selective uptake of ^{3}H-dopamine (^{3}H-DA), a gradual elevation of TH activity in the terminal field (Fig. 15), and an increase in the number of TH-containing terminals, as well as an alteration in their normal

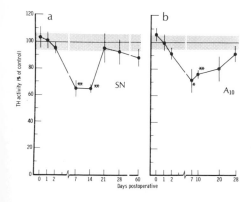

FIG. 14. Time course of changes in TH activity **A** in the substantia nigra (SN) ipsilateral to lesion of caudate nucleus, and **B** in the A10 dopamine cell group (A10) ipsilateral to a lesion in the olfactory tubercle. Note the reversible reduction in enzyme delivery. Enzyme activity is expressed as the percent of unoperated controls. Each point represents the mean ± SEM of 5–7 animals. $^*p < 0.01$; $^{**}p < 0.001$.

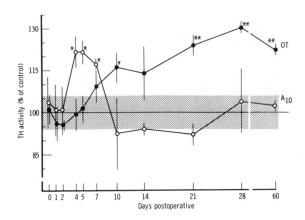

FIG. 15. Time course of changes in TH activity in cell bodies of A10 group and their terminals in the olfactory tubercle following unilateral olfactory bulbectomy. Enzyme activity is expressed as the percent of unoperated control animals. Each point represents the mean ± SEM of 6–12 animals. $*p < 0.05$; $**p < 0.005$.

pattern of distribution demonstrated by immunocytochemistry. The earliest change in the terminal field, an increase of ^{3}H-DA uptake, was one week following the lesion, followed very soon thereafter by the gradual and slow accumulation of TH.

The first event associated with removal of the olfactory bulb occurred in the A10 cell bodies in the midbrain tegmentum (Fig. 15): there was a surge of TH activity between days 3 to 7. Although the increase of enzyme activity in the A10 neurons was not sufficient in magnitude (about 30%) to permit analysis by immunotitration, an increase in immunocytochemical staining ipsilaterally suggested the presence of more enzyme protein in reacting neurons. The changes in TH in the cell body during sprouting differed in direction and timing from that seen during regenerative sprouting initiated by axonal damage (84).

SUMMARY OF SOME GENERAL NEUROLOGIC IMPLICATIONS OF STUDIES OF THE REACTION OF CENTRAL CATECHOLAMINE NEURONS TO AXONAL INJURY

The reactions of central catecholamine neurons to axonal injury reviewed in this essay not only have enlarged knowledge of the specific behaviors of NE and DA systems, but have provided new facts and provocative hypotheses with respect to the reaction of *intrinsic* neurons of the CNS to injury. Some of these hypotheses appear to have general implications with respect to the cellular dynamics of neurons during degeneration, regeneration, and development. The major hypotheses may be summarized as follows.

Reversible Reduction of the Biosynthesis of Neurotransmitter-Synthesizing Enzymes May Be a Specific Biochemical Event Associated with the Retrograde Reaction

Axonal lesions of central NE or DA neurons can lead to a reversible decrease in the activities and amounts of TH and/or DBH in the reactive cell body, most probably as a consequence of reduced biosynthesis of enzyme protein. The observation suggests that a reduction of neurotransmitter-synthesizing enzymes may be a general biochemical feature in other neuronal systems of the retrograde reaction. Supportive evidence for this generality are the observations that reduction in the activity of TH and DBH accompanies the retrograde reaction in peripheral sympathetic neurons, that amounts of choline acetyltransferase are reversibly reduced in lesions of peripheral motor neurons (which do not result in cell death) (Wooten, Park, Joh, Reis, *in preparation*), and that destruction of the terminals of central serotonergic neurons by specific neurotoxins can also result in a reversible reduction in the activity of tryptophan hydroxylase in regions containing parent cell bodies.

Biochemical Changes of the Retrograde Reaction May Occur Without Evident Morphological Changes of Chromatolysis

The absence of any evidence by light microscopy of a retrograde reaction in intrinsic neurons of the CNS, particularly small ones, is well known (55,56). Our observation that axonal lesions of NE neurons can lead to a reversible reduction in the amount of TH and DBH in locus ceruleus neurons without chromatolysis demonstrates that the biochemical and morphological changes can be dissociated. Whereas these may represent only matters of the intensity of the reaction (the biochemical events being a more sensitive indicator), they underscore the fact that the absence of chromatolysis does not mean the absence of biochemical components of the axon reaction.

Retrograde Reaction of Intrinsic Neurons of the CNS May Be Reversible

It has long been proposed (5,15,55) that intrinsic neurons of the CNS do not have the capacity to undergo retrograde responses which are reversible. It was generally believed they either underwent retrograde cell death or did not respond at all. The failure of the response was considered as possibly due to either the failure of the neuron to adequately regenerate or that in some manner intrinsic neurons of the CNS are not genetically programmed to respond in a comparable manner to their peripheral counterparts. The hypothesis with respect to an absence of reversible retrograde changes in intrinsic neurons of the CNS was entirely based on the absence of evidence of morphological changes. However the discovery that, first, a biochemical feature of the response, the reduced accumulation of neurotransmitter-synthesizing enzymes, can occur in the intrinsic NE and DA systems of brain in the absence of chromatolysis and second, can be reversible, demonstrates that the classic view is incorrect. Rather, intrinsic neurons of the CNS in fact do possess the capacity to undergo retrograde changes, and these may be reversible.

Changes in Protein Biosynthesis in the Retrograde Reaction May Be Selective

It is generally believed that during the retrograde reaction there is an increase in net protein and RNA biosynthesis (55). The evidence, entirely accrued from studies on peripheral neurons, has demonstrated an increase in nuclear RNA synthesis, nucleolar RNA content, rate of passage of newly synthesized RNA from nucleus to cytoplasm, an increase in cytoplasmic RNA content, and an increase in cytoplasmic protein content and synthesis (as determined by the incorporation of labeled amino acid into TCA-precipitable proteins or autoradiography) (55,105). These findings have suggested therefore that the retrograde reaction was primarily an anabolic event related more to the attempts of the neuron to regenerate by sprouting than to degeneration.

That the quantity of some proteins may in fact be reduced during the retrograde reaction, however, was suggested by observations that the activity of several enzymes in reactive cell bodies were depressed. However, our finding of a decrease in the synthesis of DBH in central NE neurons during the retrograde reaction, resulting in a reduction in the activity and amount of the enzyme, provides the first direct evidence of selective reordering of protein biosynthesis in neurons undergoing retrograde cell changes. The pattern of biochemical modifications suggests that the response would be characterized by an increase of proteins required for reestablishment of axonal membrane at the expense of those required for the function of the cell in neurotransmission.

Changes in the Cell Body Initiated by Damage to One Axonal Branch May Be Reflected in Uninjured Collaterals

We have demonstrated that hypothalamic lesions damaging ascending branches of a central locus ceruleus neuron initiates biochemical changes not only in the parent cell body, but in uninjured collaterals in cerebellum as well (86). This observation indicates that a whole field of innervation of a neuron is "informed" of damage to a remote collateral; thus, the cerebellum knows, through a process of intraneuronal communication, that the hypothalamus is damaged. The biological significance of such widespread impairment of neuronal functions is unknown. It could relate to a reduction in the efficacy of the neuron in chemical neurotransmission. Indeed, the widespread reduction in NE neurons following stroke lesions experimentally produced in rats (89) raises the possibility that in pathological states some of the widespread impairment of brain function (diaschesis) may be a consequence of loss of generalized reactivity of the neuron. More intriguing, however, is the possibility that the biochemical changes in remote terminals might be of importance in the recovery of physiological function following brain damage, i.e., may participate in the transfer of recovery of function from one brain area to another, leading thereby to functional compensation (86).

Neurotransmitter-Synthesizing Enzymes May Be Regulated by Axonal Integrity

One ancillary finding of our studies is the demonstration that the enzymes responsible for catecholamine neurotransmitter biosynthesis, TH and DBH, are regulated by the integrity of neuronal surface. The surface regulation is an additional mode of long-term regulation of the enzymes. In part, the regulation may relate to cell surface volume, since reduction of the field by axotomy leads to a reduced accumulation of enzyme protein, whereas an enlargement of the field during collateral sprouting will result in a transient elevation of enzyme.

ACKNOWLEDGMENTS

Research reported in this review has been supported by grants from the NIH, NIMH, NASA, and the Sloan Foundation.

REFERENCES

1. Anden, N. -E., Bedard, P., Fuxe, K., and Ungerstedt, U. (1972): Early and selective increase in brain dopamine levels after axotomy. *Experientia,* 28:300–301.
2. Anden, N. -E., Dahlstrom, A., Fuxe, K., Larsson, K., Olson, L., and Ungerstedt, U. (1966): Ascending monoamine neurons to the telencephalon and diencephalon. *Acta Physiol. Scand.,* 67:313–326.
3. Anden, N. -E., Magnusson, T., and Rosengren, E. (1965): Occurrence of dihydroxyphanylalanine decarboxylase in nerves of the spinal cord and sympathetically innervated organs. *Acta Physiol. Scand.,* 64:127–135.
4. Arbuthnott, G. W., Crow, T. J., and Spear, P. J. (1970): Functional role of an aminergic nucleus (locus coeruleus). *J. Physiol. (Lond.),* 211:28P–29P.
5. Barron, K. D., Doolin, P. F., and Oldershaw, J. B. (1967): Ultrastructural observation on retrograde atrophy of lateral geniculate body. I. Neuronal alteration. *J. Neuropath. Exp. Neurol.,* 26:300.
6. Bertler, A., and Rosengren, E. (1959): Occurrence and distribution of dopamine in brain and other tissues. *Experientia,* 15:10–11.
7. Bjerre, B., Björklund, A., and Stenevi, U. (1973): Stimulation of growth of new axonal sprouts from lesioned monoamine neurones in adult rat brain by nerve growth factor. *Brain Res.,* 60:161–176.
8. Bjerre, B., Björklund, A., and Stenevi, U. (1974): Inhibition of regenerative growth of central noradrenergic neurons by intracerebrally administered anti-NGF serum. *Brain Res.,* 74:1–18.
9. Björklund, A., Katzman, R., Stenevi, U., and West, K. (1971): Development and growth of axonal sprouts from noradrenalin and 5-hydroxytryptamine neurons in rat spinal cord. *Brain Res.,* 31:21–33.
10. Björklund, A., and Stenevi, U. (1971): Growth of central catecholamine neurons into smooth muscle grafts in the rat mesencephalon. *Brain Res.,* 31:1–20.

11. Brodal, A. (1940): Modification of Gudden method for study of cerebral localization. *Arch. Neurol. Psychiatr. (Chicago),* 43:46–58.
12. Carlsson, A. (1970): Amphetamine and brain catecholamines. In: *Amphetamines and Related Compounds,* edited by E. Costa and S. Garattini, pp. 289–300. Raven Press, New York.
13. Carlsson, A., Kehr, W., and Lindquist, M. (1974): Short term control of tyrosine hydroxylase. In: *Neuropsychopharmacology of Monoamines and Their Regulatory Enzymes, Adv. Biochem. Psychopharmacol., Vol. 12,* edited by E. Usdin, pp. 135–142.
14. Cheah, T. B., and Geffen, L. B. (1973): Effects of axonal injury on norepinephrine, tyrosine hydroxylase and monoamine oxidase levels in sympathetic ganglia. *J. Neurobiol.,* 4:443–452.
15. Cole, M. (1968): Retrograde degeneration of axon and soma in the nervous system. In: *Structure and Function of Nervous Tissue, Vol. 1,* edited by G. Bourne, pp. 269–298. Academic Press, London.
16. Coyle, J. T., and Henry, D. (1973): Catecholamines in fetal and newborn rat brain. *J. Neurochem.,* 21:61–67.
17. Cragg, B. G. (1970): What is the signal for chromatolysis? *Brain Res.,* 23:1–21.
18. Crow, T. J., Spear, P. J., and Arbuthnott, G. W. (1972): Intracranial self-stimulation with electrodes in the region of the locus coeruleus. *Brain Res.,* 36:275–287.
19. Dahlstrom, A., and Fuxe, K. (1964): Evidence for the existence of monoamine containing neurons in the central nervous system. I. Demonstration of monoamines in the cell bodies of brainstem neurons. *Acta Physiol. Scand.,* 62 (Suppl. 232): 1–55.
20. Descarries, L., and Saucier, G. (1972): Disappearance of the locus coeruleus in the rat after intra-ventricular 6-hydroxydopamine. *Brain Res.,* 37:310–316.
21. Descarries, L., Beaudet, A., and Watkins, K. C. (1975): Serotonin nerve terminals in adult rat neocortex. *Brain Res.,* 100:563–588.
22. Devor, M., and Schneider, G. E. (1975): Neuroanatomical plasticity: The principle of conservation of total axonal arborization. In: *Aspects of Neural Plasticity,* edited by F. Vital-Durand and M. Jeannerod, pp. 191–201. INSERM, Paris.
23. Dixon, J. S. (1970): Some fine structural changes in sympathetic neurons following axon section. *Acta Anat.,* 76:473–487.
24. Ehinger, B. (1977): Synaptic connections of dopaminergic retinal neurons. In: *Nonstriatal Dopaminergic Neurons, Advances in Biochemical Psychopharmacology, Vol. 16,* edited by E. Costa and G. L. Gessa, pp. 299–306. Raven Press, New York.
25. Erinoff, L., and Heller, A. (1973): Failure of catecholamine development following unilateral diencephalic lesions in the neonatal rat. *Brain Res.,* 58:489–493.
26. Freed, W. J. (1976): The role of nerve-growth factor (NGF) in the central nervous system. *Brain Res. Bull.,* 1:393–412.
27. Fuxe, K., Goldstein, M., Hokfelt, T., and Joh, T. H. (1971): Cellular localization of dopamine-β-hydroxylase and phenylethanolamine-N-methyl transferase as revealed by immunohistochemistry. *Prog. Brain Res.,* 34:127–138.
28. Geist, F. D. (1933): Chromatolysis of efferent neurons. *Arch. Neurol.,* 29:88–103.
29. Gibbs, J. W., Spector, S., and Udenfriend, S. (1967): Production of antibodies to dopamine-β-hydroxylase of bovine adrenal medulla. *Molec. Pharmacol.,* 3:473–478.
30. Gilad, G. M., and Reis, D. J. (1978): Reversible reduction of tyrosine hydroxylase enzyme protein during the retrograde reaction in mesolimbic dopaminergic neurons. *Brain Res.,* 1978 *(in press).*
31. Gilad, G. M., Joh, T. H., Pickel, V. M., and Reis, D. J. (1976): Biochemical and immunocytochemical evidences for collateral sprouting in mesolimbic dopaminergic neurons in rat brain. *Neurosci. Abst.,* 2:813.
32. Goldstein, M., Anagnoste, B., Owen, W. S., and Battista, A. F. (1966): The effects of ventromedial tegmental lesions on the biosynthesis of catecholamines in the striatum. *Life Sci.,* 5:2171–2176.
33. Grafstein, B. (1975): The nerve cell body response to axotomy. *Exp. Neurol.,* 48:32–51.
34. Halasz, N., Hokfelt, T., Ljungdahl, A., Johansson, O., and Goldstein, M. (1977): Dopamine neurons in the olfactory bulb. In: *Nonstriatal Dopaminergic Neurons, Advances in Biochemical Psychopharmacology, Vol. 16,* edited by E. Costa and G. L. Gessa, pp. 169–178. Raven Press, New York.
35. Hall, R. D., Bloom, F. E., and Olds, J. (1972): Neuronal and neurochemical substrates of reinforcement. *Neurosci. Res. Prog. Bull.,* 15:136–279.

36. Hartman, B. K. (1973): Immunofluorescence of dopamine-β-hydroxylase. Application of the peripheral and central noradrenergic nervous system. J. Histochem. Cytochem., 21:312–332.
37. Hokfelt, T., and Ungerstedt, U. (1973): Specificity of 6-hydroxydopamine induced degeneration of central central monoamine neurons: An electron and fluorescence microscopic study with special references to intracerebral injection on the nigro-striatal dopamine system. Brain Res., 60:269–297
38. Hornykiewicz, O. (1966): Metabolism of brain dopamine in human Parkinsonism: Neurochemical and clinical aspects. In: Biochemistry and Pharmacology of the Basal Ganglia, edited by E. Costa, L. Cote, and M. D. Yahr, pp. 171–186. Raven Press, New York.
39. Jaim-Etcheverry, G., Teitelman, G., and Zieher, L. M. (1975): Choline acetyltransferase activity increases in the brain stem of rats treated at birth with 6-hydroxydopa. Brain Res., 100:699–804.
40. Jenson-Holm, J., and Juul, P. (1970): The effects of guanethidine, pre- and post-ganglionic nerve division on the rat superior cervical ganglion: Cholinesterases and catecholamines (histochemistry) and histology. Acta Pharmacol. Toxicol., 28:283–298.
41. Joh, T. H., Geghman, C., and Reis, D. J. (1973): Immunochemical demonstration of increased accumulation of tyrosine hydroxylase protein in sympathetic ganglia and adrenal medulla elicited by reserpine. Proc. Natl. Acad. Sci. USA, 70:2767–2771.
42. Joh, T. H., and Reis, D. J. (1975): Different forms of tyrosine hydroxylase in central dopaminergic and noradrenergic neurons, sympathetic ganglia and adrenal medulla. Brain Res., 85:146–151.
43. Joh, T. H., Ross, R. A., and Reis, D. J. (1976): Rate of biosynthesis of dopamine-β-hydroxylase in locus coeruleus of rat brain after reserpine. Fed. Proc., 35:485.
44. Jonsson, G., and Sachs, C. (1976): Regional changes in [³H]-noradrenaline uptake, catecholamines, and catecholamine synthetic and catabolic enzymes in rat brain following neonatal administration of 6-hydroxydopamine treatment. Med. Biol., 54:286–297.
45. Katzman, R., Björklund, A., Owman, C., Stenevi, U., and West, K. (1971): Evidence for regenerative axon sprouting of central catecholamine neurons in the rat mesencephalon following electrolytic lesions. Brain Res., 25:579–596.
46. Kopin, I. J., and Silberstein, S. D. (1972): Axons of sympathetic neurons: transport of enzyme in vivo and properties of axonal sprouts in vitro. Pharmacol. Rev., 24:245–254.
47. Kostrzewa, R. M., and Garey, R. E. (1977): Sprouting of noradrenergic terminals in rat cerebellum following neonatal treatment with 6-hydroxydopa. Brain Res., 124:1–7.
48. LaVelle, A. (1964): Critical periods of neuronal maturation. Prog. Brain Res., 9:93–96.
49. LaVelle, A., and LaVelle, F. W. (1958): Neuronal swelling and chromatolysis as influenced by the state of cell development. Am. J. Anat., 102:219–241.
50. LaVelle, A., and LaVelle, F. W. (1959): Neuronal reaction to injury during development: severance of the facial nerve in utero. Exp. Neurol., 1:82–95.
51. LaVelle, A., and Sechrist, J. W. (1970): Immature and mature reaction patterns of neurons after axon section. Anat. Rec., 166:355.
52. Lewander, T. (1974): Effect of chronic treatment with central stimulants on brain monoamines and some behavioral and physiological functions in rats, guinea pigs, and rabbits. In: Neuropharmacology of Monoamines and Their Regulatory Enzymes, edited by E. Usdin, pp. 221–240. Raven Press, New York.
53. Lewander, T., Joh, T. H., and Reis, D. J. (1977): Tyrosine hydroxylase: Delayed activation in central noradrenergic neurons and induction in adrenal medulla elicited by stimulation of central cholinergic receptors. J. Pharmacol. Exp. Ther., 200:523–534.
54. Lidbrink, P. (1974): Noradrenaline nerve terminals in the rat cerebral cortex following lesion of the dorsal noradrenaline bundle: A study on the time course of their disappearance. In: Dynamics of Degeneration and Growth in Neurons. Pergamon Press, New York, pp. 141–149.
55. Lieberman, A. R. (1971): The axon reaction: a review of the principal features of perikaryal response to axon injury. Int. Rev. Neurobiol., 14:49–124.
56. Lieberman, A. R. (1974): Some factors affecting retrograde neuronal responses to axonal lesions. In: Essays on the Nervous System, edited by R. Bellairs and E. G. Gray, pp. 71–105. Clarendon Press, Oxford.
57. Lindvall, O., and Björklund, A. (1974): The organization of the ascending catecholamine neuron systems in the rat brain as revealed by the glyoxylic acid fluorescence method. Acta Physiol. Scand., (Suppl 412):1–47.

58. Lloyd, T., and Kaufman, S. (1973): Production of antibodies to bovine adrenal tyrosine hydroxy-lase: cross-reactivity with other pterin-dependent hydroxylases. *Molec. Pharmacol.*, 9:438–444.
59. Loizou, L. A. (1969): Projections of the locus coeruleus in the albino rat. *Brain Res.*, 16:563–566.
60. McGeer, E. G., Fibiger, H. C., McGeer, P. L., and Brooke, S. (1973): Temporal changes in amine synthesizing enzymes of rat extrapyramidal structures after hemitransections of 6-hy-droxy-dopamine administration. *Brain Res.*, 52:289–300.
61. Maeda, T., Tohyama, M., and Shimizu, N. (1974): Modification of postnatal development of neocortex in rat brain with experimental deprivation of locus coeruleus. *Brain Res.*, 70:515–520.
62. Malmfors, T., and Sachs, C. (1965): Direct studies on the disappearance of the transmitter and the changes in the uptake-storage mechanisms of degenerating adrenergic nerves. *Acta Physiol. Scand.*, 64:211–223.
63. Matthews, M. R., and Nelson, V. (1973): Ultrastructural changes at the synapse associated with depression of synaptic transmission in rat superior cervical ganglion after injury of post-ganglionic axons. *J. Physiol.*, 234:368–378.
64. Matthews, M. R., and Raisman, G. (1972): A light and electron microscopic study of the cellular response to axonal injury in the superior cervical ganglion of the rat. *Proc. Roy. Soc. Lond. B.*, 181:43–79.
65. Matthysse, S. W. (1977): The role of dopamine in schizophrenia. In: *Neuroregulators and Psychiatric Disorders*, edited by E. Usdin, D. A. Hamburg, and J. D. Barchas, pp. 3–13. Oxford University Press, New York.
66. Moore, R. Y., Björklund, A., and Stenevi, U. (1971): Plastic changes in the adrenergic innerva-tion of the rat septal area in response to denervation. *Brain Res.*, 33:13–35.
67. Moore, R. Y., and Heller, A. (1967): Monoamine levels and neuronal degeneration in rat brain following lateral hypothalamic lesions. *J. Pharmacol. Exp. Ther.*, 156:12–22.
68. Nissl, F. (1892): Uber die Ver. anderungen der Ganglionzellen am Facialiskern des Kaninchens nach Ausreissung der Nerven. *All. Z. Psychiatr. Ihre Grenzg.*, 48:197–198.
69. Nygren, L. -G. and Olson, L. (1977): A new major projection from locus coeruleus: The main source of noradrenergic nerve terminals in the ventral and dorsal columns of the spinal cord. *Brain Res.*, 132:85–94.
70. Nygren, L. -G., Olson, G., and Seiger, A. (1971): Regeneration of monoamine containing axons in the developing and adult spinal cord of the rat following intraspinal 6-OH-dopamine injections of transections. *Histochemie*, 28:1–15.
71. Olson, L., and Fuxe, K. (1971): On the projections from the locus coeruleus noradrenalin neurons: the cerebellar innervation. *Brain Res.*, 28:165–171.
72. Palkovits, M., and Jacobowitz, D. M. (1974): Topographic atlas of catecholamine and acetylcho-linesterase-containing neurons in the rat brain. II. Hindbrain (mesencephalon, rhomben-cephalon). *J. Comp. Neurol.*, 157:29–42.
73. Pappas, B. A., and Sobrian, S. K. (1972): Neonatal sympathectomy by 6-hydroxydopamine in the rat: no effects on behavior but changes in endogenous brain noradrenaline. *Life Sci.*, 11:653–659.
74. Pickel, V. M., Joh, T. H., and Reis, D. J. (1977): A serotonergic innervation of noradrenergic neurons in nucleus locus coeruleus: Demonstration by immunocytochemical localization of the transmitter specific enzymes tyrosine and tryptophan hydroxylase. *Brain Res.*, 131:197–214.
75. Pickel, V. M., Joh, T. H., and Reis, D. J. (1976): Monoamine synthesizing enzymes in central dopaminergic, noradrenergic, and serotonergic neurons: Immunocytochemical localization by light and electron microscopy. *J. Histochem. Cytochem.*, 24:792–806.
76. Pickel, V. M., Joh, T. H., Field, P. M., Becker, C. G., and Reis, D. J. (1975): Cellular localization of tyrosine hydroxylase by immunohistochemistry. *J. Histochem. Cytochem.*, 23:1–12.
77. Pickel, V. M., Joh, T. H., and Reis, D. J. (1975): Ultrastructural localization of tyrosine hydroxylase in noradrenergic neurons of brain. *Proc. Natl. Acad. Sci. USA*, 72:659–663.
78. Pickel, V. M., Segal, M., and Bloom F. E. (1974): A radioautographic study of the efferent pathways of the nucleus locus coeruleus. *J. Comp. Neurol.*, 155:15–42.
79. Pickel, V. M., Segal, M., and Bloom, F. E. (1974): Axonal proliferation following lesions of cerebellar peduncles. A combined fluorescence microscopic and radioautographic study. *J. Comp. Neurol.*, 155:43–60.

80. Poirier, L. J., and Sourkes, T. L. (1965): Influence of the substantia nigra on the catecholamine content of the striatum. *Brain,* 88:181–192.

81. Potter, L. T., Cooper, T., Willman, V. L., and Wolfe, D. E. (1965): Synthesis, binding, release and metabolism of norepinephrine in normal and transplanted hearts. *Circ. Res.,* 16:468–481.

82. Raisman, G. (1969): Neuronal plasticity in the septal nuclei of the adult rat. *Brain Res.,* 14:25–48.

83. Raisman, G., and Field, P. M. (1973): A quantitative investigation of the development of collateral reinnervation after partial deafferentation of the septal nuclei. *Brain Res.,* 50:241–264.

84. Reis, D. J., Gilad, G., Pickel, V. M., and Joh, T. H. (1978): Reversible changes in the activities and amounts of tyrosine hydroxylase in dopamine neurons of the substantia nigra in response to axonal injury: As studied by immunochemical and immunocytochemical methods. *Brain Res. (in press).*

85. Reis, D. J., and Molinoff, P. B. (1972); Brain dopamine-β-hydroxylase: regional distribution and effects of lesions and 6-hydroxydopamine on activity. *J. Neurochem.,* 19:195–204.

86. Reis, D. J., and Ross, R. A. (1973): Dynamic changes in brain dopamine-β-hydroxylase activity during anterograde and retrograde reaction to injury of central noradrenergic axons. *Brain Res.,* 57:307–326.

87. Reis, D. J., Ross, R. A., and Joh, T. H. (1974): Some aspects of the reaction of central and peripheral noradrenergic neurons to injury. In: *Dynamics of Degeneration and Growth in Neurons,* edited by K. Fuxe, pp. 109–125. Pergamon Press, Oxford.

88. Reis, D. J., Joh, T. H., and Ross, R. A. (1975): Effects of reserpine on activities and amounts of tyrosine hydroxylase and dopamine-β-hydroxylase in catecholaminergic neuronal systems in rat brain. *J. Pharmacol. Exp. Ther.,* 193:775–784.

89. Robinson, R. G., Shoemaker, W. J., Schlumpf, M., Valk, T., and Bloom, F. E. (1975): Experimental cerebral infarction in rat brain: Effect on catecholamines and behavior, *Nature,* 255:332–334.

90. Romanes, G. J. (1946): Motor localization and the effects of nerve injury on the ventral horn cells of the spinal cord. *J. Anat.,* 80:117–131.

91. Ross, R. A., Joh, T. H., and Reis, D. J. (1975): Reversible changes in the accumulation and activities of tyrosine hydroxylase and dopamine-β-hydroxylase in neurons of nucleus locus coeruleus during the retrograde reactions. *Brain Res.,* 92:57–72.

92. Ross, R. A., and Reis, D. J. (1974): Effects of lesions of locus coeruleus on regional distribution of dopamine-β-hydroxylase activity in rat brain. *Brain Res.,* 73:161–166.

93. Roth, R. H., Walters, J. R., and Morgenroth, V. H., III (1974): Effects of alterations in impulse flow on transmitter metabolism in central dopaminergic neurons. In: *Neuropsychopharmacology of Monoamines and Their Regulatory Enzymes, Adv. Biochem. Psychopharmacol., Vol. 12,* edited by E. Usdin, pp. 369–384.

94. Roussel, B., Buguet, A., Bobillies, P., and Jouvet, M. (1967): Locus coeruleus, sommeil paradoxal, et noradrenaline cerebrale. *C. R. Soc. Biol.,* 161:2537–2541.

95. Sachs, C., and Jonsson, G. (1972): Degeneration of central noradrenaline neurons after 6-hydroxydopamine in newborn animals. *Res. Commun. Chem. Path. Pharmacol.,* 4:203–220.

96. Sachs, C., and Jonsson, G. (1975): Effects of 6-hydroxydopamine on central noradrenaline neurons during ontogeny. *Brain Res.,* 99:277–291.

97. Schildkraut, J. J., Orsulak, P. J., Gudeman, J. E., Schatzberg, A. F., Rohde, W. A., LaBrie, R. A., Cahill, J. F., Cole, J. O., and Frazier, S. H. (1977): Recent studies of the role of catecholamines in the pathophysiology and classification of depressive disorders. In: *Neuroregulators and Psychiatric Disorders,* edited by E. Usdin, D. A. Hamburg, and J. D. Barchas, pp. 122–128. Oxford University Press, New York.

98. Sedvall, G. C., and Kopin, I. J. (1967): Influence of sympathetic denervation and nerve impulse activity on tyrosine hydroxylase in the rat submaxillary gland. *Biochem. Pharmacol.,* 16:39–46.

99. Singh, B., and De Champlain, J. (1972): Altered ontogenesis of central noradrenergic neurons following neonatal treatment with 6-hydroxy-dopamine. *Brain Res.,* 48:432–437.

100. Stenevi, U., Björklund, A., and Moore, R. Y. (1972): Growth of intact central adrenergic axons in the denervated lateral geniculate body. *Exp. Neurol.,* 35:290–299.

101. Tassin, J. P., Velley, L., Stinus, L., Blanc, G., Glowinski, J., and Thierry, A. M. (1975): Development of cortical and nigro-neostriatal dopaminergic systems after destruction of central noradrenergic neurones in foetal or neonatal rats. *Brain Res.,* 83:93–106.

102. Tennyson, V. M., Heikkila, R., Mytilineou, C., Cote, L., and Cohen, G. (1974): 5-Hydroxydopa-mine "tagged" neuronal boutons in rabbit neostriatum: interrelationship between vesicles and axonal membrane. *Brain Res.,* 82:341–348.
103. Ungerstedt, U. (1971): Stereotaxic mapping of the monoamine pathways in the rat brain. *Acta Physiol. Scand.,* 82 (Suppl 367):1–48.
104. Watson, W. E. (1976): *Cell Biology of Brain,* John Wiley and Sons, Inc., New York.
105. Watson, W. E. (1974): Cellular responses to axotomy and to related procedures. *Brit. Med. Bull.,* 30:112–115.
106. Wise, C. D. and Stein, L. (1973): Dopamine-β-hydroxylase deficits in the brains of schizophrenic patients, *Science,* 181:344–347.
107. Zigmond, M. J., Chalmers, J. P., Simpson, J. R., and Wurtman, R. J. (1971): Effect of lateral hypothalamic lesions on uptake of norepinephrine by brain homogenates. *J. Pharmacol. Exp. Ther.,* 179:20–28.

Neuronal Plasticity, edited by
Carl W. Cotman.
Raven Press, New York © 1978.

Reactive Synaptogenesis in the Hippocampus

Carl W. Cotman and J. Victor Nadler

Department of Psychobiology, University of California at Irvine, Irvine, California 92717

It is now generally recognized that many neurons in the adult CNS can reorganize their synaptic connections or form entirely new ones in response to lesions or other perturbations. We shall refer to this process as reactive synaptogenesis (26) in order to emphasize that it is a reaction to some stimulus and is not part of the normal developmental process. Reactive synaptogenesis may involve axon sprouting, but the use of this term can lead to inappropriate or premature mechanistic inferences where actual knowledge is absent or irrelevant. Essentially all studies on reactive synaptogenesis have made use of lesions to investigate this phenomenon and its mechanisms, even though other stimuli may also be effective. Ultimately, these studies are expected to elucidate mechanisms by which central neurons connect with one another, those involved in recovery of function after brain damage, and perhaps mechanisms concerned with the adaptive properties of normal brain. Before these expectations can be realized, however, we must know a great deal more about the factors which regulate this process.

Reactive synaptogenesis can probably either facilitate or prevent recovery of function after brain damage. In all instances a clearly aberrant pattern of connections is created, and in some cases this appears to produce abnormal behavior (79,119). However, other studies strongly indicate that reactive synaptogenesis underlies the restitution of normal behavior (35,59,90,117,135). The outcome depends most obviously on the type of lesion and the nature of the pre- and postsynaptic neurons involved. Different populations of fibers in the deafferented area can react very differently to a given lesion and some do not react at all. On the other hand, a particular afferent can react in different ways to different lesions. It is the cellular and molecular bases for these differences with which we will be concerned here.

The rat hippocampal formation has proved a very suitable model system for the study of morphological plasticity after lesions. Its structure is relatively simple for a cortical region, being composed primarily of two well-segregated neuronal types innervated by fibers arranged in parallel, well-defined laminae (Fig. 1). Additionally, the major afferents have been well characterized and are readily accessible to manipulation. Since the hippocampal formation evidently serves associative functions and the dentate granule cells develop mainly after birth (2,9,10,118), one might expect *a priori* that the operation of this region would be readily modeled by postnatal experience and that the synaptic specifications need not be so restrictive as in sensory or motor areas. Indeed a number of physiological adaptations, such as habituation (1,78,146) and long-term potentiation (1,17,18,33,120) can be elicited easily at synapses in the hippocampal formation. Moreover, numerous investigations in our laboratory and in others have shown that this plasticity extends to the anatomical, as well as the physiological, aspects of connectivity (26,63). When one set of connections is removed, others replace it. As we will describe, this reinnervation process produces a

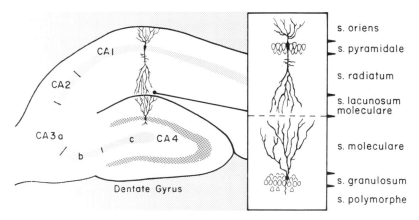

FIG. 1. Diagrammatic cross section of the rat hippocampal formation. **Left:** Subfields are denoted according to Lorente de Nó (60). **Right:** Laminae of area CA1 and dentate gyrus according to Ramón y Cajal (109) shown in relation to a schematic pyramidal (CA1) or granule (dentate gyrus) cell.

pattern of afferent connections as rigidly laminated as the normal pattern. Some of our recent studies have provided clues to the rules which determine how reactive growth shall take place. They will be discussed in relation to two questions: What treatments will initiate the growth response, and what factors determine the revised pattern of connections?

The detection and interpretation of changes in hippocampal circuitry produced by a partial deafferentation depend on a detailed knowledge of the normal circuitry, including the cells of origin, topographic organization, and the role of each projection in the physiological function of hippocampal regions. Therefore before we describe our experimental results, we will briefly summarize the relevant morphology of the dentate gyrus and area CA1, hippocampal regions that we have used as models for studies of reactive synaptogenesis.

NORMAL ANATOMY OF THE HIPPOCAMPUS

Dentate Gyrus

The cellular architectonics of the hippocampal formation were clearly described by Ramón y Cajal at the turn of the century (109) (Fig. 1). In the dentate gyrus a single row of granule cell bodies (stratum granulosum, granule cell layer) forms an arch enclosing the free end of hippocampus regio inferior. The region thus enclosed is termed the hilus of the dentate gyrus. The granule cells send their apical dendrites into the molecular layer (stratum moleculare) perpendicular to the layer of cell bodies and their axons (mossy fibers) into the regio inferior, where they contact the pyramidal cells. Between the granule cell layer and the pyramidal cells within the hilus lies an area of variously shaped interneurons (stratum polymorphe, layer of polymorph cells). The granular and molecular layers together form the fascia dentata. Blackstad, considering the polymorph cell layer an integral part of this structure, has used the term "area dentata" (dentate gyrus) to include all three layers (13).

The afferents to the dentate gyrus (Fig. 2) may be divided into four classes:

A. Extrinsic cortical connections (perforant path and crossed perforant path). The major extrinsic input to the dentate gyrus, indeed to the entire hippocampal formation, originates in the entorhinal cortex. It is particularly important for the studies to be described, because its removal has served as the major stimulus for reactive synaptogenesis in the dentate gyrus. This paleocortical structure lies immediately posterior and ventral to the hippocampal formation and has been divided into medial and lateral subregions (Brodmann areas) on cytoarchitectonic grounds. The input from entorhinal cortex to dentate gyrus originates mainly or entirely from the layer II "stellate" cells (136). The axons of the layer II cells (perforant-path fibers) pass into the angular bundle, ascend a variable distance, and cross the subiculum and hippocampal fissure in a direction perpendicular to the pyramidal cell layers. Upon entering the dentate gyrus, the fibers branch and form boutons *en passant* with small dendritic spines (55, 74,96) in the outer 70% of the molecular layer (44,46,105,130). Studies of termi-

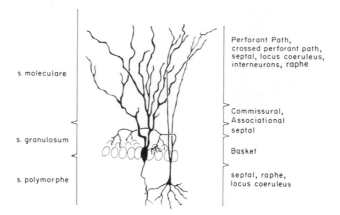

s. moleculare

Perforant Path,
crossed perforant path,
septal, locus coeruleus,
interneurons, raphe

Commissural,
Associational
septal

s. granulosum

Basket

s. polymorphe

septal, raphe,
locus coeruleus

FIG. 2. Innervation of the dentate gyrus. Lamination of afferents is depicted in relation to a granule and basket cell. The major projections to a given zone are capitalized. The dentate gyrus is divided into laminae as in Fig. 1.

nal degeneration with the electron microscope show that 86% of the boutons in this zone are derived from perforant-path fibers (74). Cells in the most medial portion of the entorhinal cortex project to the deepest portion of the perforant-path terminal zone, while successively more laterally placed cells project to progressively more superficial portions (44,46,130).

Whereas the entorhinal projection to the dentate gyrus was long considered an entirely ipsilateral one, a small crossed perforant path has been discovered in rats (37) and rabbits (48). These fibers also arise from the layer II stellate cells (131,136), probably as collaterals of the ipsilateral fibers, cross the midline by an as yet uncertain route, and merge with the perforant-path fibers.

The perforant-path fibers provide a powerful excitatory drive to the dentate granule cells (6,71). Excitatory postsynaptic potentials can also be recorded upon stimulation of the crossed perforant path, but this input is apparently too sparse to drive the granule cells (149). Current evidence suggests that glutamate is the transmitter of the perforant-path fibers (94,150).

B. Connections from ipsilateral (associational) and contralateral (commissural) regio inferior pyramidal cells. Pyramidal cells of hippocampus regio inferior send a modest bilateral projection to the granule cells of the dentate gyrus. It now appears very likely that only axons of pyramidal cells lying within the hilus (area CA4) contribute to this projection (38,47,65). Fibers from the contralateral pyramids (commissural fibers) run into the fimbria, cross the midline in the ventral psalterium, and enter the fimbria of the opposite side. Fibers from the ipsilateral pyramids (associational fibers) pass mainly around the free edge of the granule cell layer and enter the molecular layer.

Both CA4-derived projections provide excitatory input to the proximal portion of the granule cell dendrite (4,31,137), on which their terminal zones overlap (13,38,47,65,154). Their thick fiber plexus is a prominent feature of the inner third of the molecular layer (64,115) and may be used to localize these projections and follow their response to lesions. The associational and commissural projections do not mix with the overlying entorhinal afferents.

C. Extrinsic connections from the septum and brain stem. The perforant path and commissural-associational projections provide dense excitatory innervation to the granule cell dendrites and thus can readily be studied by conventional anatomical and electrophysiological techniques. In contrast, the extrinsic afferents from lower brain centers are comprised of relatively few fibers whose zones of termination are not nearly so finely delimited. As a result, less conventional morphology and few electrophysiological studies have been done on them. Fortunately, the transmitters used by these afferents have been rather well established. Many studies of their distribution within the dentate gyrus have thus involved histochemical or biochemical localization of the transmitter itself or its related enzymes.

The cholinergic septohippocampal tract arises from cell bodies in the medial (medial septal nucleus), ventral (nucleus of the diagonal band), and intermediolateral regions of the septum (81). Septohippocampal fibers which originate from cell bodies lying adjacent to the midline pass into the dorsal fornix and innervate the septal third of the hippocampal formation. Those arising from increasingly laterally placed cell bodies project to increasingly temporal levels *via* the fimbria. The projection is largely ipsilateral, but a small crossed component has been demonstrated (123). The septohippocampal fibers appear particularly reactive to a variety of lesions and other treatments (see below).

Acetylcholinesterase (AChE) histochemistry serves as a convenient method for the localization of septohippocampal fibers. By this technique cholinergic fiber bundles can be seen immediately above and below the granule cell layer and in the hilus (57,76,125,142). Lighter staining in the outer 70% of the molecular layer suggests a sparse distribution of cholinergic fibers in this area. All studies of septohippocampal terminals have demonstrated a moderate number just below the granule cell layer and deeper in the hilus and fewer in the molecular layer (83,88,112,126). The infragranular fibers probably innervate hilar interneurons, particularly the basket cells (see below).

The septohippocampal tract is generally considered an excitatory input, since acetylcholine depolarizes the granule cells when it is applied to them iontophoretically (16,153), but electrophysiological confirmation has been difficult to obtain. These fibers may excite the granule cells without producing an excitatory postsynaptic potential (EPSP) (3).

Rather sparse inputs to the dentate gyrus originate in the midbrain raphe nuclei and the nucleus locus coeruleus (123). Within the dentate gyrus the noradrenergic locus coeruleus (49,54,101,145) and serotonergic raphe projections (21,87) are similarly distributed. The innervation is densest in the hilus, especially immediately below the granule cell layer. Many fewer fibers and varicosities are scattered diffusely in the granular and molecular layers. From the localization of their terminals, it would appear that both brainstem afferents innervate primarily interneurons, particularly basket cells. They are probably inhibitory, since stimulation of these fibers inhibits the firing of hippocampal pyramidal cells (121,122). Thus projections to the dentate gyrus from lower brain centers appear to exert antagonistic effects on the postsynaptic cells; the septohippocampal fibers mediating excitation and the two brainstem inputs mediating inhibition.

D. Intrinsic connections from interneurons. Ramón y Cajal (109) described numerous short axon neurons in the dentate gyrus. For the most part their connections and role in the operation of this region remain unknown. The only interneuron about which we know anything of consequence is the basket cell. The basket cells are situated immediately beneath the granule cell layer and among the deepest granule cells. Their axons originate from one of the apical dendrites just above the granule cell layer, run parallel to this layer, and send numerous branches into it. Each basket-cell axon forms synapses on the soma and dendritic shaft of many granule cells (8), hundreds according to the electro-physiological evidence (6). These synapses mediate a powerful and long-lasting inhibition through release of GABA (95,139,141). Aside from inputs which originate in lower brain centers, the basket cell receives excitatory input from collaterals of the mossy fibers (6,14). The connections between granule and basket cells thus form a recurrent inhibitory circuit.

GABAnergic boutons have also been localized in the molecular layer, particularly in the outer third (8). These must be derived from intrinsic interneurons (139), though not necessarily from the basket cells. The few polymorphic cells of the molecular layer (109) would seem the most likely source of GABAnergic input to the distal dendritic region.

Area CA1

We have recently investigated reactive synaptogenesis in area CA1 in order to compare responses to denervation in hippocampal regions which receive similar innervation, but contain different postsynaptic cells.

The small pyramidal cells of area CA1 (regio superior of Ramón y Cajal) form a narrow, closely packed layer (60,109) (Fig. 1). Their basal dendrites are directed toward the alvear surface of the hippocampal formation and ramify in a distinct layer (stratum oriens). The apical dendrites are directed oppositely. Their long, relatively smooth shafts travel over a distance of several hundred micrometers before branching extensively. The layer of apical dendritic shafts is referred to as stratum radiatum and the shorter layer of extensive branching as stratum lacunosum-moleculare. No distinct stratum lacunosum (zone of Schaffer collaterals) can be identified in the rat, in contrast to many other mammals. However, a thin zone of fibers from the septum and raphe nuclei within the innermost part of stratum lacunosum-moleculare (76,87) could be considered to define a rudimentary stratum lacunosum. The axons of the pyramidal cells pass through stratum oriens to the alveus, a fiber tract that covers the dorsal surface of the hippocampal formation. They terminate mainly in the subiculum and the lateral septum (82,144). Interneurons, including basket cells, are found in stratum oriens and in lesser numbers in other layers, but they are far less numerous than the pyramidal cells.

Area CA1 receives innervation from essentially the same sources as the dentate gyrus, but important differences have been identified (Fig. 3). Again the apical dendritic layer is divided between terminal zones of excitatory projections which originate in the entorhinal cortex and regio inferior. In area CA1, as in the dentate gyrus, fibers from regio inferior form synapses on a more proximal region of the dendrite than cortical fibers. However, the fibers which project to area CA1 and those from the same region which project to the dentate gyrus originate from different cell groups, and the relative partitioning of the dendritic layer differs.

A. Connections from ipsilateral (Schaffer collaterals) and contralateral (commissural) regio inferior pyramidal cells. Ipsilateral (45,60) and contralateral (38) afferents from regio inferior arise from pyramidal cells in areas CA3a, b, and c, lateral to those which project to the dentate gyrus. The ipsilateral fibers that project to the apical dendrites, the Schaffer collaterals, branch from the ascending axon trunk in stratum radiatum and run horizontally into area CA1. These are believed to constitute the major innervation of area CA1. A second ipsilateral projection originates in the same parts of regio inferior (from the same cells?) and passes through the alveus to terminate in stratum oriens of area CA1 *(unpublished observations)*. Commissural fibers originate in the same region of the contralateral hippocampus. These fibers run through the contralateral fimbria and ventral psaltcrium then pass via the ipsilateral fimbria to the hippocampus. They terminate in strata radiatum and oriens similarly to ipsilat-

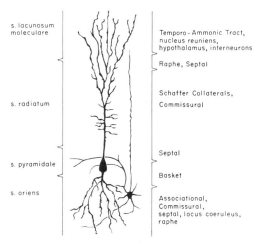

s. lacunosum moleculare — Temporo-Ammonic Tract, nucleus reuniens, hypothalamus, interneurons

Raphe, Septal

Schaffer Collaterals, Commissural

s. radiatum

Septal

s. pyramidale

Basket

s. oriens

Associational, Commissural, septal, locus coeruleus, raphe

FIG. 3. Innervation of area CA1. Lamination of afferents is depicted in relation to a pyramidal and basket cell. The major projections to a given zone are capitalized. Area CA1 is divided into laminae as in Fig. 1.

eral fibers. Thus the CA1 pyramidal cells receive a dense bilateral innervation from CA3 cells on both their apical and basal dendrites.

B. Extrinsic cortical connections. The entorhinal afferents (temporo-ammonic tract) arise from the pyramidal cells of layer III (136). These cells project bilaterally to stratum lacunosum-moleculare of area CA1 via the angular bundle and dorsal psalterium (130). Pyramidal cells in the most medial entorhinal area project to the portion of area CA1 nearest the CA2 transition, whereas those in the most lateral entorhinal area project to area CA1 where it adjoins the subiculum.

C. Extrinsic connections from the septum and brain stem. Cholinergic septo-hippocampal fibers (83,88) and serotonergic (21,87) fibers from the midbrain raphe nuclei terminate mainly in stratum oriens and the proximal part of stratum lacunosum-moleculare. A smaller number of fibers terminates in stratum radiatum, where they overlap a minor adrenergic projection from nucleus locus coeruleus (49). Histochemical data suggest that the cholinergic fibers in stratum radiatum primarily lie adjacent to the pyramidal cell layer (76,138), but this has not been confirmed by more traditional anatomical methods. The inputs from lower brain centers in area CA1 may operate as they do in the dentate gyrus, although they appear to provide even a sparser innervation.

D. Intrinsic connections from interneurons. As in the dentate gyrus, glutamate decarboxylase-containing boutons have been localized to the pyramidal cell somata and the distal portion of the apical dendrites (8), where they probably form inhibitory synapses (5). Electrophysiological evidence suggests that those on or near the somata are formed by axons of the basket cells and constitute a link in the recurrent inhibitory circuit. Inhibitory synapses on the distal apical dendrites most likely originate from intrinsic interneurons (139,141), possibly the few indigenous to stratum lacunosum-moleculare.

Recently, area CA1 has been shown to receive projections from certain thalamic (42) and hypothalamic (99,100) nuclei. Both terminate in stratum lacunosum-moleculare. In the temporal half of the hippocampal formation the portion of stratum lacunosum-moleculare adjacent to the subiculum receives a small cholinergic projection, which originates only in part from the septum (139). The source of the remaining cholinergic fibers is presently unknown. None of these projections peculiar to area CA1 has been investigated electrophysiologically.

PLASTICITY AFTER SELECTIVE LESIONS

Unilateral ablation of the entorhinal cortex in adult rats removes 86% of the synapses from the distal 70% of the ipsilateral granule cell dendrites (74). The synaptic reorganization which results from this massive denervation has been reviewed in detail (26). Briefly, reactive synaptogenesis restores the perforant-path terminal zone to its normal synaptic density (75). The width of this zone decreases by about 20%, however. Thus only about 80% of the synapses which degenerate are replaced. The commissural- , associational- , crossed-perforant path, and septohippocampal fibers participate in reinnervation of this zone (Fig. 4). The commissural-associational fiber system expands outward by about 30 to 40 μm (64,115), and new synapses made by these afferents replace those derived from the most medial perforant-path fibers (65,69). Septohippocampal (66) and crossed-perforant path (133,134) fibers proliferate in the remainder of the denervated area. In doing so, these fibers may actually abandon the zone reinnervated by commissural and associational fibers (Fig. 5). GABAnergic interneurons increase their synthetic enzyme levels (91) and the amount of GABA released (95). We feel these signs most likely represent a change in the efficacy of preexisting boutons (see ref. 95), but cannot entirely rule out the formation of additional inhibitory synapses. Locus coeruleus fibers do not react anatomically (R. Y. Moore, *personal communication*). Thus an entorhinal lesion alters the density and lamination of some afferents to the dentate molecular layer.

A similar lesion during development also produces a laminar pattern of reor-

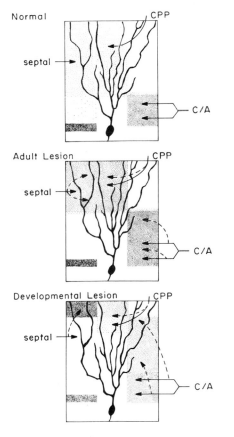

FIG. 4. Schematic diagrams showing the laminar distribution of septohippocampal, crossed perforant-path (CPP), and associational-commissural projections in the dentate gyrus. *Dark shading,* heavy projection; *light shading,* sparse to moderate projection; *no shading,* lack of projection. *Solid arrows* indicate normal projection; *broken arrows* indicate growth induced by an ipsilateral entorhinal lesion.

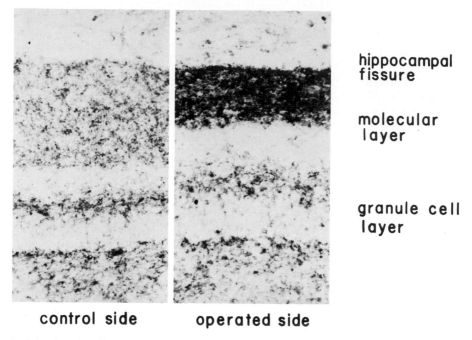

hippocampal
fissure

molecular
layer

granule cell
layer

control side   operated side

FIG. 5. Acetylcholinesterase staining of the dentate gyrus after a unilateral entorhinal lesion in an adult rat. Note the intensification of staining in the outer two-thirds of the denervated area and virtual lack of staining in the inner portion. This result indicates growth and relocation of cholinergic septohippocampal fibers (92). Magnifications: control side, X218; operated side, X272.

ganization, but differing markedly in detail (Fig. 4). The commissural fibers grow out nearly to the superficial edge of the molecular layer (67,155), and the associational fibers may actually reach the edge (155). Septohippocampal fibers form a dense plexus along the outer edge of the molecular layer superficial to the commissural fibers (27,92). Crossed perforant-path fibers proliferate in approximately the outer half of the molecular layer (132), but the exact dimensions of this area have not been reported. Neither has the degree of reinnervation been determined in developing rats, but a comparison of sections from animals with an entorhinal lesion made during development and in adulthood suggests little difference. This impressive fiber growth can even be obtained with small entorhinal lesions, although in such cases a correspondingly smaller portion of the molecular layer is denervated and growth is confined to this precise area (93,157).

It is important to note that the afferents examined thus far probably do not account for all the reinnervation which follows an entorhinal lesion. In particular, it seems unlikely that the very sparse septohippocampal and crossed perforant-path inputs could entirely replace the lateral perforant path. Experiments to identify additional reactive afferents are required.

In contrast to the dramatic effect of an entorhinal lesion, removal of innervation derived from hippocampal pyramidal cells has rather less effect. Removal of the commissural fibers does not affect the lamination of perforant-path (70) or septohippocampal fibers (93,140). The commissural zone does become reinnervated, however (80), probably by its ipsilateral homologues, the associational fibers. Even the sectioning of most commissural and associational fibers together produces no unequivocal growth of perforant-path fibers into the denervated area (70; and *unpublished observations*), although other intact fibers might reinnervate in this situation (156).

A similar rigidity seems to prevail in area CA1 of the hippocampus. Removal of 75% of the innervation from the commissural-Schaffer collateral terminal zone with a hippocampal transection fails to induce growth of the temporo-ammonic fibers into the denervated area (Goldowitz et al., *in preparation*). The sparse septohippocampal innervation also fails to respond to this lesion. Reinnervation does occur, however, to the extent of 80% replacement. The new synapses may be supplied by the few undamaged commissural fibers and Schaffer collaterals which remain.

We have recently examined the reinnervation of area CA1 after selective destruction of CA3 pyramidal cells with kainic acid. This agent, unlike a hippocampal transection, does not damage fibers directly or cause nonspecific destruction of tissue substance. The synaptic density of stratum radiatum is reduced by kainic acid treatment to 17% of normal. Again the denervated area becomes reinnervated, but the septohippocampal and temporo-ammonic fibers do not participate to any measurable extent. Thus translaminar growth, so easily induced in areas innervated by perforant-path fibers, is not readily elicited by interrupting inter- and intrahippocampal connections.

TIME COURSE OF EVENTS IN REACTIVE SYNAPTOGENESIS

We have carried out detailed studies on the time course of degeneration and reinnervation processes in the dentate molecular layer after an entorhinal lesion in adult rats. In this situation, the sequence and timing of events is precise and stereotyped. By 2 days after operation, fibers and synapses display an extensive degeneration reaction. Synaptic counts show that a large percentage of perforant-path synapses have already been lost. Terminal degeneration proceeds rapidly for the first 10 days and at a slower rate thereafter. Even 8 months after operation, some degenerating synapses are still present. Preterminal fibers are removed much more rapidly. Finally, many of the dendritic spines degenerate along with the presynaptic element or are resorbed into the dendritic shaft (74).

The period of rapid degeneration coincides with the development of an impressive glial reaction. Astrocytes in the molecular layer hypertrophy within the first day or two after operation, orient their processes toward the denervated area, and actually migrate part way into this zone (68,113). At the same time,

microglia proliferate to three times their preoperative numbers within 4 days
(68). For the first few days then, degeneration and events concerned with removal
of its products are the most prominent morphological effects of the lesion. Also
in this initial period the vascular bed in the outer molecular layer reorients
from primarily a vertical alignment to one which is largely horizontal (Fig. 6)
(Scheff et al., *in preparation*).

The first clear signs of reactive growth are seen 4 or 5 days after operation.

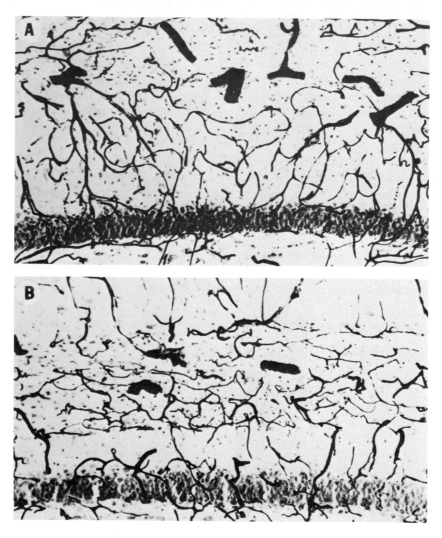

FIG. 6. Vasculature of the dentate gyrus demonstrated by perfusion with India ink after a
unilateral entorhinal lesion. Control side at **top** (A); operated side at **bottom** (B). Note the
change from a vertical to a horizontal alignment in the inner part of the denervated area.
Calibration bar, 50 μm.

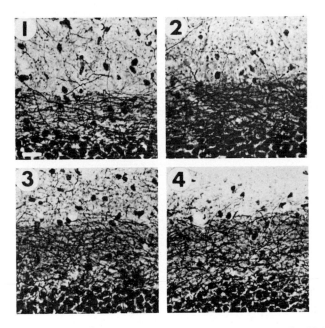

FIG. 7. Afferent fibers in the dentate molecular layer demonstrated by the Holmes method after an ipsilateral entorhinal lesion. Crossed perforant-path fibers were removed 2 days previously to facilitate accurate measurement of the associational-commissural plexus (immediately above the granule cells). 1, normal; 2, 5 days after operation; 3, 6 days after operation; 4, 30 days after operation. Note the outward expansion of this plexus induced by the lesion. Calibration bar, 25 μm.

Septohippocampal fiber growth becomes histochemically detectable (27,92), and associational and commissural fibers begin to invade the denervated area (Figs. 7 and 8) (64,116). These reactive fibers require about 12 to 15 days to reach their final state. Some new synapses appear to be formed very soon after the reactive fibers start to grow, but the most rapid phase of synaptogenesis occurs

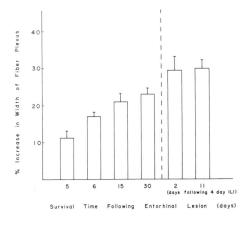

FIG. 8. Increase in width of the associational-commissural fiber plexus at various times after a complete ipsilateral entorhinal lesion or serial lesion. (From ref. 116.)

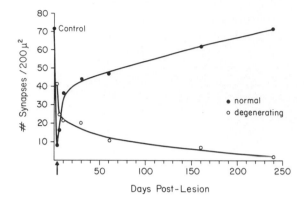

FIG. 9. Time course of degeneration and reinnervation in the perforant-path terminal zone after an ipsilateral entorhinal lesion. Note the delay in formation of new synaptic contacts and the inverse relationship between the two processes once reactive synaptogenesis begins. (Modified from refs. 74, 75.)

between 9 and 30 days (56,75). Electrophysiological studies on the commissural afferents and crossed perforant path show that nascent synapses first become functional at 9 days after operation, and nearly all are functional at 15 days survival (133,134,148). Removal of degeneration products and synaptogenesis proceed more rapidly in the zone invaded by associational and commissural fibers than in the rest of the denervated area (74,75). Thus within a given denervated area new synapses form at a rate proportional to the removal of degenerating synapses (Fig. 9).

TYPES OF RESPONSES IN REACTIVE SYNAPTOGENESIS

Conceptually, reactive afferents could form new synapses in a number of ways (26) (Fig. 10). In the peripheral nervous system existing axons grow new branches which invade the denervated target organ and establish synaptic contact. This has been called collateral sprouting. Some evidence of its occurrence

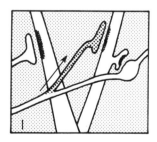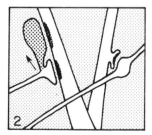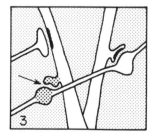

FIG. 10. Schematic representation of possible mechanisms in reactive synaptogenesis. Dotted areas *(arrows)* denote new growth. 1, collateral sprouting; 2, paraterminal sprouting; 3, contact synaptogenesis.

in the central nervous system (CNS) has also been reported, but collateral sprouting would appear uneconomical in the case of an afferent already in contact with the partially denervated portion of a target cell. In these cases new boutons may bud off existing ones or from the immediately adjacent portion of the axon and form a new synaptic contact close to that already present. Instances of this so-called paraterminal sprouting have been reported mainly in the CNS. The two forms of sprouting are distinguished experimentally by the location of the branch point, when this can be seen, and by the distance over which the growth occurs. Finally, a reactive fiber which contacts a denervated cell could simply form new synapses at points of apposition where there were none previously or the formation of new synapses could follow a shift in position of axon or postsynaptic process, creating new points of apposition. Axonal growth might not be required. This presently hypothetical possibility has been referred to as contact synaptogenesis.

In the CNS it is often difficult to distinguish these responses, since it is impossible to follow the behavior of a single fiber or even a group of similar fibers over time. However, it is possible to assess the likely contribution of each in particular instances. In the hippocampus afferents already present in the denervated area could reinnervate the granule cells more economically by paraterminal sprouting or contact synaptogenesis than by forming collateral sprouts. The same may also be true in area CA1 after a lesion of Schaffer collaterals and commissural fibers, a situation in which translaminar growth has not been detected. In contrast, the associational and commissural fibers grow into the perforant-path terminal zone from another lamina. This extension would seem to require collateral sprouting. However, the formation of sprouts has not been demonstrated, and there is evidence the reaction may be quite complex. In the degeneration-free associational-commissural terminal zone there occurs a temporary, rather slight reduction of synaptic contacts and a corresponding increase in bare postsynaptic sites (74). It may be that some associational and/or commisural fibers abandon their former synaptic sites and create new ones in the denervated zone. Perhaps some axons simply shift to more superficial locations. In recent autoradiographic studies we have obtained results consistent with this hypothesis. Commissural fibers were labeled with tritiated amino acid up to 30 days prior to the entorhinal lesion, and autoradiography was performed after these fibers had spread into the denervated area. The entire fiber plexus was uniformly labeled, indicating that preexisting axonal protein was used. This result would be expected if existing fibers had spread into the denervated area, but not if axon sprouts had been formed. However, nothing is known so far about the underlying mechanisms of sprouting, and it may be that axonal components extensively redistribute during the process. AChE histochemistry suggests that the septohippocampal fibers might also vacate their synaptic sites deep within the denervated area and assume a more superficial location. The synapses that are formed after these postulated axonal shifts could most easily arise by contact synaptogenesis. To restore the synaptic densities of all zones to normal, axonal growth would be required at some point, but our evidence indicates the participation of other processes as well.

We should also note in considering types of responses that the size of individual synaptic contacts appears slightly greater after an entorhinal lesion than before (75). Enlargement of existing synapses may be yet another means of compensating for a synaptic loss without the need of axonal growth. But since this response does not involve new synapse formation, it will not be discussed further.

From a mechanistic point of view, it is important to distinguish among these possible means of reinnervation. For example, an axon collateral will have to locate its target in some fashion, but if collaterals are not formed, axonal guidance probably would not be a consideration. Unfortunately, it is very difficult to do this experimentally. We have therefore chosen the term "reactive synaptogenesis" to refer to the formation of synapses in reaction to a stimulus. This usage avoids any mechanistic implication, such as is conveyed by the commonly employed term "sprouting." It also clearly distinguishes the process from developmental synaptogenesis, which takes place in an altogether different milieu and may employ different mechanisms.

INITIATION

What factors initiate reactive synaptogenesis? Most studies of the factors that influence axonal growth have utilized developing systems, either *in vivo* or in tissue culture. These investigations have yielded a large amount of information which may be applicable to the problem of reactive synaptogenesis, particularly with regard to the involvement of humoral factors. In our studies, however, we are dealing for the most part with fiber populations that have already entered the hippocampal formation and assumed their final lamination. When we refer to axonal growth after a lesion, we really mean extension, branching, or relocation of the axon followed by formation of new contacts. This process is distinct from that of axon formation during development, in that in reactive synaptogenesis the neurons are already differentiated. In reactive synaptogenesis, the first manifestation of selectivity can appear at the time when growth is initiated. The factors involved may be very selective; some afferents may simply not respond to the growth signal. In this section we summarize our results and those of other workers which bear on the subject of growth-initiating factors in the hippocampal formation.

General Properties

Is growth evoked only by particular types of lesions? At a general level one might consider whether growth of a particular afferent is initiated by a lesion of any neighboring afferent or by a lesion of only certain afferents. If the latter is the case, this would constitute strong evidence that some afferents selectively influence the growth of others. We have already mentioned the striking contrast between extensive translaminar growth after removal of perforant-path fibers and the very limited, or even negligible, translaminar growth evoked by a lesion of afferents from regio inferior. In a recent experiment along this line, we removed large numbers of regio inferior afferent fibers by destroying their cell bodies of origin with intraventricular kainic acid. This treatment reduced the synaptic density in stratum radiatum of area CA1 by 83% and in the inner molecular layer on the external leaf of the dentate gyrus by 70%. In confirmation of previous results, neither perforant-path nor temporo-ammonic fibers could be seen to grow into the denervated area. The septohippocampal fibers also reacted very little; certainly their response was nothing like the obvious reaction to perforant-path lesions. We cannot exclude the possibility that translaminar growth would occur if the dendrites were totally denuded of synapses derived from regio inferior afferents. However, even partial removal of the perforant-path fibers initiates a substantial growth response. Thus at least the septohippocampal fibers respond solely to a perforant-path lesion and whereas associational and commissural fibers react to a lesion of the perforant path, the converse reaction was not obtained. Curiously enough, this ability of perforant-path fibers to evoke reactive growth does not extend to the temporo-ammonic tract in area CA1, which originates from a separate layer of cells in the entorhinal cortex. Unilateral removal of the entorhinal cortex induces very little, if any, growth of commissural or septohippocampal fibers into stratum lacunosum-moleculare (67,69,92). We have also found similar results from septohippocampal, commissural, and Schaffer collateral projections after a bilateral entorhinal lesion (93; and *unpublished observations*) which denervates stratum lacunosum-moleculare more completely. On the basis of these studies it appears that perforant-path degeneration or something associated with it encourages growth of heterologous afferents, whereas degeneration of the other afferents does not. Lesions of regio inferior afferents must provide some sort of growth signal, since reinnervation does take place, but the heterologous afferents examined to date respond only weakly, if at all.

Results from several lines of investigation indicate that powerful attractants are involved at the stage of initiation and that these can operate over some distance. Pertinent to this consideration are studies performed in our laboratory on the regenerative growth of fimbrial fibers (25; and Goldowitz et al., *in preparation*). The fimbria carries most of the fibers which pass to or from the hippocampal formation and can easily be exposed by removing the overlying cortex and part of the striatum. These fibers do not regenerate or sprout to any significant extent when they are cut. However, a freeze lesion, which is presumably less traumatic, initiates the development of a branch at the point where the cold probe is applied. The same result has recently been obtained by applying colchicine to the fimbria. This treatment blocks axoplasmic flow, resulting in a damming up of transported substances proximal to the site of application. Most remarkably, even the application of saline initiates formation of the branch in some cases (Fig. 11). It seems that any chemical or mechanical

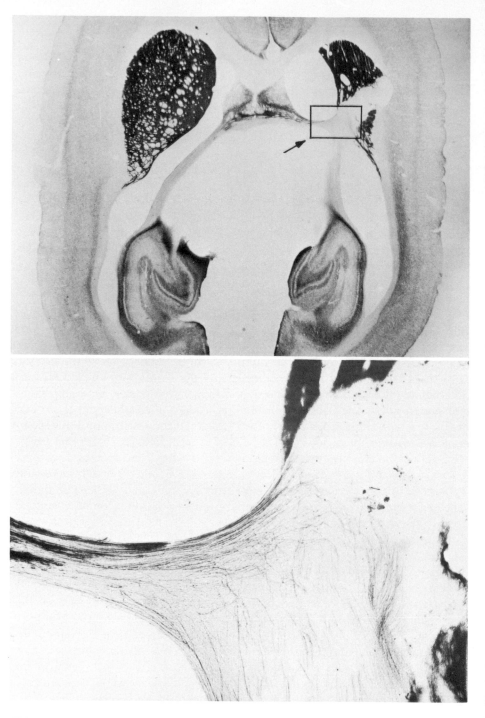

FIG. 11. Acetylcholinesterase histochemistry 60 days after application of saline-soaked cotton to the fimbria. **Top:** Horizontal section through the brain at the level of the fimbria. Treated side is on the *right*. Note the development of a branch crossing the ventricle *(box and arrow)*. Magnification, X9. **Bottom:** High-power view of the fimbrial branch showing cholinergic fibers projecting toward the striatum. Magnification, X90

disturbance of the fimbria can initiate axonal growth. Perhaps the interruption of axoplasmic flow itself induces growth at that point, as though it were an axon terminal. AChE histochemistry has demonstrated involvement of the septo-hippocampal fibers in fimbrial branching. Noncholinergic fibers apparently also participate, but we are uncertain of their identity. Invariably, the branch appears on the lateral surface of the fimbria and eventually bridges the lateral ventricle to contact the striatum. Although we have no evidence that the fimbrial fibers actually come to innervate striatal neurons, they are clearly drawn toward them and never toward thalamic neurons which are actually closer. The reason for this specificity may lie in the necessity of removing much striatal tissue to expose the fimbria. Since the remaining striatal neurons have been deprived of much of their cholinergic innervation, septohippocampal fibers could be induced to grow not only by the mechanical or chemical injury, but also by the availability of unoccupied synaptic sites on cholinoceptive cells. Because of the distance involved, such information could probably only be transmitted by a humoral attractant.

Several other studies suggest that factors can entice regenerating or growing fibers toward particular targets (11,12,50,124,143). For example, if implants of fetal hippocampus are placed into the anterior chamber of the rabbit eye, the hippocampal pyramidal cells survive, aggregate into a layer, and become functionally innervated by sympathetic and parasympathetic nerves (97). Again, because of the distance involved, the initiation factor must be a humoral substance, and peripheral nerves are receptive to this stimulus. The postulated initiation factors presumably induce the metabolic changes required for axonal growth, similar to the well-characterized nerve growth factor. Direct evidence on this point must, however, await their isolation.

Most studies assume that axonal growth must be triggered, in the case of lesions, by initiation factors released in the course of degeneration. However, Diamond and co-workers (32) have reported convincing evidence that substances released by nerve terminals restrain the growth of adjacent nerves. In these studies the application of colchicine, which blocks axoplasmic flow but not conduction, to one of the sensory nerves innervating a salamander limb triggered the growth of other nerves into the treated nerve's receptive field. Since growth was initiated in the absence of degeneration, the authors suggested that colchicine blocked the flow of some growth-retarding trophic substance toward the axon terminals. Their results further imply that mature axons would grow continuously, but are prevented from doing so by the action of externally supplied growth retardants.

Similar experiments in our laboratory have extended this observation to the mammalian brain (36). Colchicine applied to the fimbria inhibited axoplasmic transport within the commissural fibers, but did not interfere with conduction of electrical impulses or cause terminal degeneration. Synaptic counts performed on the commissural terminal zone in the dentate gyrus showed a highly significant increase when compared to saline-treated controls (Table 1). No change in synap-

TABLE 1. *Synaptic density in the inner molecular layer at various times following colchicine treatment* [c]

Group	Synapses/100 μm^2
Control	28.7 ± 1.0
4 days	28.2 ± 0.6
11 days	32.3 ± 0.4 [a]
60 + days	34.4 ± 0.9 [b]

[a] p, < 0.05.
[b] p, < 0.005 two-tailed Students t-test.
[c] From Goldowitz et al., *in preparation*.

tic density was found in the perforant-path terminal zone. It seems likely that these new synapses were formed by a converging afferent, probably the associational fibers. This result suggests that the commissural fibers normally prevent adjacent fibers from extending their synaptic territory by a mechanism dependent on axoplasmic flow, perhaps by releasing a growth retardant. Thus functional denervation, whether created by loss of synaptic connections or by disruption of axoplasmic flow, may be a sufficient condition for the initiation of reactive synaptogenesis. The pre- and postsynaptic elements may either emit growth-initiating factors or cease to provide growth retardants.

Initiation with Minimal Growth

A recent series of studies conducted in our laboratory has shown that a lesion can initiate the events required for subsequent growth, even if it itself is not extensive enough to permit significant growth. These studies were based on the observation that animals recover more rapidly and completely from small multiple lesions made in stages than from a single large lesion. If reactive synaptogenesis underlies recovery of function, serial lesions should also enhance this process. Exactly this result was obtained. A small priming lesion of the most medial entorhinal cortex was followed 4 or 13 days later by removal of the remaining entorhinal cortex. The priming lesion induced minimal septohippo-campal fiber growth and little or no extension of associational and commissural fibers into the denervated area. However, the response to completion of the lesion was greatly accelerated. Ordinarily, reactive fiber growth is not clearly detected for 4 to 5 days after an entorhinal lesion, but in this case it was demonstrated within 2 days. Moreover, the ultimate extent of associational-commissural growth was significantly greater than that which follows a complete, single-stage entorhinal lesion. The priming effect was limited in time, being erased by a 30-day interlesion interval and was not significant when the interval was shorter than 4 days (Fig. 12). Thus we conclude that denervation, whether or not it is sufficient to trigger significant growth, can prepare reactive afferents for subsequent growth, possibly by altering their metabolism. If a second, more

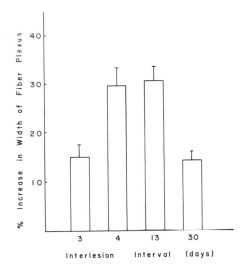

FIG. 12. Increase in width of the associational-commissural fiber plexus 2 days after serial entorhinal lesions. Animals received a small lesion of the most medial ipsilateral entorhinal cortex and then the remaining entorhinal cortical tissue was removed after the interval indicated. Note the lesser effectiveness of short and long interlesion intervals. (From ref. 116.)

extensive, lesion makes large numbers of synaptic sites available within 2 weeks or so, the conditioned afferents can respond without the normal delay (115,116).

One of the more significant findings in these studies was the unexpectedly stringent requirements of the successful priming lesion. Only subtotal perforant-path lesions accelerated the subsequent reactive growth. Even a lesion of the lateral entorhinal cortex, which denervated only the distal dendritic region, primed the associational-commissural response to removal of the remaining entorhinal cortex. (A lateral entorhinal lesion induced no growth of these fibers, however, probably because an intact region lay between them and the denervated area.) Thus as seen in other situations, the initiation signal operated over some distance. An initial lesion of the crossed perforant-path was ineffective, however, and a commissurotomy did not accelerate the response of associational fibers to an entorhinal lesion. This result raises the possibility that the priming response sensitizes the reactive fibers only to degeneration of the originally damaged pathway. If so, a different growth signal must be emitted by each degenerating system.

What Provides the Initiation Stimulus?

The initiation stimulus could conceivably be provided by any of the tissue elements involved in degeneration, including the degenerating fibers themselves, the denervated postsynaptic element and glial phagocytes, or from outside the region altogether through the circulation or CSF. It would be difficult, however, to explain the specificity of, for example, the priming signal on the basis of a factor released by glia or of a growth hormone. Glial proliferation, changes in the vasculature, and increased secretion of anabolic hormones would be expected to follow any lesion, and there is no obvious mechanism by which the identity of the degenerating fibers could be communicated through these events. This leaves the degenerating fibers themselves and the denervated postsynaptic elements. If the signal arises from the denervated cell, our studies on serial lesions indicate it must be specific to particular afferents. However, selectivity in the response to lesions could be mediated more easily by factors emanating from the degenerating elements. Degeneration products appear to initiate sprouting in partially deafferented sympathetic ganglia (151).

How these hypothetical initiation factors operate once they reach the potentially reactive afferent is presently a matter of conjecture. In view of the evidence that axons and terminals have minimal capacity to synthesize proteins, it would appear that the growth signal must reach the cell body, which in the case of denervated hippocampus is far removed from the locus of degeneration. This could be accomplished by retrograde axonal transport from the terminals, as has been shown for nerve growth factor. The reactive cells must assemble the components required for new axonal membrane and presynaptic constituents. This preparatory step might very well be responsible for the lag period between the lesion and the beginning of reactive growth. If so, the serial lesion effect can probably be explained by the prior accomplishment of this step before the second lesion.

In summary, we are beginning to understand the general properties of the growth initiation process. Humoral factors appear to provide the stimulus, and these are endowed with a high degree of specificity. In the normal state, they may be opposed by growth-retarding substances. The next step in studying initiation must include a direct search for such factors.

SPECIFICITY OF GROWTH

After lesions of hippocampal afferents, the postsynaptic neuron becomes densely reinnervated in a pattern as rigidly laminated as normal. We will now consider the factors which govern this specificity once reactive growth has been initiated. This problem closely resembles that of synaptogenesis during development, and similar mechanisms might be involved in both processes. In the case of reactive synaptogenesis, however, any growth would have to take place within or very close to the denervated area, amid both normal structures and a phagocytic reaction. Also the option of contact synaptogenesis is inapplicable to developing systems. We might add that it is usually much more difficult to distinguish between factors which initiate the response and those which determine the number and position of new synapses in reactive synaptogenesis than in development.

Quantitative Restraints

It is well known that the density of synapses in a given brain area varies little from animal to animal. For example, in the dentate molecular layer the density of synapses on the internal (ventral) leaf (35/100 μm^2) varies by less than 10% (74,75; and *unpublished observations*). Does this quantitative precision also apply to reactive synaptogenesis?

In the dentate molecular layer after an entorhinal lesion either in adulthood (75) or during development *(unpublished observations)*, reinnervation proceeds until the normal synaptic density is reached. There seems to be a slightly lower density in the outer part of the denervated area and a hyperinnervation of the inner part, but the average density of synapses along the granule cell dendrite returns to normal. The same can be said for reinnervation of CA1 pyramidal cells after a commissurotomy (Goldowitz et al., *in preparation*). A similar result has also been reported in a quantitative electron microscopic study on the septum denervated by a fimbrial transection (106).

We have, however, found one instance in which granule cells become hyperinnervated. As discussed previously, application of colchicine to the fimbria increased the synaptic density of the inner third of the dentate molecular layer by 20% (Table 1), presumably by blocking the axoplasmic transport of a growth-retarding factor within the commissural fibers. Since there was no change in the synaptic density of the remainder of the molecular layer, the granule cells must have become hyperinnervated. The granule cells may, however, have regarded their commissural synapses as abnormal in this situation because of their deficiency in constituents which can be supplied only from the cell body.

In the studies on lesions described above, the postsynaptic cell regained its normal density of innervation despite a decrease in the number of afferents. Would hyperinnervation occur if a normal number of afferents encountered fewer target cells? We have tested this possibility by use of rats whose hippocampi were X-irradiated during the postnatal period. Such treatment reduced the number of granule cells by about 82%. In these animals the density of synapses in the dentate molecular layer was normal, whether expressed relative to cross-sectional area or linear dendritic length. The dendritic configuration was also relatively unaffected, except for a broadening and shortening of the dendritic tree in some cases. Present evidence thus supports the view that postsynaptic neurons determine how densely they will be innervated, and changes in the proportion of afferents to neurons have little or no effect.

One might then ask whether the density of innervation is genetically fixed or susceptible to alteration by external factors. In favor of the first possibility is the observation that the postsynaptic sites on cerebellar Purkinje cells appear to develop independently of synaptic connections (41,43,58,127). There may be an innate genetic control over the amount of postsynaptic material which can be produced. On the other hand, increasing evidence indicates that information conveyed retrogradely by a neuron's own terminals influences the number of connections it receives. These studies have shown that neurons lose most of their synapses when their axons are cut (103). Regeneration of the axon to its target organ partially restores synaptic input. At least in sympathetic ganglia, regulation of synaptic input seems to depend on a trophic substance accumulated by the terminals and not by impulse flow through the circuit, since application of colchicine to the postganglionic trunk produces the same denervation effect as axotomy, but does not interfere with conduction (102,103). Perhaps the genes determine only the maximum synaptic complement, whereas a trophic substance(s) determines the proportion of the total which can be sustained at any given time. It is unclear from these studies whether the target organ supplies the trophic substance.

We have now obtained some preliminary evidence of synapse shedding in the hippocampal formation. In these experiments large numbers of CA3 and CA4 pyramidal cells were destroyed with kainic acid, a treatment which spares the dentate granule cells that project to them. Synaptic counts in the perforant path terminal zone in the dentate molecular layer showed about a one-third reduction from normal without any evidence of presynaptic degeneration. Whereas other explanations have not been rigorously excluded, this result is consistent with the idea that postsynaptic targets supply some factor necessary to maintain maximum innervation of the presynaptic neuron.

Knowledge of the manner in which the number of inputs to a cell is controlled is of major importance to an understanding of the rewiring which follows brain damage. For example, regeneration of cut fibers may be aborted in some cases simply because the denervated cells have already received new connections from undamaged fibers and have thus exhausted their capacity to receive input (104). Indeed collateral sprouting in the peripheral nervous system can retard the reestablishment of normal innervation by regenerating fibers (111) and in some instances can even reduce the effectiveness of those normal synapses which do form (40).

Qualitative Specificity

The reactive formation of aberrant contacts raises the question of whether these contacts are also ultrastructurally aberrant or whether they resemble those they replace. In some regions with a normally varied synaptic population, such as the nuclei of the visual system, some workers have found a shift in the proportion of each synaptic class after denervation and reinnervation (62,152). In the dendritic regions of the hippocampal formation, however, the great majority of synapses have an asymmetric appearance and are located on spines. Since both degenerating and reinnervating afferents terminate similarly, one might expect the reinnervated area to look much like normal, and indeed exactly that result has been obtained.

In the best-studied case, that of the dentate molecular layer after a unilateral entorhinal lesion, a normal proportion of asymmetric contacts is seen at survival times when reinnervation is essentially complete (Fig. 13). The postsynaptic densities, size, and appearance of the synaptic cleft and clustering of presynaptic vesicles at the junction all appear perfectly normal. Only a very few clearly aberrant structures are evident. These include a few synapses which retain a remnant of the old presynaptic membrane in the synaptic cleft, some boutons which seem to contain abnormally few synaptic vesicles, and some partially or completely vacant postsynaptic densities (75).

Despite the extensive loss of dendritic spines after the lesion (74,98), nearly all synapses in the reinnervated molecular layer are again located on spines. These spines must be newly created, a finding which brings up a point too often neglected in studies of reactive synaptogenesis: reinnervation requires growth of both pre- and postsynaptic elements. Since few boutons on dendritic shafts degenerate, few new ones make contact at this location. Particular spine configurations usually characterize a given region of brain and are good indices of normal structure. In the normal dentate molecular layer cup-shaped or w-shaped synapses are distinctive features (74). These are recreated when reinnervation occurs, along with the much larger number of simple contacts. However, there is some increase in the number of multiple-contact terminals. In the normal neuropil a single bouton generally contacts not more than three postsynaptic elements in a single cross section, whereas in the reinnervated neuropil a few boutons make five, six, or even nine synaptic contacts (75). This may serve to increase input from certain afferents which contribute only a few reinnervating fibers, such as the crossed perforant path (Fig. 14) (24).

In summary, our studies on the recovery from an entorhinal lesion show, despite creation of a few aberrant structures, that reactive synaptogenesis can reproduce the normal ultrastructure of a denervated area. Less complete studies of recovery from lesions of other hippocampal afferents agree entirely with this conclusion (Goldowitz et al., *in preparation* and *unpublished observations*). Both pre- and postsynaptic elements probably contribute to the reconstitution of normal synapses. The monotonous ultrastructure of the hippocampal formation makes it difficult to decide which element primarily determines synaptic structure. In other regions, however, available evidence favors the postsynaptic cell as the major determinant (89), and this is most likely true also for the dentate molecular layer (75).

Specificity of Synapse Position

Whereas synaptic density and ultrastructure appear very similar in normal and reinnervated areas, reactive synaptogenesis may create a very abnormal pattern of connections. Reactive fibers form more synapses than usual, and translaminar growth may be initiated. At least in the case of entorhinal lesions, homologous afferents possess no advantage in replacing the lost synapses; neither reinnervation by the crossed perforant-path nor residual ipsilateral perforant-path fibers excludes heterologous reinnervation of the denervated area (24). In accounting for the peculiar specificities of reactive synaptogenesis in the hippocampal formation, we have attributed some aspects to the selective action of initiation factors. The remainder, which appear to arise from interactions that follow initiation of growth, will be considered in this section. We must emphasize,

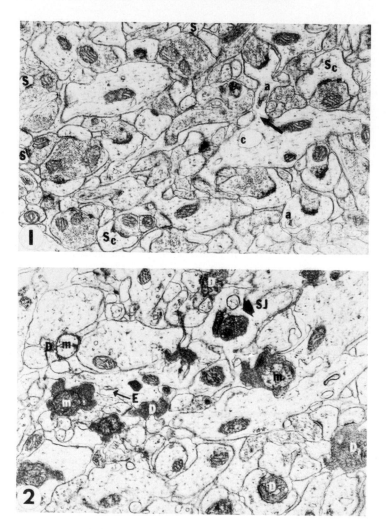

FIG. 13. Ultrastructure of the middle portion of the rat dentate molecular layer. **1:** A field from the contralateral side 240 days after an entorhinal lesion showing normal synaptic relationships. S, simple spine; S_c, complex spine; a, spine apparatus; c, dendritic cisterna. *Arrow* indicates a spine emerging from a dendritic shaft. Magnification, X15,700. **2:** A similar area of the operated side 4 days after an entorhinal lesion. D, electron dense degenerating bouton; m, altered mitochondrion within a degenerating bouton; E, vacated postsynaptic specialization; SJ, degenerating synaptic junction being engulfed by an astrocytic process. Magnification, X15,700. **3:** A field from the operated side 240 days after an entorhinal lesion showing return of normal ultrastructure. S, simple spine; S_c, complex spine; B_p, bouton en passant; MC, multiple contact terminal; E′, partially vacated postsynaptic specialization. *Arrow* indicates a synapse in an unusual position on the side of a spine stalk. Magnification, X20,700. (From refs. 74, 75.)

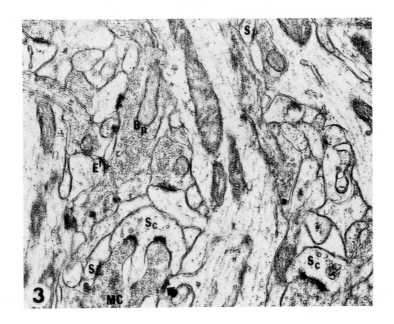

however, that it is usually impossible to assign the mechanism of selectivity to the initiation or synaptogenesis phase with any firm assurance. In most cases we are merely presented with a final pattern of connections for which we must account. For example, when an afferent population lies adjacent to a denervated zone and does not grow into that zone it is difficult to determine whether the degeneration process failed to provide a suitable growth signal or whether growth was initiated but new connections could not be made. It must be shown that

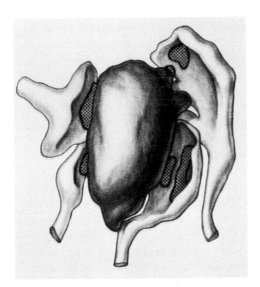

FIG. 14. Reconstruction from serial electron microscopic sections of a multiple-contact terminal formed by a crossed perforant-path fiber in the dentate molecular layer after an ipsilateral entorhinal lesion. The synaptic contacts are drawn slightly opened to show the number and type of synaptic contacts. *Stippled zones* represent postsynaptic sites. (From ref. 24.)

the afferent is, in fact, reactive. A distinction must obviously rest on studies of reinnervation kinetics, but, unfortunately, few such studies have been reported.

We have recently been able to dissociate the influences of initiation and selectivity on reinnervation of the dentate molecular layer by septohippocampal fibers. The septohippocampal fibers show a highly selective response to removal of converging afferents. It proliferates after an entorhinal lesion, but not after an associational-commissural lesion. To determine whether this is due solely to a selective initiation of growth by perforant-path fibers, we made a unilateral entorhinal lesion and injected kainic acid bilaterally to remove 70% of the associational and commissural innervation from the external leaf. Septohippocampal fiber growth was initiated by the entorhinal lesion, and these fibers proliferated in the perforant-path terminal zone, but they did not enter the associational-commissural terminal zone. Therefore it seems unlikely that the failure of an associational-commissural lesion to initiate growth could account for the selective response of septohippocampal fibers. It follows that there must be a mechanism of selectivity at a time after growth is initiated.

In considering the mechanisms which control reinnervation, it is convenient to separate this process into two phases, one of axonal elongation, branching, or movement and another of formation of synaptic connections. There is little to be said about the first phase, except in cases of translaminar growth. This is a rare event in the hippocampal formation, occurring only in the dentate molecular layer after an entorhinal lesion and only in the associational-commissural system. Although regenerating peripheral nerves are guided back to their target organs (108), we cannot say whether fibers in the central nervous system, which start growing much closer to the denervated cells, also require guidance. If so, guidance could be most easily provided by degenerating sheaths or by glial processes. The former appear to be important in directing growth of regenerating and sprouting peripheral nerves and the latter in guiding axonal growth in the developing cerebellum (107). Neither form of guidance seems adequate to explain the spread of associational and commissural fibers into the denervated area. Reactive astrocytes form a layer within the denervated area and direct their processes away from the granule cell layer. In contrast, the associational and commissural fibers do not appear to grow predominantly in a vertical direction. In addition, these fibers invade a zone normally relatively free of myelinated axons, and those which are present run at an angle toward the granule cell layer, not away from it. Thus the mechanism of axonal guidance in translaminar growth remains elusive. We do not even know whether a "track" must be provided.

One of the key issues in studies of reactive synaptogenesis is the means by which the new synaptic sites are chosen (Fig. 15). Most investigators once assumed that reactive afferents simply located and occupied the vacated postsynaptic sites. In this simplistic hypothesis, the postsynaptic cell plays only a passive role in reinnervation. Our evidence, however, indicates an active role for the postsynaptic element. We have already discussed the formation of new dendritic

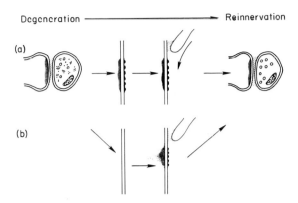

FIG. 15. Schematic diagram of reinnervation by **(a)** occupation of a vacant postsynaptic site or **(b)** induction of a postsynaptic site *de novo*. (See ref. 22, 26.)

spines by denervated granule cells. In addition, we have obtained strong evidence for the creation of new postsynaptic sites.

Shortly after an entorhinal lesion the sum of intact and degenerating asymmetric synapses and vacant postsynaptic densities totaled only about half the normal value (Table 2). As reinnervation proceeded, the number of asymmetric postsynaptic sites returned to normal (75). This indicates the assembly of new postjunctional complexes *de novo*. We could not tell, of course, whether the contact zones on the postsynaptic side had disappeared along with the postsynaptic density (the only visible postsynaptic constituent). This seems likely, however, in light of the current belief that the postsynaptic density anchors receptors and molecules involved in recognition or adhesion at a particular site (53). Without the postsynaptic density, these membranous particles would probably disperse. There was also some indication that the postsynaptic element was sometimes phagocytized along with the degenerating bouton (74).

Thus the postsynaptic cell actively participates in reactive synaptogenesis.

TABLE 2. *Loss and reappearance of postsynaptic densities in the molecular layer of the dentate gyrus at various times after a unilateral entorhinal lesion*[b]

	Zone	Days survival		Control
		4	240	
Synaptic sites/ 100 μm linear dendritic surface	Inner	28 ± 1	30 ± 2	27 ± 3
	Denervated	12 ± 2	26 ± 2	36 ± 1
Total synaptic sites[a]	Inner	48	50	45
	Denervated	57	90	97

[a]Degenerating synapses, vacant postsynaptic densities, and normal synapses in a 10-μm wide zone from top of granule cell layer to the edge of the molecular layer.

[b]Data from refs. 74,75.

This suggests the further possibility that it may be capable of selecting among the available reactive afferents.

Finally, we must consider the mechanisms which govern the lamination of reactive afferents. Aside from controls at the levels of initiation and axonal growth, laminar specificity must also be governed by interactions among afferents or between afferents and the denervated cell. The most prominently suggested mechanisms involve competitive interactions, dendritic growth, and chemoaffinity.

The rigid lamination of reactive afferents itself first suggested the possibility that newly available synaptic sites might be divided among reactive afferents on the basis of competitive interactions. After an entorhinal lesion during development or in adulthood, the septohippocampal and crossed perforant-path fibers on the one hand and the associational and commissural fibers on the other seem to occupy mutually exclusive portions of the former perforant-path terminal zone. We and others reasoned that the two groups of afferents grew until they contacted one another, the line of contact being determined by the proximity of each to the denervated area, comparative growth rates, and the size of each projection (26). In this context, competition implies no inherent preference of the postsynaptic site for any afferent over any other.

On the basis of present evidence, competition seems an unlikely mechanism. For one thing, competitive interactions should lead to graded boundaries between afferents rather than the sharp boundaries found in the normal and reinnervated hippocampal formation. In addition, a competitive mechanism cannot readily account for the failure of septohippocampal fibers to replace the medial perforant path after an entorhinal lesion in developing rats, despite the fact that some of these reactive fibers are initially in contact with the denervated dendritic area (93). Also studies of reinnervation after a bilateral entorhinal lesion show that associational and commissural fibers occupy no more of the denervated area than they do after a unilateral lesion, despite the absence of crossed perforant-path fibers with which they might compete (65; and *unpublished observations*). Finally, one could cite the apparently equally intense reaction of septohippocampal fibers to a partial or complete entorhinal lesion (93). In the case of a partial lesion, one might expect little septohippocampal growth according to a competitive model, since residual perforant-path fibers are in much greater abundance.

The competitive model predicts that proximity to degenerating fibers necessarily insures growth in or into the denervated area. This is clearly not the case in the hippocampal formation. We have discussed a number of negative results in preceding sections, and these need not be repeated. Our arguments do not, however, rule out some involvement of proximity and competition in determining the number and location of new synapses. Indeed, reactive afferents have never been shown to traverse an undamaged zone in order to invade a denervated one. Competitive interactions may be important in determining the relative success of homologous afferents, such as the associational and commissural fibers.

Storm-Mathisen (140) has suggested that, after an entorhinal lesion in adult rats, the granule cell dendrites grow from the base, carrying their attached fibers with them. If so, the idea of translaminar growth could be discarded. This attractively simple hypothesis could readily account for the sharp boundary which separates reactive septohippocampal and associational-commissural plexuses and the rapid disappearance of degeneration products from the inner part of the denervated area. Moreover, developmental evidence suggests that such a mechanism would be quite reasonable. The dentate molecular layer becomes laminated very early in development, when the granule cell dendrites are only one-third their mature length. As the dendrites grow, the laminae expand, but maintain the same relation to one another (61).

Recent electron microscopic evidence appears to rule out the dendritic growth model, however. In the area reinnervated by associational and commissural fibers, degenerating and apparently newly formed synapses are found intermixed, often on the same dendrite (56). In addition, this hypothesis predicts that expansion of the associational-commissural fiber plexus and appearance of new synapses in the reinnervated area should follow the same time course. Actually, the fibers grow out faster than new synapses form (64,115,116). It would appear that dendritic growth could account for the lamination of reactive afferents only if the areas of membrane contacted by associational and commissural fibers were moved selectively. Whereas this mechanism seems unlikely on its face, a sufficiently fluid membrane might permit such selective movement. If this does occur, the dendritic branch points might also be displaced outward. We are currently examining this possibility as a further test of the dendritic growth model.

Chemoaffinity between afferent and postsynaptic targets has been advanced as a mechanism underlying the specificity of connections formed during development (128). It is envisaged that macromolecular components on the growing axon and the presumptive postsynaptic site recognize each other and bind together, thus initiating the development of a mature synapse. The advantages and difficulties of this hypothesis have been argued at length (34,85).

The best evidence for the involvement of chemoaffinity in determining the lamination of reactive afferents in the hippocampal formation comes from experiments of Björklund and co-workers (12,129), in which the entorhinal cortex was removed and replaced with various implants containing monoaminergic neurons. Fibers grew into the hippocampal formation from all these implants, but their patterns of termination were strikingly different. If a source of serotonergic fibers or dopaminergic (normally exceedingly sparse in the hippocampal formation) fibers was implanted, the fibers invaded part of the perforant-path terminal zone. However, implantation of a source of noradrenergic fibers resulted only in replacement of the normal locus coeruleus projection. (The normal locus coeruleus input had been removed along with the entorhinal cortex.) Even though the noradrenergic fibers had experienced the same environment as the others, they grew directly past available synaptic sites in the perforant-path terminal zone. The growth of a reactive afferent past a denervated target would seem to imply a lack of chemoaffinity. It has also been found that noradrenergic fibers from the locus coeruleus do not react to an entorhinal lesion (R. Y. Moore, *personal communication*), but in this study one could not tell whether they were simply unreceptive to initiation factors or lacked an affinity for the denervated sites.

The reaction of septohippocampal fibers to an entorhinal lesion during development may also provide evidence for the importance of chemoaffinity. These fibers initially react throughout the denervated area, but within a short time the reactive fibers become concentrated along the outer edge of the molecular layer (92). Some factor must prevent the septohippocampal fibers, once they have begun to grow, from making anomalous connections in much of the denervated area. The lack of a necessary chemoaffinity seems to offer the best explanation.

Chemoaffinity, however, is not so specific as to be restricted to hippocampal tissue. Cut monoaminergic or cholinergic hippocampal afferents will selectively invade implants of peripheral effector organs. Septohippocampal fibers and fibers from the locus coeruleus can invade an iris or portal vein implanted in the brain and form functional connections (11,143). This situation differs somewhat from those we have investigated, since it involves regenerative, rather than reactive growth. Presumably, the availability of newly exposed receptor sites encourages regeneration in a manner selective for the transmitter, rather than for the particular fibers. Our previously cited studies of fimbrial growth toward the striatum further support this notion. However, reactive synaptogenesis need not be transmitter specific. For example, the septohippocampal fibers can replace the noncholinergic perforant-path fibers.

At present, chemoaffinity seems to be the only obvious mechanism which could explain the laminar pattern of reinnervation. The major problem with the chemoaffinity hypothesis is that it requires respecification of distinct dendritic regions when denervation occurs, at least in the few cases of translaminar growth. What mechanism could account for this, and why does it operate only when perforant-path connections are disrupted? These questions can only be answered by investigations of synapse formation at the molecular level. In particular, one must explain how the postulated selective affinities are modified by age, denervation, and the availability of particular afferents.

In summary, reactive synaptogenesis in response to denervation restores the neuropil to a state very much like normal, except that the number and position of synapses made by individual afferents is altered. No satisfactory mechanism governing these changes emerges from the work that has been done to date. Neither competitive interactions, axonal guidance, nor dendritic growth seems capable of explaining selective reinnervation, and we know too little about chemoaffinity, particularly on the molecular level, to judge whether it will explain the current data any better.

Molecular Considerations

The molecular events of synaptogenesis can be considered in terms of a recognition stage, during which pre- and postsynaptic elements make appropriate contacts and a subsequent adhesive stage involving the formation of a synaptic junction. Accordingly, a number of studies have concentrated on an analysis of the molecular basis of recognition. These have been concerned primarily with the retinotectal system (72,73,84,114). Other investigations, such as those of our laboratory, have focused on the molecular composition and structure of mature synaptic junctions, since it is necessary to identify the components of synapses before one can analyze the process by which they are assembled. To characterize synaptic junctions and their components, pure fractions must be available. Accordingly, we and others have developed methods to isolate synaptic junctions (28,30,77,147) and postsynaptic densities (20,23).

Glycoproteins have been shown to play a critical role in cellular recognition in a variety of systems. We now know that the external surface of the postsynaptic membrane within the cleft is characterized by a unique array of glycoproteins. These molecules can be identified at synapses by their ability to bind lectins (proteins with a selective affinity for particular carbohydrates). Lectins can be conjugated to ferritin, allowing the localization of binding sites at the electron microscopic level. Ferritin conjugates of Concanavalin A (Con A) and Ricinus communis agglutinin (RCA) bind to the external surface of the postsynaptic membrane just overlying the PSD on several neuronal types in brain (53). Since these binding sites also are present in isolated synaptic junctions, their molecular characteristics can be studied *in vitro* (29). The Con A-binding molecules are glycoproteins which have molecular weights of 95,000, 100,000, 123,000 and 160,000, with the most prevalent component being the 123,000 species (52). These glycoproteins are minor components of the synaptic junction. Their molecular weights and isoelectric points do not appear to vary significantly among brain cell types, such as hippocampal pyramidal and granule cells, and caudate neurons *(unpublished observations)*. Thus the basic characteristics of these glycoproteins appear similar throughout the mature CNS. We do not know, however, whether their carbohydrate compositions or sequences are distinct, as would be expected if these glycoproteins played a role in recognition.

In order to function as recognition factors, these glycoproteins must be present in newly formed synapses. In preliminary experiments we have found that Con A-binding molecules, similar in molecular weight to those in mature junctions, are present in synaptic junctions isolated from immature brain during the period of rapid synaptogenesis *(unpublished observations)*. Such surface glycoproteins could be involved either in synaptic recognition or adhesion (29,53). Their identification paves the way for an analysis of molecular interaction between pre- and postsynaptic membranes during synaptogenesis.

It is not yet known how these membranes initially establish and then secure the contact. We do know, however, that once a synapse is formed the union between pre- and postsynaptic membranes is very strong. Synaptic junctions from either the mature or neonatal brain are able to withstand various harsh treatments designed to dissociate noncovalent and some covalent bonds. These treatments have included incubation of brain slices or isolated synaptosomes in solutions which disrupt ionic interactions (concentrated salt solutions or solutions of alkaline pH), coordinate bonds (EDTA, EGTA), weak hydrophobic bonds (urea, triton X-100), and disulfide bonds (mercaptoethanol) (22; and *unpublished observations*).

It appears that shortly after the initial contact is made the internal postsynaptic surface of excitatory synapses becomes morphologically differentiated by the presence of a postsynaptic density, and the presynaptic interior surface shows a similar differentiation (110). At both immature and mature synapses recent ultrastructural studies have identified an intimate relationship between components of the cytoskeletal network, such as microtubules, and synaptic membranes (39). Postsynaptic densities isolated from mature brain contain proteins of the cytoskeletal network, such as actin, tubulin, and brain filament protein (19,-52,147; and *unpublished observations*). The predominant protein, however, does not correspond to any known fibrous protein (Fig. 16). It appears to be very insoluble and may serve a structural role, perhaps in joining the cytoskeletal proteins firmly to the plasma membrane (7,52). Disulfide bonds may aid in joining these proteins together, creating a durable structure well-suited for anchoring synapses in place and linking the synapse with cytoplasmic organelles (51). The manner in which fibrous proteins are assembled and the synaptic site determined is unknown. However, we can now say that creation of the postsynaptic structure depends on an interaction of cytoskeletal components with the plasma membrane, perhaps culminating in the insertion of the major postsynaptic density protein.

The processes of synaptic recognition and assembly of the junction are likely to be the same in both developmental and reactive synaptogenesis. In order to understand these processes, we particularly need more information on the molecular basis of recognition and on the earliest events of synaptogenesis immediately following recognition. The recent information on the composition and structure of mature synaptic junctions provides a solid basis for these studies.

CONCLUSION

Reactive synaptogenesis, like developmental synaptogenesis, is an exceedingly complex process. From the present evidence, the sequence of steps is as follows: (a) release of initiation factor; (b) reception of the growth signal by responsive fibers and conveyance to the cell body; (c) anabolic biochemical response by reactive fibers; (d) axonal extension, branching or relocation; and (e) formation of new synapses. We have discussed the possibilities for regulation at most of these steps; selectivity could be mediated by factors operating at any of them. It is evident that one can derive from the present evidence few general rules governing reinnervation, even in a single region like the hippocampal formation, since different lesions or chemical treatments evoke markedly different responses. Fibers homologous to those which were removed appear sometimes to have a significant advantage in reinnervation, but in other instances they do not. For example, in area CA1 the remaining Schaffer collateral and commissural fibers may selectively recapture their lost synaptic territory after the great majority are removed, but in the dentate gyrus the remaining perforant-path fibers are unable to regain the entire denervated area after a partial entorhinal lesion. Similarly, variable selectivity has been found in cases of reinnervation by fibers which use the same transmitter as those which degenerated. Yet even when homology and transmitter identity confer no advantage, as in the dentate molecular layer denervated by removal of the perforant-path fibers, not all converging afferents participate in reinnervation. The bases for this selectivity are not understood. At least in one case, that of implanted aminergic fibers invading a dentate gyrus devoid of perforant-path input, specific chemoaffinities seem to be involved. In other cases initiation factors may, for some reason, trigger a growth response in only certain fibers.

Reactive synaptogenesis may be selective in the sense that nearby fibers which do not normally project to the denervated cells have never been shown to reinnervate them. For example, the crossed temporo-ammonic tract, which innvervates area CA1, does not replace the perforant-path fibers in the dentate gyrus after a unilateral entorhinal lesion (131). Further studies, however, are needed to determine the generality of this notion. During development, growing fibers can innervate denervated foreign postsynaptic cells (119).

Despite the differences in response to various types of denervation, some principles seem to be universally applicable: (a) the rate of reinnervation depends on the rate of degeneration; (b) the onset of functional recovery at physiological and behavioral levels coincides with the onset of reactive synaptogenesis; (c) the density of synaptic sites on a given cell is primarily determined by the cell itself, and reactive synaptogenesis can restore this value to normal; (d) growth is initiated by factors released from the degenerating elements or denervated cells and which can operate over a considerable distance. Their action may be opposed by growth-retarding substances; (e) reactive synaptogenesis takes place mainly at newly created sites, rather than at vacated sites. Thus both pre- and postsynaptic elements actively participate in reinnervation; and (f) proximity to a denervated zone is a necessary, but insufficient, condition for reactive growth.

Additional principles may yet be found generally applicable. However, the variation in reinnervation patterns is considerably more impressive than the consistencies, even in an area such as the hippocampal formation, where the major inputs do not differ markedly from one another. Perhaps the mechanisms underlying these processes are so flexible that only the most general selection rules apply and each treatment brings into play a unique set of processes. Similar considerations apply to the formation of neural circuitry during development. Certain principles appear to be universally applicable, but in specific cases

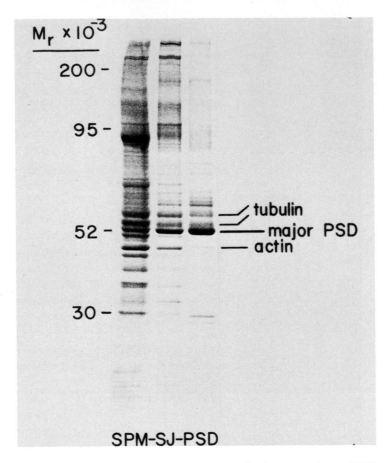

FIG. 16. SDS-polyacrylamide gel electrophoresis of synaptic plasma membrane (SPM), synaptic junction (SJ), and postsynaptic density (PSD) fractions. Position on the gel and molecular weight of identified proteins are indicated.

some features play a greater role in creating the pattern of innervation than others. Reactive synaptogenesis therefore seems to follow rather few selection rules, being influenced to a great extent by the organization and inherent plasticity of the particular region.

Further progress in this area requires investigation at both cellular and molecular levels. Up to this point the most useful studies have involved the placement of a variety of lesions or combinations of lesions and the transplantation of the hippocampus or of the cells which innervate it. These manipulations of pre- and postsynaptic elements, similar to those carried out in other systems, have been discussed in this chapter. The results of such studies have provided the general rules given above, but also the variable responses which are presently difficult to fit into any coherent scheme. Whereas future studies along these lines may clarify the situation to some extent, it seems certain that the most basic rules governing reactive synaptogenesis can be uncovered only through a molecular approach. For example, elucidation of the process by which denervation elicits a growth response requires isolation and identification of the initiation factors whose existence is so strongly implied by studies at the cellular level. Several groups have established tissue culture systems for testing these substances, and thus some progress in this effort can be expected shortly. In addition, assuming that selective chemoaffinities determine the final pattern of hippocampal connectivity, it will be necessary to characterize the surface macromolecules involved. If the pattern of "recognition molecules" determines laminar boundaries, as presently seems possible, one might then be able to follow such changes and determine the manner in which they are regulated. Such studies are in their infancy, and it is not clear that any of the constituents identified in synaptic membranes to date participates in recognition of synaptic sites. One profitable avenue of future work might be a quantitative and qualitative comparison of synaptic membrane constituents in developing, mature, and reinnervating hippocampi.

With regard to the clinical applicability of these studies, one can only hope that sufficient homology exists among mammals to permit the admittedly tenuous extrapolation from rodents to man. It is encouraging, however, that the time course of reinnervation obtained from model studies on rats corresponds rather well to the time course of recovery from brain damage, as exemplified by coma, (Fig. 17) in man. This does not necessarily imply, of course, that reactive synaptogenesis underlies recovery of function, but it certainly justifies further pursuit of the possible relationship. The preliminary behavioral work in animals has also been encouraging. In this regard, studies on primates may be particularly worthwhile.

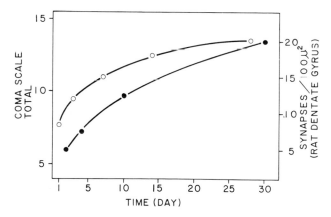

FIG. 17. Rate of recovery from coma in patients with head injuries compared to rate of reinnervation of rat dentate molecular layer after an entorhinal lesion. (○) Depth of coma; (●) recovery of synapses in molecular layer. Reinnervation data from ref. 75. Clinical data courtesy of Dr. S. Galbraith who pointed out this relationship to us.

Whereas it is rather more difficult to test recovery of function after hippocampal damage than after lesions of the spinal cord or visual system, this region deserves to be a focus of work in this area because of its extreme vulnerability to a number of conditions in which neurons are lost. Indeed, loss of hippocampal pyramidal cells with development of a glial scar is one of the most common forms of brain damage encountered clinically, being a prominent histopathological finding in such diverse conditions as status epilepticus, anoxia, and senile dementia (15,86). One requires a means of producing similar lesions in experimental animals. We have recently found that kainic acid, a potent convulsant structurally related to glutamic acid, reproduces in rats this very form of hippocampal damage (Nadler et al., *in preparation*). Despite the difficulty in determining when functional recovery has occurred, investigation of reactive synaptogenesis after kainic acid lesions would be very important, given the frequency of equivalent lesions in man. Possibly such model damage may help to explain the behavioral role of the hippocampus, thus allowing for rational tests of functional recovery.

In our view then, the study of reactive synaptogenesis must shortly move from the essentially phenomenological studies at the cellular level to both molecular approaches and behavioral studies with use of more clinically relevant lesions. It is only at the molecular level that we are likely to uncover the bases for the few consistencies and many variabilities in the response to denervation. In addition, one can gain control over this process only by knowing the chemical and physical interactions by which reinnervation is achieved. Knowing the histological consequences of selective brain damage, it should now be possible to relate our findings more definitively to the clinical situation. Such correlations would greatly enhance the value of this work and give a greater impetus to the more basic companion studies.

We contend that studies on reactive synaptogenesis are not only relevant to an understanding of recovery of function, but probably also reveal important adaptive capacities of normal brain circuitry. Studies on reactive synaptogenesis clearly show that the mature brain possesses an innate capacity to form new synapses in a highly selective manner. It would be surprising if this ability were used only for the purpose of repair. Indeed, the finding that growth can be induced in the absence of denervation may signify that neuronal circuitry continuously remodels itself according to the balance of trophic materials in the environment. It seems likely that in denervation studies we are revealing an extreme expression of the inherent plastic properties of the adult brain. Thus, studies on reactive synaptogenesis, as the term implies, should provide insights into the capacity of the mature brain to react to a vast number of perturbations, both normal and pathological.

ACKNOWLEDGMENTS

We thank Ms. Julene Mueller for secretarial skills and Ms. Maureen Killackey for the illustrations. This work was supported in part from NIH Research grant

NS 08597, NIMH Research grant MS 19691, and NSF Research grant BNS 7609973.

REFERENCES

1. Alger, B. E., and Teyler, T. J. (1976): Long-term and short-term plasticity in the CA1, CA3 and dentate regions of the rat hippocampal slice. *Brain Res.,* 110:463–480.
2. Altman, J., and Das, G. D. (1965): Autoradiographic and histological evidence of postnatal hippocampal neurogenesis in rats. *J. Comp. Neurol.,* 124:319–336.
3. Alvarez-Leefmans, F. J., and Gardner-Medwin, A. R. (1975): Influences of the septum on the hippocampal dentate area which are unaccompanied by field potentials. *J. Physiol.,* 249:14P–15P.
4. Andersen, P. (1959): Interhippocampal impulses. I. Origin, course and distribution in cat, rabbit and rat. *Acta Physiol. Scand.,* 47:63–90.
5. Andersen, P., Eccles, J. C., and Løyning, Y. (1964): Pathway of postsynaptic inhibition in the hippocampus. *J. Neurophysiol.,* 27:608–619.
6. Andersen, P., Holmqvist, B., and Voorhoeve, P. E. (1966): Entorhinal activation of dentate granule cells. *Acta Physiol. Scand.,* 66:448–460.
7. Banker, G., Churchill, L., and Cotman, C. W. (1974): Proteins of the postsynaptic density, *J. Cell Biol.,* 63:456–465.
8. Barber, R., and Saito, K. (1976): Light microscopic visualization of GAD and GABA-T in immunocytochemical preparations of rodent CNS. In: *GABA in Nervous System Function,* edited by E. Roberts, T. N. Chase, and D. B. Tower, pp. 113–132. Raven Press, New York.
9. Bayer, S. A., and Altman, J. (1974): Hippocampal development in the rat: cytogenesis and morphogenesis examined with autoradiography and low-level X-irradiation. *J. Comp. Neurol.,* 158:55–80.
10. Bayer, S. A., and Altman, J. (1975): Radiation-induced interference with postnatal hippocampal cytogenesis in rats and its long-term effects on the acquisition of neurons and glia. *J. Comp. Neurol.,* 163:1–20.
11. Björklund, A., and Stenevi, U. (1971): Growth of central catecholamine neurones into smooth muscle grafts in the rat mesencephalon, *Brain Res.,* 31:1–20.
12. Björklund, A., Stenevi, U., and Svendgaard, N. A. (1976): Growth of transplanted mono-aminergic neurones into the adult hippocampus along the perforant path. *Nature,* 262:787–790.
13. Blackstad, T. W. (1956): Commissural connections of the hippocampal region in the rat, with special reference to their mode of termination. *J. Comp. Neurol.,* 105:417–537.
14. Blackstad, T. W., Brink, K., Hem, J., and Jeune, B. (1970): Distribution of hippocampal mossy fibers in the rat. An experimental study with silver impregnation methods. *J. Comp. Neurol.,* 138:433–450.
15. Blackwood, W., and Corsellis, J. A. N., (editors) (1976): *Greenfield's Neuropathology.* Edward Arnold, London.
16. Bland, B. H., Kostopoulos, G. K., and Phillis, J. W. (1974): Acetylcholine sensitivity of hippocampal formation neurons. *Can. J. Physiol. Pharmacol.,* 52:966–971.
17. Bliss, T. V. P., and Gardner-Medwin, A. R. (1973): Long-lasting potentiation of synaptic transmission in the dentate area of the unanaesthetized rabbit following stimulation of the perforant path. *J. Physiol.,* 232:357–374.
18. Bliss, T. V. P., and Lømo, T. (1973): Long-lasting potentiation of synaptic transmission in the dentate area of the anaesthetized rabbit following stimulation of the perforant path. *J. Physiol.,* 232:331–356.
19. Blomberg, F., Cohen, R. S., and Siekevitz, P. (1977): The structure of postsynaptic densities isolated from dog cerebral cortex. II. Characterization and arrangement of some of the major proteins within the structure. *J. Cell Biol.,* 74:204–225.
20. Cohen, R. S., Blomberg, F., Berzins, K., and Siekevitz, P. (1977): The structure of postsynaptic densities isolated from dog cerebral cortex. I. Overall morphology and protein composition. *J. Cell Biol.,* 74:181–203.
21. Conrad, L. C. A., Leonard, C. M., and Pfaff, D. W. (1974): Connections of the median and dorsal raphe nuclei in the rat: an autoradiographic and degeneration study. *J. Comp. Neurol.,* 156:179–206.

22. Cotman, C. W. (1976): Lesion-induced synaptogenesis in brain: a study of dynamic changes in neuronal membrane specializations. *J. Supramolec. Str.,* 4:319–327.
23. Cotman, C. W., Banker, G., Churchill, L., and Taylor, D. (1974): Isolation of postsynaptic densities from rat brain. *J. Cell Biol.,* 63:441–455.
24. Cotman, C. W., Gentry, C., and Steward, O. (1977): Synaptic replacement in the dentate gyrus after unilateral entorhinal lesion: electron microscopic analysis of the extent of replacement of synapses by the remaining entorhinal cortex. *J. Neurocytol.,* 6:455–464.
25. Cotman, C. W., Hyatt, H., Kaups, P., and Lynch, G. (1975): On the regeneration of CNS axons. *Neurosci. Abstr.,* 1:499.
26. Cotman, C. W., and Lynch, G. S. (1976): Reactive synaptogenesis in the adult nervous system: the effects of partial deafferentation on new synapse formation. In: *Neuronal Recognition,* edited by S. Barondes, pp. 69–108. Plenum Press, New York.
27. Cotman, C. W., Matthews, D. A., Taylor, D., and Lynch, G. (1973): Synaptic rearrangement in the dentate gyrus: histochemical evidence of adjustments after lesions in immature and adult rats. *Proc. Natl. Acad. Sci. USA,* 70:3473–3477.
28. Cotman, C. W., and Taylor, D. (1972): Isolation and structural studies on synaptic complexes from rat brain. *J. Cell Biol.,* 55:696–711.
29. Cotman, C. W., and Taylor, D. (1974): Localization and characterization of Concanavalin A receptors in the synaptic cleft. *J. Cell Biol.,* 62:236–242.
30. Davis, G., and Bloom, F. E. (1970): Proteins of synaptic junctional complexes. *J. Cell Biol.,* 47:46a.
31. Deadwyler, S. A., West, J. R., Cotman, C. W., and Lynch, G. S. (1975): A neuro-physiological analysis of commissural projections to dentate gyrus of the rat. *J. Neurophysiol.,* 38:167–184.
32. Diamond, J., Cooper, E., Turner, C., and Macintrye, L. (1976): Trophic regulation of nerve sprouting. *Science,* 193:371–377.
33. Douglas, R. M., and Goddard, G. V. (1975): Long-term potentiation of the perforant path-granule cell synapse in the rat hippocampus. *Brain Res.,* 86:205–215.
34. Gaze, R. M., and Keating, M. J. (1972): The visual system and "neuronal specificity." *Nature,* 237:375–378.
35. Goldberger, M. E., and Murray, M. (1974): Restitution of function and collateral sprouting in the cat spinal cord: the deafferented animal. *J. Comp. Neurol.,* 158:37–54.
36. Goldowitz, D., and Cotman, C. W. (1977): Does neurotrophic material control synapse formation in the adult rat brain? *Neurosci. Abstr.,* 3:534.
37. Goldowitz, D., White, W. F., Steward, O., Cotman, C., and Lynch, G. (1975): Anatomical evidence for a projection from the entorhinal cortex to the contralateral dentate gyrus of the rat. *Exp. Neurol.,* 47:433–441.
38. Gottlieb, D. I., and Cowan, W. M. (1973): Autoradiographic studies of the commissural and ipsilateral association connections of the hippocampus and dentate gyrus of the rat. *J. Comp. Neurol.,* 149:393–422.
39. Gray, E. G., and Westrum, L. E. (1976): Microtubules associated with nuclear pore complexes and coated pits in the CNS. *Cell Tiss. Res.,* 168:445–453.
40. Grinnell, A. D., Rheuben, M. B., and Letinsky, M. S. (1977): Mutual repression of synaptic efficacy by pairs of foreign nerves innervating frog skeletal muscle. *Nature,* 265:368–370.
41. Hanna, R. B., Hirano, A., and Pappas, G. D. (1976): Membrane specializations and dendritic spines and glia in the weaver mouse cerebellum: a freeze fracture study. *J. Cell Biol.,* 68:403–410.
42. Herkenham, M. A. (1976): A thalamo-hippocampal connection in the rat. *Neurosci. Abstr.,* 2:387.
43. Hirano, A., and Dembitzer, H. M. (1973): Cerebellar alterations in the weaver mouse. *J. Cell Biol.,* 56:478–486.
44. Hjorth-Simonsen, A. (1972): Projection of the lateral part of the entorhinal area to the hippocampus and fascia dentata. *J. Comp. Neurol.,* 146:219–232.
45. Hjorth-Simonsen, A. (1973): Some intrinsic connections of the hippocampus in the rat: an experimental analysis. *J. Comp. Neurol.,* 147:145–162.
46. Hjorth-Simonsen, A., and Jeune, B. (1972): Origin and termination of the hippocampal perforant path in the rat studied by silver impregnation. *J. Comp. Neurol.,* 144:215–232.
47. Hjorth-Simonsen, A., and Laurberg, S. (1977): Commissural connections of the dentate area in the rat. *J. Comp. Neurol.,* 174:591–606.

48. Hjorth-Simonsen, A., and Zimmer, J. (1975): Crossed pathways from the entorhinal area to the fascia dentata. I. Normal in rabbits. *J. Comp. Neurol.,* 161:57–70.
49. Jones, B. E., and Moore, R. Y. (1977): Ascending projections of the locus coeruleus in the rat. II. Autoradiographic study. *Brain Res.,* 127:23–53.
50. Katzman, R., Björklund, A., Owman, C. H., Stenevi, U., and West, K. H. (1971): Evidence for regenerative axon sprouting of central catecholamine neurons in the rat mesencephalon following electrolytic lesions. *Brain Res.,* 25:579–596.
51. Kelly, P. T., and Cotman, C. W. (1976): Intermolecular disulfide bonds at central nervous system synaptic junctions. *Biochem. Biophys. Res. Comm.,* 73:858–864.
52. Kelly, P. T., and Cotman, C. W. (1977): Identification of glycoproteins and proteins at synapses in the central nervous system. *J. Cell Biol.,* 252:786–793.
53. Kelly, P. T., Cotman, C. W. Gentry, C., and Nicolson, G. L. (1976): Distribution and mobility of lectin receptors on synaptic membranes of identified CNS neurons. *J. Cell Biol.,* 71:487–496.
54. Koda, L. Y., and Bloom, F. E. (1977): A light and electron microscopic study of noradrenergic terminals in the rat dentate gyrus. *Brain Res.,* 120:327–335.
55. Laatsch, R. H., and Cowan, W. M. (1966): Electron microscopic studies of the dentate gyrus of the rat I. Normal structure with special reference to synaptic organization. *J. Comp. Neurol.,* 128:359–396.
56. Lee, K., Stanford, E., Cotman, C. W., and Lynch, G. S. (1977): Ultrastructural evidence for bouton sprouting in the adult mammalian brain. *Exp. Brain Res.,* 29:475–485.
57. Lewis, P. R., and Shute, C. C. D. (1967): The cholinergic limbic system: projection to hippocampal formation, medial cortex, nuclei of the ascending cholinergic reticular system, and the subfornical organ and supraoptic crest. *Brain,* 90:521–540.
58. Llinas, R., Hielman, D., and Precht, W. (1973): Neuronal circuit reorganization in mammalian agranular cerebellar cortex. *J. Neurobiol.,* 4:69–94.
59. Loesche, J., and Steward, O. (1977): Behavioral correlates of denervation and reinnervation of the hippocampal formation of the rat: recovery of alternation performance following unilateral entorhinal cortex lesions. *Brain Res. Bull.,* 2:31–39.
60. Lorente de Nó, R. (1934): Studies on the structure of the cerebral cortex. II. Continuation of the study of the ammonic system. *J. Psychol. Neurol. (Lpz.),* 46:113–177.
61. Loy, R., Cotman, C. W., and Lynch, G. S. (1977): The development of afferent lamination in the fascia dentata of the rat *Brain Res.,* 121:229–243.
62. Lund, R. D., and Lund, J. S. (1971): Synaptic adjustment after deafferentation of the superior colliculus of the rat. *Science,* 171:804–807.
63. Lynch, G., and Cotman, C. W. (1975): The hippocampus as a model for studying anatomical plasticity in the adult brain. In: *The Hippocampus, Vol. 1,* edited by R. L. Isaacson and K. H. Pribram, pp. 123–155. Plenum Press, New York.
64. Lynch, G., Gall, C., and Cotman, C. (1977): Temporal parameters of axon "sprouting" in the brain of the adult rat. *Exp. Neurol.,* 54:179–183.
65. Lynch, G., Gall, C., Rose, G., and Cotman, C. W. (1976): Changes in the distribution of the dentate gyrus associational system following unilateral or bilateral entorhinal lesion in the adult rat. *Brain Res.,* 110:57–71.
66. Lynch, G. S., Matthews, D. A., Mosko, S., Parks, T., and Cotman, C. W. (1972): Induced acetylcholinesterase-rich layer in rat dentate gyrus following entorhinal lesions. *Brain Res.,* 42:311–318.
67. Lynch, G. S., Mosko, S., Parks, T., and Cotman, C. W. (1973): Relocation and hyperdevelopment of the dentate gyrus commissural system after entorhinal lesions in immature rats. *Brain Res.,* 50:174–178.
68. Lynch, G., Rose, G., Gall, C., and Cotman, C. W. (1975): The response of the dentate gyrus to partial deafferentation. In: *Golgi Centennial Symposium Proceedings,* edited by M. Santini, pp. 505–517. Raven Press, New York.
69. Lynch, G., Stanfield, B., and Cotman, C. W. (1973): Developmental differences in post-lesion axonal growth in the hippocampus. *Brain Res.,* 59:155–168.
70. Lynch, G., Stanfield, B., Parks, T., and Cotman, C. W. (1974): Evidence for selective post-lesion axonal growth in the dentate gyrus of the rat. *Brain Res.,* 69:1–11.
71. Lømo, T. (1971): Patterns of activation in a monosynaptic cortical pathway: the perforant path input to the dentate area of the hippocampal formation. *Exp. Brain Res.,* 12:18–45.

72. Marchase, R. B. (1977): Biochemical investigations of retinotectal adhesive specificity. *J. Cell Biol.,* 75:237–257.
73. Marchase, R. B., Barbera, A. J., and Roth, S. (1975): A molecular approach to retinotectal specificity. In: *Cell Patterning, Ciba Foundation Symposium, Vol. 15.* A.S.P., Amsterdam.
74. Matthews, D. A., Cotman, C. W., and Lynch, G. (1976): An electron microscopic study of lesion-induced synaptogenesis in the dentate gyrus of the adult rat. I. Magnitude and time course of degeneration. *Brain Res.,* 115:1–21.
75. Matthews, D. A., Cotman, C., and Lynch, G. (1976): An electron microscopic study of lesion-induced synaptogenesis in the dentate gyrus of the adult rat. II. Reappearance of morphologically normal synaptic contacts. *Brain Res.,* 115:23–41.
76. Matthews, D. A. Nadler, J. V., Lynch, G. S., and Cotman, C. W. (1974): Development of cholinergic innervation in the hippocampal formation of the rat. I. Histochemical demonstration of acetylcholinesterase activity. *Develop. Biol.,* 36:130–141.
77. Matus, A. I., Walters, B. B., and Jones, D. H. (1975): Junctional ultrastructure in isolated synaptic membranes. *J. Neurocytol.,* 4:357–367.
78. Mays, L. E., and Best, P. J. (1975): Hippocampal unit activity to tonal stimuli during arousal from sleep and in awake rats. *Exp. Neurol.,* 47:268–279.
79. McCouch, G. P., Austin, G. M., Liu, C. -N., and Liu, C. Y. (1958): Sprouting as a cause of spasticity. *J. Neurophysiol.,* 21:205–216.
80. McWilliams, J. R., and Lynch, G. S. (1978): Terminal proliferation and synaptogenesis following partial deafferentation. *J. Comp. Neurol. (in press).*
81. Meibach, R. C., and Siegel, A. (1977): Efferent connections of the septal area in the rat: an analysis utilizing retrograde and anterograde transport methods. *Brain Res.,* 119:1–20.
82. Meibach, R. C., and Siegel, A. (1977): Efferent connections of the hippocampal formation in the rat. *Brain Res.,* 124:197–224.
83. Mellgren, S. I., and Srebro, B. (1973): Changes in acetylcholinesterase and distribution of degenerating fibres in the hippocampal region after septal lesions in the rat. *Brain Res.,* 52:19–36.
84. Merrell, R., Gottlieb, D. I., and Glaser, L. (1976): Membranes as a tool for the study of cell surface recognition. In: *Neuronal Recognition,* edited by S. Barondes, pp. 249–273. Plenum Press, New York.
85. Meyer, R. L., and Sperry, R. W. (1974): Explanatory models for neuroplasticity in retinotectal connections. In: *Plasticity and Recovery of Function in the Central Nervous System,* edited by D. G. Stein, J. J. Rosen, and N. Butters, pp. 45–63. Academic Press, New York.
86. Minckler, J., (editor) (1971): *Pathology of the Nervous System, Vol. 2.* McGraw-Hill, New York.
87. Moore, R. Y., and Halaris, A. E. (1975): Hippocampal innervation by serotonin neurons of the midbrain raphe in the rat. *J. Comp. Neurol.,* 164:171–184.
88. Mosko, S., Lynch, G. S., and Cotman, C. W. (1973): The distribution of septal projections to the hippocampus of the rat. *J. Comp. Neurol.,* 152:163–174.
89. Mugnaini, E. (1970): Neurons as synaptic targets. In: *Excitatory Synaptic Mechanisms,* edited by P. Andersen and J. K. S. Jansen, pp. 149–169. Universitetsforlag, Oslo, Norway.
90. Murray, M., and Goldberger, M. E. (1974): Restitution of function and collateral sprouting in the cat spinal cord: the partially hemisected animal. *J. Comp. Neurol.,* 158:19–36.
91. Nadler, J. V., Cotman, C. W., and Lynch, G. S. (1974): Biochemical plasticity of short-axon interneurons: increased glutamate decarboxylase activity in the denervated area of rat dentate gyrus following entorhinal lesion. *Exp. Neurol.,* 45:403–412.
92. Nadler, J. V., Cotman, C. W., and Lynch, G. S. (1977): Histochemical evidence of altered development of cholinergic fibers in the rat dentate gyrus following lesions. I. Time course after complete unilateral entorhinal lesion at various ages. *J. Comp. Neurol.,* 171:561–588.
93. Nadler, J. V., Cotman, C. W., Paoletti, C., and Lynch, G. S. (1977): Histochemical evidence of altered development of cholinergic fibers in the rat dentate gyrus following lesions. II. Effects of partial entorhinal and simultaneous multiple lesions. *J. Comp. Neurol.,* 171:589–604.
94. Nadler, J. V., Vaca, K. W., White, W. F., Lynch, G. S., and Cotman, C. W. (1976): Aspartate and glutamate as possible transmitters of excitatory hippocampal afferents. *Nature,* 260:538–540.
95. Nadler, J. V., White, W. F., Vaca, K. W., and Cotman, C. W. (1977): Calcium-dependent

γ-aminobutyrate release by interneurons of rat hippocampal regions: lesion-induced plasticity. *Brain Res.*, 131:241–258.

96. Nafstad, P. H. J. (1967): An electron microscope study of the termination of the perforant path fibres in the hippocampus and the fascia dentata. *Z. Zellforsch.*, 76:532–542.
97. Olson, L., Freedman, R., Seiger, Å., and Hoffer, B. J. (1977): Electrophysiology and cytology of hippocampal formation transplants in the anterior chamber of the eye. I. Intrinsic organization. *Brain Res.*, 119:87–106.
98. Parnavelas, J. G., Lynch, G., Brecha, N., Cotman, C. W., and Globus, A. (1974): Spine loss and regrowth in hippocampus following deafferentation. *Nature*, 248:71–73.
99. Pasquier, D. A., and Reinoso-Suarez, F. (1976): Direct projections from hypothalamus to hippocampus in the rat demonstrated by retrograde transport of horseradish peroxidase. *Brain Res.*, 108:165–169.
100. Pasquier, D. A., and Reinoso-Suarez, F. (1977): The differential efferent connections of the brain stem to the hippocampus in the cat. *Brain Res.*, 120:540–548.
101. Pickel, V. M., Segal, M., and Bloom, F. E. (1974): A radioautographic study of the efferent pathways of the nucleus locus coeruleus. *J. Comp. Neurol.*, 155:15–42.
102. Purves, D. (1976): Functional and structural changes in mammalian sympathetic neurons following colchicine application to post-ganglionic nerve. *J. Physiol.*, 259:159–175.
103. Purves, D. and Njå, A. (1978): Trophic maintenance of synaptic connections in autonomic ganglia. In: *Neuronal Plasticity*, edited by C. Cotman. Raven Press, New York.
104. Raisman, G. (1969): Neuronal plasticity in the septal nuclei of the adult rat. *Brain Res.*, 14:25–48.
105. Raisman, G., Cowan, W. M., and Powell, T. P. S. (1965): The extrinsic afferent, commissural and association fibres of the hippocampus. *Brain*, 88:963–998.
106. Raisman, G., and Field, P. (1973): A quantitative investigation of the development of collateral reinnervation after partial deafferentation of the septal nuclei. *Brain Res.*, 50:241–264.
107. Rakic, P. (1971): Neuron-glia relationship during granule cell migration in developing cerebellar cortex. A Golgi and electron microscopic study in Macacus rhesus. *J. Comp. Neurol.*, 141:283–312.
108. Ramón y Cajal, S. (1968): *Degeneration and Regeneration of the Nervous System*, translated by R. M. May. Hafner, New York.
109. Ramón y Cajal, S. (1968): *The Structure of Ammon's Horn*, translated by L. M. Kraft. Charles C Thomas, Springfield, Illinois.
110. Rees, R. P., Bunge, M. B., and Bunge, R. P. (1976): Morphological changes in the neurite growth cone and target neuron during synaptic junction development in culture. *J. Cell Biol.*, 68:240–263.
111. Roper, S. (1976): Sprouting and regeneration of synaptic terminals in the frog cardiac ganglion. *Nature*, 261:148–149.
112. Rose, A. M., Hattori, T., and Fibiger, H. C. (1976): Analysis of the septohippocampal pathway by light and electron microscopic autoradiography. *Brain Res.*, 108:170–174.
113. Rose, G., Lynch, G., and Cotman, C. W. (1976): Hypertrophy and redistribution of astrocytes in the deafferented dentate gyrus. *Brain Res. Bull.*, 1:87–92.
114. Roth, S., and Marchase, R. B. (1976): An *in vitro* assay for retinotectal specificity. In: *Neuronal Recognition*, edited by S. Barondes, pp. 227–248. Plenum Press, New York.
115. Scheff, S., Benardo, L., and Cotman, C. (1977): Progressive brain damage accelerates axon sprouting in the adult rat. *Science*, 197:795–797.
116. Scheff, S. W., Benardo, L. S., and Cotman, C. W. (1978): Effect of serial lesions on sprouting in the dentate gyrus: onset and decline of the catalytic effect. *Brain Res. (in press)*.
117. Scheff, S. W., and Cotman, C. W. (1977): Recovery of spontaneous alternation following lesions of the entorhinal cortex in adult rats: possible correlation to axon sprouting. *Behav. Biol.*, 21:286–293.
118. Schlessinger, A. R., Cowan, W. M., and Gottlieb, D. I. (1975): An autoradiographic study of the time of origin and the pattern of granule cell migration in the dentate gyrus of the rat. *J. Comp. Neurol.*, 159:149–176.
119. Schneider, G. E. (1973): Early lesions of superior colliculus: factors affecting the formation of abnormal retinal projections. *Brain Behav. Evol.*, 8:73–109.
120. Schwartzkroin, P. A., and Wester, K. (1975): Long-lasting facilitation of a synaptic potential following tetanization in the *in vitro* hippocampal slice. *Brain Res.*, 89:107–119.

121. Segal, M. (1975): Physiological and pharmacological evidence for a serotonergic projection to the hippocampus: *Brain Res.,* 94:115–131.
122. Segal, M., and Bloom, F. E. (1974): The action of norepinephrine in the rat hippocampus. II. Activation of the input pathway. *Brain Res.,* 72:99–114.
123. Segal, M., and Landis, S. (1974): Afferents to the hippocampus of the rat studied with the method of retrograde transport of horseradish peroxidase. *Brain Res.,* 78:1–15.
124. Seiger, Å., and Olson, L. (1977): Reinitiation of directed nerve fiber growth in central monamine neurons after intraocular maturation. *Exp. Brain Res.,* 29:15–44.
125. Shute, C. C. D., and Lewis, P. R. (1963): Cholinesterase-containing systems of the brain of the rat. *Nature,* 199:1160–1166.
126. Shute, C. C. D., and Lewis, P. R. (1966): Electron microscopy of cholinergic terminals and acetylcholinesterase-containing neurones in the hippocampal formation of the rat. *Z. Zellforsch.,* 69:334–343.
127. Sotelo, C. (1973): Permanence and fate of paramembranous synaptic specializations in mutants and experimental animals. *Brain Res.,* 62:345–352.
128. Sperry, R. W. (1963): Chemoaffinity in the orderly growth of nerve fiber patterns and connections. *Proc. Natl. Acad. Sci. USA,* 50:703–710.
129. Stenevi, U., Björklund, A., and Svendgaard, N. -A. (1976): Transplantation of central and peripheral monoamine neurons to the adult rat brain: techniques and conditions for survival. *Brain Res.,* 114:1–20.
130. Steward, O. (1976): Topographic organization of the projections from the entorhinal area to the hippocampal formation of the rat. *J. Comp. Neurol.,* 167:285–314.
131. Steward, O. (1976): Reinnervation of dentate gyrus by homologous afferents following entorhinal cortical lesions in adult rats. *Science,* 194:426–428.
132. Steward, O., Cotman, C. W., and Lynch, G. S. (1973): Re-establishment of electrophysiologically functional entorhinal cortical input to the dentate gyrus deafferented by ipsilateral entorhinal lesions: innervation by the contralateral entorhinal cortex, *Exp. Brain Res.,* 18:396–414.
133. Steward, O., Cotman, C. W., and Lynch, G. S. (1974): Growth of a new fiber projection in the brain of adult rats: reinnervation of the dentate gyrus by the contralateral entorhinal cortex following ipsilateral entorhinal lesions. *Exp. Brain Res.,* 20:45–66.
134. Steward, O., Cotman, C., and Lynch, G. (1976): A quantitative autoradiographic and electrophysiological study of the reinnervation of the dentate gyrus by the contralateral entorhinal cortex following ipsilateral entorhinal lesions. *Brain Res.,* 114:181–200.
135. Steward, O., Loesche, J., and Horten, W. C. (1977): Behavioral correlates of denervation and reinnervation of the hippocampal formation of the rat: open field activity and cue utilization following bilateral entorhinal cortex lesions. *Brain Res. Bull.,* 2:41–48.
136. Steward, O., and Scoville, S. A. (1976): Cells of origin of entorhinal cortical afferents to the hippocampus and fascia dentata of the rat. *J. Comp. Neurol.,* 169:347–370.
137. Steward, O., White, W. F., and Cotman, C. W. (1977): Potentiation of the excitatory synaptic action of commissural, associational and entorhinal afferents to dentate granule cells, *Brain Res.,* 134:551–560.
138. Storm-Mathisen, J. (1970): Quantitative histochemistry of acetylcholinesterase in rat hippocampal region correlated to histochemical staining. *J. Neurochem.,* 17:739–750.
139. Storm-Mathisen, J. (1972): Glutamate decarboxylase in the rat hippocampal region after lesions of the afferent fibre systems. Evidence that the enzyme is localized in intrinsic neurones. *Brain Res.,* 40:215–235.
140. Storm-Mathisen, J. (1974): Choline acetyltransferase and acetylcholinesterase in fascia dentata following lesion of the entorhinal afferents. *Brain Res.,* 80:181–197.
141. Storm-Mathisen, J. (1976): Distribution of the components of the GABA system in neuronal tissue: cerebellum and hippocampus—effects of axotomy. In: *GABA in Nervous System Function,* edited by E. Roberts, T. N. Chase, and D. B. Tower, pp. 149–168. Raven Press, New York.
142. Storm-Mathisen, J., and Blackstad, T. W. (1964): Cholinesterase in the hippocampal region. *Acta Anat.,* 56:216–253.
143. Svendgaard, N. -A., Björklund, A., and Stenevi, U. (1976): Regeneration of central cholinergic neurones in the adult brain. *Brain Res.,* 102:1–22.
144. Swanson, L. W., and Cowan, W. M. (1977): An autoradiographic study of the organization of the efferent connections of the hippocampal formation in the rat. *J. Comp. Neurol.,* 172:49–84.

145. Swanson, L. W., and Hartman, B. K. (1975): The central adrenergic system. An immunofluorescence study of the location of cell bodies and their efferent connections in the rat utilizing dopamine-β-hydroxylase as a marker. *J. Comp. Neurol.,* 163:467–506.

146. Teyler, T. J., and Alger, B. E. (1976): Monosynaptic habituation in the vertebrate forebrain. The dentate gyrus examined *in vitro. Brain Res.,* 115:413–425.

147. Therien, H. M., and Mushinski, W. E. (1976): Isolation of synaptic junctional complexes of high structural integrity from rat brain. *J. Cell Biol.,* 71:807–822.

148. West, J. R., Deadwyler, S. A., Cotman, C. W., and Lynch, G. S. (1975): Time-dependent changes in commissural field potentials in the dentate gyrus following lesions of the entorhinal cortex in adult rats. *Brain Res.,* 97:215–233.

149. White, W. F., Cotman, C. W., Goldowitz, D., and Lynch, G. S. (1976): Electrophysiological analysis of the projection from the contralateral entorhinal cortex to the dentate gyrus in normal rats. *Brain Res.,* 114:201–209.

150. White, W. F., Nadler, J. V., Hamberger, A., Cotman, C. W., and Cummins, J. T. (1977): Glutamate as transmitter of the hippocampal perforant path. *Nature,* 270:356–357.

151. Williams, T. H., Jew, J., and Palay, S. L. (1973): Morphological plasticity in the sympathetic chain. *Exp. Neurol.,* 39:181–203.

152. Wong-Riley, M. T. T. (1972): Changes in the dorsal lateral geniculate nucleus of the squirrel monkey after unilateral ablation of the visual cortex. *J. Comp. Neurol.,* 146:519–548.

153. Yamamoto, C., and Kawai, N. (1967): Presynaptic action of acetylcholine in thin sections from the guinea pig dentate gyrus *in vitro. Exp. Neurol.,* 19:176–187.

154. Zimmer, J. (1971): Ipsilateral afferents to the commissural zone of the fascia dentata, demonstrated in decommissurated rats by silver impregnation. *J. Comp. Neurol.,* 142:393–416.

155. Zimmer, J. (1973): Extended commissural and ipsilateral projections in postnatally deentorhinated hippocampus and fascia dentata demonstrated in rats by silver impregnation. *Brain Res.,* 64: 293–311.

156. Zimmer, J. (1974): Proximity as a factor in the regulation of aberrant axonal growth in postnatally deafferented fascia dentata. *Brain Res.,* 72:137–142.

157. Zimmer, J., and Hjorth-Simonsen, A. (1975): Crossed pathways from the entorhinal area to the fascia dentata. II. Provokable in rats. *J. Comp. Neurol.,* 161:71–102.

Neuronal Plasticity, edited by
Carl W. Cotman.
Raven Press, New York © 1978.

Effects of Cortical Denervation and Stimulation on Axons, Dendrites, and Synapses

L. T. Rutledge

Department of Physiology, University of Michigan, Ann Arbor, Michigan 48109

In the clinical literature it has been known for some time that recovery can occur following injury to certain regions of the human CNS (21), but until recently considerations of compensatory mechanisms revolved entirely around aspects of clinical recovery with little understanding of the underlying basic processes. Rosner (21) cites four recent developments which have aided in understanding the mechanism underlying the recovery of function: a rediscovery of the use of seriatim lesions, considerations of supersensitivity in denervated receptors in the CNS, use of drugs to facilitate recovery, and observations of axonal growth in damaged CNS neurons. In my opinion these do not represent equally fruitful approaches for revealing the mechanisms underlying recovery of function. We must be ultimately concerned with finding means to facilitate compensatory processes following lesions whether it is by injecting certain drugs, by specific retraining, or by using direct electrical stimulation.

Our studies have been directed toward the investigation of the effect of electrical stimulation on the reorganization of structure and function in the partially neuronally isolated cerebral cortex. This preparation originally investigated by Cajal (3) provides a means to investigate plasticity in a sophisticated brain area and to manipulate it experimentally. Our studies have provided good evidence that experimental excitation of neural elements by direct electrical stimulation has distinctive structural and perhaps beneficial effects.

UNDERCUT CORTEX PREPARATION

Various methods have been used to partially or completely isolate a portion of neocortex. One or more gyri in an experimental animal may be completely neuronally isolated by undercutting at a desired depth and introducing subpial cuts to maintain pial blood supply. A modification of this technique, which is perhaps less traumatic, is to undercut some or all cortical layers such that gray matter bridges are left intact at the ends of the undercut area. We have used the latter procedure since slab stimulation apparently can result in activation of nonundercut cortex via the intact ends (24).

We undercut the cerebral cortex in cats by entering the cortex on the lateral aspect of the cerebral hemisphere, in the most lateral edge of the suprasylvian gyrus (or in ectosylvian gyrus), and passing a dull cutting tool 4 to 5 mm under the cortex to the midline for a length of 20 mm. Bipolar stimulating and recording electrodes could be implanted in or over the undercut tissue (marginal gyrus). Two procedures have been used to study the effects of chronic electrical stimulation to the slab. In one procedure the undercut area is stimulated daily. Daily stimulation usually consisted of 20 2-sec trains of symmetric biphasic pulses (0.5 msec each direction) at 50 Hz and spaced at 1-min intervals. Total

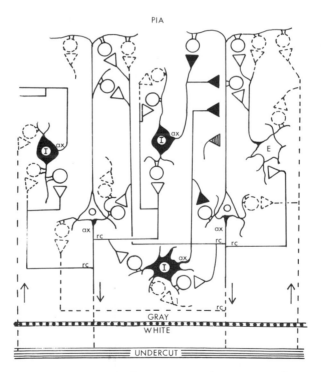

FIG. 1. Effects of cortical undercutting. Only two types of neurons are shown, pyramidal cells and generalized stellate cells. Excitatory elements, clear; inhibitory, darkened or hatched. Degenerated structures indicated by *dashed lines*. Note marked postsynaptic spine loss, some presynaptic elements not identifiable (e.g., 1, *lower center*). The hatched, inhibitory terminal on pyramidal cell dendritic shaft *(right center)* is a new synaptic element, but presynaptic source is unknown. Arrows depict afferent and efferent axons. ax, Axon; rc, recurrent collateral. I, inhibitory stellate cells. E, excitatory stellate cell.

stimulation was about 400 pulses at 0.6 mA, 400 at 0.8 mA, and 200 at 1.0 mA, all constant current. In the other procedure the cat was trained to make foot flexion responses to a conditional electrical stimulus (CS) when the CS was brain stimulation. The cat was trained to the CS then, following undercut surgery, retraining was started. As far as the excitable properties of undercut cortex were concerned, prevention of supersensitivity and hyperexcitability occurred with or without training (27). Because of these and other observations, effects of stimulation were studied without behavioral training.

Figure 1 shows some of the effects of cortical undercutting of several months duration upon neuronal structure. All afferent axons and their synaptic elements had degenerated. This included at least some of the receptive postsynaptic processes served by the incoming axon terminals. Retrograde degeneration of efferent axons adversely affected some neurons to the point of death and resorption, while others showed persistent chromatolysis.

The more subtle degenerative changes to be described in detail below will be called those of "denervation," which includes deafferentation and deefferentation. It is likely that stability of cortical neuronal structure, at least for those elements that have been studied, is reached in 2 months (33) or less (11). However, in terms of functional stability partially isolated frontal cortex may continue to develop "more supersensitivity" for many months (7). We have no evidence that excitability changes continue to increase in undercut marginal or suprasylvian gyri beyond about 2 months.

LIGHT MICROSCOPY

Effect of Denervation

Using a Golgi-Cox method of tissue impregnation, several distinct features of neurons in chronic undercut cortex have been described (22,39). Most obvious were the contorted, beady dendritic shafts which were usually deficient in dendritic spines (Fig. 2). These features were readily seen on small- to medium-sized pyramidal neurons in the upper cortical layers. There were large losses of dendritic spines on the major vertical dendrites and apical terminal dendrites of the pyramidal cells (average 41%, Table 1) (Fig. 1). In an independent study a 43% spine loss was found on apical dendrites of layers II, III, and IV (2). In our subsequent work approximately 50% of apical dendritic spines disappeared in layer II (26). Undoubtedly much of this spine loss occurred as a result of deafferentation. The loss was mainly on pyramidal cell basal dendrites, apical dendritic shaft branches, and terminals and stellate cells (Fig. 1). Spines also receive synapses from the intrinsic axons of stellate cells and axon recurrent collaterals (rc) of pyramidal cells. Consequently a study of the pyramidal cell axon rc's was later undertaken to determine the extent of loss resulting from deafferentation and retrograde degeneration (25). Three measures of pyramidal cell axon rc's in cells of layers II and III were made: the average length of

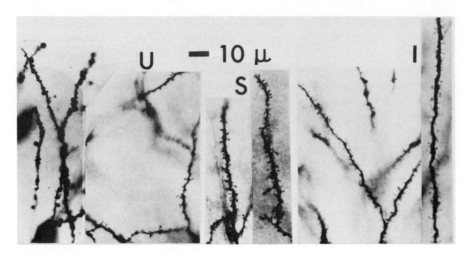

FIG. 2. Terminal twigs of apical dendrites of layer II pyramidal cells. Undercut, U; stimulated undercut, S; intact, I. Modified Golgi-Cox preparation (From Rutledge (22). Copyright © 1969, Little, Brown.)

the two longest collaterals, the number of collaterals, and the number of branch points. Only the latter proved to be reliable. Undercutting resulted in a significant loss of axon rc branch points (Table 2). Suggested locations of these losses are shown in Fig. 1, but it is not known what portion of the 29% loss represents loss of rc terminals on interneurons, apical dendritic spines, or spines on basal dendrites.

Effects of Denervation and Stimulation

From the conditioning experiments, it was apparent that an electrical CS applied to undercut cortex over many weeks produced significant functional

TABLE 1. *Dendritic spines in intact, undercut, and stimulated undercut cortex*

	Spines/10 μm	Comparisons	% Difference	*p*
Major vertical dendrites				
I	6.2	I–UC	42	0.001
UC	3.6	I–UCS	32	0.001
UCS	4.2	UC–UCS	17	0.02
Apical terminal dendrites				
I	11.5	I–UC	40	0.001
UC	6.9	I–UCS	7	0.001
UCS	10.7	UC–UCS	55	0.001

I, intact; UC, undercut; UCS, stimulated undercut cortex.
p, Significance level of mean differences.

TABLE 2. *Measurement of pyramidal cell axon recurrent collateral branch points in intact, undercut, and stimulated undercut cortex*

	Number of branches	Comparisons	% Difference	p
I	4.2	I–UC	29	<0.01
UC	3.0	I–UCS	17	NS
UCS	3.5	UC–UCS	17	NS

Abbreviations as in Table 1.
p, Significance level; NS, not significant.

changes (24). Histology using Nissl and Weil stains gave no clue as to possible structural alterations. With the Golgi method important quantitative and qualitative differences were found in stimulated undercut cortex (Tables 1, 2; Fig. 2). The loss of spines on major vertical dendrites was 10% less than with no stimulation, but still significantly below the value for normal, intact cortex. For spines on apical dendritic terminals the loss, with stimulation, was only 7%, as compared with 40% in the unstimulated undercut cortex (Table 1). Thus, chronic electrical stimulation, on the average, prevented all but 7% of the apical dendritic spine loss expected with undercutting alone.

It is not known what proportion of the 40% apical dendritic spine loss in undercut cortex is caused by loss of primary afferents, but it is very likely to be more than 7%. This is an important consideration since if electrical stimulation preserves only those apical terminal spines receiving intrinsic axons then the proportion of afferent axons can be no more than 7% of those lost with undercutting. Any "preservation" greater than this must represent in part not preservation but rather the appearance of new spines! To clarify this interpretation further, consider an example in which one-half of the apical spines remaining after undercutting had previously contacted afferent axons (20% afferent loss, 20% intrinsic loss). If there is only a 7% afferent loss with stimulation, then 13% (20 minus 7) must be accounted for as a result of stimulation. Thus allowing that the full 20% of the intrinsic spines were lost following surgery, then 13% of the spines "preserved" were actually new spines. Any assumption of more than 7% afferents (out of the 40% lost) to apical dendritic terminals must represent the portion of newly created spines as a result of chronic stimulation. This interpretation will be discussed again with the electron microscopic observations below.

Chronic electrical stimulation also had a "preservative" effect upon branches of pyramidal cell axon rc's (Table 2). There was a 17% (statistically insignificant) loss of collateral branches, compared with a 29% loss without stimulation. Stimulation then prevented at least 12% of the "expected" loss which occurred with undercutting alone. If axon collateral branches were preserved, it might be thought that total collateral lengths would be maintained, yet we have found no solid quantitative evidence for this. The Golgi procedure is probably an

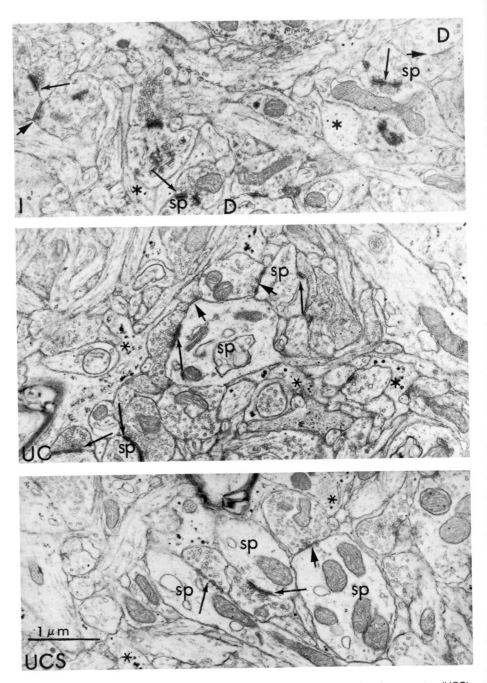

FIG. 4. Electron micrographs of intact (I), undercut (UC), and stimulated undercut cortex (UCS), all from the upper 750 μm. Areas were selected to show common synaptic elements for comparisons. D, dendritic shaft; sp, spine; *, neuroglial processes. *Long arrows,* asymmetric membrane contacts; *arrowheads,* symmetric contacts. Approximately ×19,000.

tric membrane contacts and more synapses on dendritic shafts. Chronic stimulation of denervated cortex resulted in more symmetric membrane contacts, more flat- and mixed vesicle-containing terminals, larger terminal boutons, more synapses on dendritic shafts and spines, and longer asymmetric and symmetric synaptic membrane contacts. The expected decrease in asymmetric contacts was prevented.

Qualitative Observations

Major differences among the three types of tissues were not found. This is apparent in the electron micrographs of Fig. 4 from intact, undercut, and stimulated undercut cortex. Synaptic elements appear to be about the same in all three. Round vesicle-containing terminals associated with asymmetric membrane appositions and flat vesicle profiles with symmetric membrane contacts were found in all tissues. Normal appearing synapses were prevalent, and they were located on readily identifiable dendritic spines and shafts.

It was our impression that terminal boutons in undercut and stimulated undercut cortex contained more vesicles, whether round, flat or mixed, than did those in intact cortex. There were regions where boutons in undercut and stimulated undercut cortex seemed to be especially large, some exceeding 1.75 μm in diameter. Few boutons in intact cortex were larger than 1.25 μm. It was also our impression that in stimulated undercut cortex bouton profiles containing flat vesicles were the largest seen anywhere in cortex, about 2.0 μm in diameter. None of these unusually large boutons were selected for the micrograph in Fig. 4.

Finally, neuroglial processes were more prevalent in undercut cortex, chronically stimulated or not. Small, dark opacities, probably glycogen granules, were readily found in these elements (Fig. 4). Marked gliosis was most noticeable within about 50 μm from the pial surface in undercut cortex.

In general the qualitative appearance of cortical ultrastructure in undercut cortex was not remarkably different from intact. Subtle changes, as described, could only be determined after careful measurements.

DISCUSSION

The electron microscopic data illustrate that neural reorganization occurs in chronically undercut cortex. There was an increase in bouton area associated with synapses having symmetric membrane contacts and an increase in the number of contacts on dendritic shafts. These findings can be interpreted as evidence of reactive synaptogenesis (6). Larger terminals with flat vesicles are indicative of continued vesicle and terminal membrane production. Although this could be prompted by continued spontaneous neuronal electrical activity, this is unlikely because the spontaneous electrical activity of chronically undercut cortex is much reduced compared with that in intact. A 62% increase in synapses

14. Larramendi, L. M. H., Fickenscher, L., and Lemkey-Johnston, N. (1967): Synaptic vesicles of inhibitory and excitatory terminals in the cerebellum. *Science,* 156:967–969.
15. Lund, R. D., and Westrum, L. E. (1966): Synaptic vesicle differences after primary formalin fixation. *J. Physiol. (Lond.),* 185:7–9.
16. Lynch, G. S., Mosko, S., Parks, T., and Cotman, C. W. (1973): Relocation and hyperdevelopment of the dentate gyrus commissural system after entorhinal lesions in immature rats. *Brain Res.,* 50:174–178.
17. Matthews, D. A., Cotman, C., and Lynch, G. (1976): An electron microscopic study of lesion-induced synaptogenesis in the dentate gyrus of the adult rat. II. Reappearance of morphologically normal synaptic contacts. *Brain Res.,* 115:23–41.
18. Møllgaard, K., Diamond, M. C., Bennett, E. L., Rosenzweig, M. R., and Lindner, B. (1971): Quantitative synaptic changes with differential experience in rat brain. *Int. J. Neurosci.,* 2:113–128.
19. Moore, R. Y., Björklund, A., and Stenevi, U. (1974): Growth and plasticity of adrenergic neurons. In: *The Neurosciences: Third Study Program,* edited by F. O. Schmitt and F. G. Worden, pp. 961–977. M.I.T. Press, Cambridge.
20. Raisman, G., and Field, P. M. (1973): A quantitative investigation of the development of collateral reinnervation after partial deafferentation of the septal nuclei. *Brain Res.,* 50:241–264.
21. Rosner, B. S. (1974): Recovery of function and localization of function in historical perspective. In: *Plasticity and Recovery of Function in the Central Nervous System,* edited by Donald G. Stein, Jeffrey J. Rosen, and Nelson Butters, pp. 1–29. Academic Press, Inc., New York.
22. Rutledge, L. T. (1969): Effects of stimulation on isolated cortex. In: *Basic Mechanisms of the Epilepsies,* pp. 349–355. Little, Brown, and Company, Inc., Boston.
23. Rutledge, L. T. (1976): Synaptogenesis: effects of synaptic use. In: *Neural Mechanisms of Learning and Memory,* edited by M. R. Rosenzweig and E. L. Bennett, pp. 329–339. M.I.T. Press, Cambridge.
24. Rutledge, L. T., and Doty, R. W. (1962): Surgical interference with pathways mediating responses conditioned to cortical stimulation. *Exp. Neurol.,* 6:478–491.
25. Rutledge, L. T., Duncan, J. A., and Beatty, N. (1969): A study of pyramidal cell axon collaterals in intact and partially isolated adult cerebral cortex. *Brain Res.,* 16:15–22.
26. Rutledge, L. T., Duncan, J. A., and Cant, N. (1972): Long-term status of pyramidal cell axon collaterals and apical dendritic spines in denervated cortex. *Brain Res.,* 41:249–262.
27. Rutledge, L. T., Ranck, J. B., Jr., and Duncan, J. A. (1967): Prevention of supersensitivity in partially isolated cerebral cortex. *Electroencephalogr. Clin. Neurophysiol.,* 23:256–262.
28. Rutledge, L. T., Wright, C., and Duncan, J. A. (1974): Morphological changes in pyramidal cells of mammalian neocortex associated with increased use. *Exp. Neurol.,* 44:209–228.
29. Sharpless, S., and Halpern, L. (1962): The electrical excitability of chronically isolated cortex studied by means of permanently implanted electrodes. *Electroencephalogr. Clin. Neurophysiol.,* 14:224–255.
30. Stenevi, U., Björklund A., and Moore R. Y. (1973): Morphological plasticity of central adrenergic neurons. *Brain Behav. Evol.,* 8:110–134.
31. Steward, O., Cotman, C. W., and Lynch, G. S. (1974): Growth of a new fiber projection in the brain of adult rats: Re-innervation of the dentate gyrus by the contralateral entorhinal cortex following ipsilateral entorhinal lesions. *Exp. Brain Res.,* 20:45–66.
32. Steward, O., Cotman, C. W., and Lynch, G. S. (1976): A quantitative autoradiographic and electrophysiological study of the reinnervation of the dentate gyrus by the contralateral entorhinal cortex following ipsilateral entorhinal lesions. *Brain Res.,* 114:181–200.
33. Szentágothai, J. (1965): The synapses of short local neurons in the cerebral cortex. *Symp. Biol. Hung.,* 5:251–276.
34. Uchizono, K. (1968): Inhibitory and excitatory synapses in vertebrate and invertebrate animals. In: *Structure and Function of Inhibitory Neuronal Mechanisms,* edited by C. von Euler, S. Skoglund, and U. Söderberg, pp. 33–58. Pergamon Press, New York.
35. Ulmar, G., Vickers, G., Dowdall, M. J., and Neuhoff, V. (1976): Pre-fractionation of rat cortical nerve endings by experimental deafferentation. *Exp. Brain Res.,* 24:22.
36. Van Harreveld, A., and Fifkova, E. (1975): Swelling of dendritic spines in the fascia dentata after stimulation of the perforant fibers as a mechanism of post-tetanic potentiation. *Exp. Neurol.,* 49:736–749.

37. Walberg, F. (1968): Morphological correlates of postsynaptic inhibitory processes. In: *Structure and Function of Inhibitory Neuronal Mechanisms,* edited by C. von Euler, S. Skoglund, and U. Söderberg, pp. 7–12. Pergamon Press, New York.
38. Wall, P. D., and Egger, M. D. (1971): Formation of new connexions in adult rat brains after partial deafferentation. *Nature,* 232:542–545.
39. Westrum, L. E., White, L. E. Jr., and Ward, A. A. Jr. (1964): Morphology of the experimental epileptic focus. *Neurosurgery,* 21:1033–1046.

Neuronal Plasticity, edited by
Carl W. Cotman.
Raven Press, New York © 1978.

Developmental Biology of Brain Damage and Experience

*Patricia S. Goldman and **†Michael E. Lewis

*Laboratory of Neuropsychology, National Institute of Mental Health, Bethesda, Maryland 20014; and **†Section on Intermediary Metabolism, Laboratory of Developmental Neurobiology, National Institute of Child Health and Human Development, Bethesda, Maryland 20014*

INTRODUCTION

The importance of experience for the development of behavior and for the maturation of the central nervous system in normal individuals is widely recognized (for reviews, see refs. 1,31,93). Only recently, however, it has become clear that experience may play an equally important though as yet poorly defined role in neuropathological development. A growing number of studies have provided evidence that recovery of function following brain injury in early life does not necessarily occur spontaneously but rather depends on the opportunities that the environment provides for stimulation during the course of postoperative development. The recognition that environmental stimulation may be a potent factor governing an organism's capacity to compensate for brain injury raises certain hopes for the treatment of brain injury and also poses some basic questions about the mechanisms by which functions are restored in a damaged nervous system (125). The aim of this chapter is to review briefly some of the evidence relating to the effects of experience on recovery of function with emphasis on findings from recent research on infrahuman primates, to consider a number of explanations that have been proposed to account for behavioral plasticity, and finally to propose a neurobiological framework for analyzing the processes by which experience during formative periods of growth could influence the physiological substrates of recovery.

---

† Present Address: The Psychological Laboratory, University of Cambridge, Cambridge, England.

EVIDENCE THAT EXPERIENCE FACILITATES
RECOVERY OF FUNCTION

The influence of environmental stimulation on recovery from brain damage is discussed in recent reviews (125). In what follows here, we limit ourselves to the special case of surgical lesions performed in immature animals and to the effects of experience given during the course of their postoperative development. The first experimental studies relating early experience to symptomology following brain injury were performed at McGill University nearly 25 years ago in the laboratory of D. O. Hebb. Hebb was concerned with the surprising observation that IQ scores often remained normal in patients that had undergone various forms of neurosurgery, including frontal lobotomy. He postulated that those forms of intelligence that permit an organism to approach a problem in different ways were the product of varied experience during development and relatively resistant to brain injury (49). As part of a broad program of research on the contributions of experience to intelligence, Lansdell (64) subjected rats to anterior or posterior cortical ablations as infants or as adults and kept them in enriched environments for 3 months to determine if such rearing would offset the expected behavioral deficits. Smith's (108) later investigations in the same laboratory analyzed the effects of cortical lesions in rats raised under impoverished conditions as compared with enriched environments. Taken together, the two studies provided support for the idea that enriched rearing conditions could ameliorate behavioral deficits following bilateral cortical lesions performed in weanling rats; later the finding that experience offset brain injuries was extended to rats incurring cortical lesions at birth (103,127) and to young animals with subcortical lesions (17,54).

The salutary impact of experience appears to depend upon a number of factors possibly including the extent to which there is a match between the postoperative environment and the measures used to assess subsequent behavioral status. Beneficial consequences of environmental complexity have been most clearly shown in studies in which brain-injured rats were raised in enriched environments and then subsequently tested on maze problems (64,103,108,127,128). In contrast, rearing in enriched environments does not benefit visual discrimination performance after total visual cortical lesions (5), and dark- or light-rearing is likewise inconsequential for performance on a pattern discrimination task (118). The evidence that enriched environments provide a postoperative milieu more conducive to maze learning than to discrimination learning led Greenough et al. (41) to suggest that the effects of experience are highly specific, i.e., depend upon the extent to which skills acquired in the rearing environment can be carried over to the test situation.

A number of studies on adult animals, however, have pointed to a nonspecific function for the postoperative sensory environment. Of special interest are the findings of Harrell et al. (48) that rats with hypothalamic lesions recover feeding behavior more quickly if exposed to daily 1-hr episodes of low-level electrical stimulation through lesion electrodes. Likewise there is evidence that recovery of visuomotor functions can be enhanced by centrally active drugs given postoperatively (72,79,126) or between serially imposed lesions (10). Recovery of visual functions has followed experiences as dissimilar as noise (10,56) and light (10, 56,76). All of these studies provide evidence for the importance of a general level of CNS activation in resilience to brain injury. However, since age of subject, type and size of lesion, rearing history, and behavioral task are all confounded in the research that has been conducted to date, an evaluation of the features of experience that are critical for protecting against brain injury must await further experimentation.

Experimental evidence on the role of early experience in recovery from local brain damage has come predominantly from studies of rodents (41). These studies have provided evidence that experience counteracts brain trauma, but in general, the environmental effects have not been impressive in magnitude. Recently, evidence that early experience may have profound effects on the course of recovery from brain damage has been obtained in rhesus monkeys whose cerebral organization, parameters of development, and capacity for complex behavior are more similar to those of man. Accordingly, special emphasis is given here to the studies on infrahuman primates. The major findings from these studies may be summarized as follows.

First, the return of some abilities after brain injury in early life depends heavily upon experience. Rhesus monkeys given orbital prefrontal cortical lesions as adults typically exhibit severe impairments on a spatial alternation test (29, 57,80). However, rhesus monkeys given the same lesion as infants can perform as well as normal monkeys when they reach two years of age, but *only* if they have received prior training on a series of cognitive tasks during development (32). Without such prior test experience, monkeys given the equivalent lesions as infants fail to learn the delayed alternation task when they reach two years of age (Fig. 1). For the conditions under review, the effect is all-or-none.

Second, the impact of formal test experience in promoting recovery is directly related to the age of the subject when the brain injury is sustained (32). If equivalent postoperative experience is provided for monkeys operated as infants or as adults, recovery of function is exhibited only by those operated as infants. Again, the effect is all-or-none (Fig. 2).

Third, the effectiveness of experience in promoting recovery appears to be related to the age at which it is given (32). Monkeys whose orbital prefrontal cortex was resected at 2 months of age tend to achieve higher recovery scores on the spatial task if the same kind and amount of experience is allowed earlier, rather than later, in the course of their postoperative development (Fig. 3). It is not known, however, if the greater effectiveness of the earlier experience is due to its temporal proximity to the injury or whether, in absolute terms, there exist sensitive or critical periods for these effects.

Fourth, if brain damage is extensive or includes critical areas, recovery does not occur in spite of the opportunity for extensive postoperative test experience

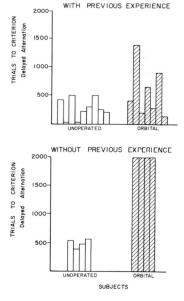

FIG. 1. Upper: Trials-to-criterion scores on a spatial delayed alternation test of 2-year-old monkeys that were raised in a primate colony from infancy and tested on a variety of cognitive tests between 12–18 months of age. **Lower:** Trials-to-criterion scores on the same task of monkeys reared under identical circumstances as those shown in the upper panel except that they were not previously tested on the cognitive tasks. *Open bars,* unoperated monkeys. *Striped* bars, monkeys given bilateral orbital prefrontal lesions at about 50 days of age.

(29). A striking example is given by the finding that monkeys whose dorsolateral prefrontal cortex is removed along with the orbital cortex (prefrontal lobectomy) do not exhibit any sign of learning spatial tasks at maturity, even when given the same kind and amount of experience as that which induces recovery following orbital prefrontal resections alone (29). Such findings indicate that the dorsola-

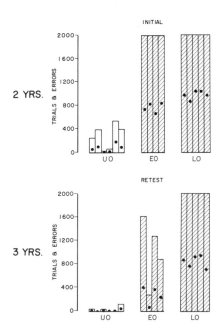

FIG. 2. Upper: Trials-to-criterion *(bars)* and errors-to-criterion *(dots)* of monkeys on the spatial delayed alternation task after orbital prefrontal lesions at around 50 days of age (EO) or after comparable lesions at around 18 months of age (LO). Unoperated controls are designated UO. The monkeys were about 27 months of age when initially tested on delayed alternation. Note that both early-operated and late-operated monkeys exhibit severe impairments at initial testing. **Lower:** Retest performance of the same groups 9–12 months later. Recovery of function was exhibited only by the early-operated group. The late-operated monkeys apparently did not benefit from prior test experience. Note that these animals were given a total of 4,000 trials—ample opportunity to exhibit improvement. (From ref. 32).

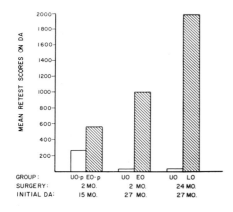

FIG. 3. Average trials-to-criterion scores on a *retest* of delayed alternation as a function of age at surgery and age at initial test. *Open bars,* unoperated controls. *Striped bars,* monkeys given bilateral orbital prefrontal lesions. Note that the retest performance of monkeys initially tested on delayed alternation at 15 months is better than that of monkeys initially tested at 27 months in spite of the fact that both groups were operated at the same age. Also noteworthy is the finding that prior experience on delayed alternation at 27 months is helpful only to the monkeys operated upon in infancy. (From ref. 32).

teral prefrontal area may be a critical neural substrate for mediating the environmentally facilitated recovery of function. Anatomical and physiological studies designed to examine this possibility are now in progress.

Finally, the salutary effects of experience on recovery are not reducible to training effects. To determine if the positive consequences of early experience are due to its specific content, monkeys with orbital prefrontal lesions and unoperated controls were trained on a nonspatial task as infants and examined on both a spatial and a nonspatial task as juveniles (35). As the nonspatial task was identical to that given in early life, the opportunity for savings as a result of direct experience was optimized for this test. The performance of the experienced monkeys was compared to that of operated and unoperated monkeys who had not received early training. Performance on both classes of tasks was predictably impaired by orbital lesions; however, in spite of the opportunity for test-retest savings, postoperative training in infancy ameliorated the spatial but not the nonspatial deficits caused by orbital prefrontal lesions (Fig. 4). The evidence that recovery of spatial functions can be fostered by a variety of different training histories, including one which actually reinforces nonspatial strategies, indicates that experience may act nonspecifically to offset deficits caused by circumscribed brain damage in primates. Therefore the effects of experience in these studies do not seem to be a simple matter of specific training or incidental learning related to familiarity with the testing situation.

The evidence that environmental stimulation may act nonspecifically is at variance with the hypothesis advanced by Greenough et al. (41) concerning the relationship between experience and its behavioral consequences. As mentioned, these authors suggested that experience acts by providing direct opportunities for training. Their review of the literature, however, was based largely on data from rats and on evidence from studies of adults as well as infants. Although there have been too few studies to decide these issues, it is possible that the degree of similarity between the postoperative milieu and the tests used to index recovery may be more critical for rodents than for primates, or alternatively, animals suffering brain injury as adults may have a greater depen-

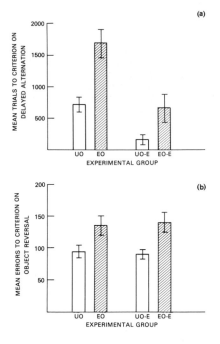

FIG. 4. Average performance of 15–18 month old monkeys on **(A)** the spatial delayed alternation task and **(B)** an object discrimination reversal task. UO, unoperated. EO, early-operated (prefrontal orbital lesions at 50 days). UO-E, unoperated with previous experience on the object reversal task. EO-E, early-operated with the same previous object reversal experience. The experienced groups (UO-E,EO-E) perform better than the inexperienced groups (UO,EO) on spatial delayed alternation. Experience does not benefit performance on the object reversal problem in spite of the opportunity for test-related savings. This finding and its interpretation is discussed further in Goldman and Mendelson, 1977. (From ref. 35).

dence on stimulus-response learning than animals in formative stages of their development. Methodological differences between the studies on rodents and primates may also give rise to different results. Experience, for example, takes quite different forms in the two classes of study. Stimulation in enriched environments is more global, but less control exists over which aspects of the environment or which experiences within it are enriching for brain-damaged animals. In the studies on primates, in contrast, experience is confined to specified cognitive tests, given under standardized conditions in which each animal must meet uniformly imposed requirements. These studies thus provide more control over the experiential variable and assure more commonality in the experience of individual subjects. Perhaps some of these factors account in part for differences in the impact of experience in studies on rodents and primates.

Although further investigations are clearly needed to unravel the relevant parameters of experience that encourage restitution of function, the evidence available from studies on both rats and monkeys indicates that experiential factors do play a role in minimizing the behavioral effects of focal brain injury sustained in early life. The studies on primates in particular suggest that the effects of experience can be powerful and that experience may produce its beneficial effects by providing a general level of stimulation rather than by encouraging the entrainment of specific habits. This evidence for a nonspecific facilitatory function of experience may provide a clue to some of the neural mechanisms involved in neurobehavioral plasticity.

EFFECTS OF DIFFERENTIAL EARLY EXPERIENCE
ON BRAIN MEASURES

The effects of early environmental experience on a variety of morphological and biochemical measures have been extensively reviewed (e.g., 1,81,93,124). This section will briefly cover findings which may be of particular interest from the viewpoint of behavioral recovery after brain damage. A later section will discuss these findings in relation to the effects of early experience on behavioral recovery.

The cerebral cortex of rats reared in enriched environments is heavier and thicker than the cortex of rats reared under less stimulating conditions (95). This overall difference has been attributed, in enriched rats, to increased glial cell number (15), enlarged neuronal cell bodies and nuclei (14), and augmented dendritic branch and spine formation (27,51,100). These morphological changes imply considerable activation of ribonucleic acid (RNA) and protein synthesis in the brains of rats exposed to enriched environments. In fact, such experience results in higher brain RNA content (21,94) and increased RNA diversity (43,121). Levitan, Mushynski, and Ramirez (66) reported that the incorporation of ^{3}H-leucine into four nuclear protein fractions from brain was increased in enriched rats, effects which may be related to genome expression. Whereas these biochemical studies only begin to hint at the central metabolic effects of enriched experience, the morphological studies clearly imply increased synthesis of structural proteins. Increased synthesis of enzymatic proteins may also occur, but further studies are required to examine this possibility.

The strongest evidence for environmental influences on brain development have come from the study of selective stimulation or deprivation in a single sensory modality. Although neural (and behavioral parameters) have been shown to be altered by perturbation of virtually every sense (for review, see ref. 81), the most striking results have been obtained in studies of the visual system. The functional and anatomical modifications resulting from alteration of visual input have been amply documented and are reviewed elsewhere (1,3,4,41,42, 53,85; see also Pettigrew, *this volume*). From the early demonstration by Chow et al. (7) that retinal ganglion cells of chimpanzees degenerate as a consequence of dark-rearing to the most recent evidence for anatomical alterations in the width of ocular dominance stripes in the striate cortex of monkeys that have been subjected to monocular deprivation (53), there exists overwhelming evidence that the early visual environment can modify the structure and function of connections in various regions of the mammalian visual system.

The results decribed thus far were obtained from experiments with unoperated animals. To date, there is little information on the effects of differential experience on brain anatomy or chemistry in brain-damaged organisms. However, in two recent studies of environmental influences on the effects of occipital cortical lesions in rats, enrichment was found to promote behavioral recovery and increase hemispheric length (127) and the ratio of RNA to deoxyribonucleic acid

(DNA) in ventral cortex (128). Since the quantity of DNA per cell is constant, and since lesion size between groups was reported to be the same, the altered RNA/DNA ratio may indicate increased synthesis (or decreased degradation) of RNA. The lengthening of the cerebral hemispheres, which is especially notable for having occurred only in operated, enriched rats, and not in unoperated controls, is likewise suggestive of increased metabolic activity.

In sum, there is morphological, physiological, and biochemical evidence for alteration of neural tissue in the brains of mammals subjected to a variety of environments during development. As will be discussed, this evidence has implications for mechanisms by which experience could affect the outcome of brain injury.

THEORIES OF RECOVERY

A variety of explanations have been offered to account for behavioral recovery after brain damage (e.g., 22,39,60,65,82). These explanations can be broadly categorized as behavioral or physiological, stressing, however, that such classification is more one of convenience than a valid description of processes that are in actuality dichotomous.

Behavioral explanations of recovery tend to emphasize that brain-damaged organisms can learn to employ alternate strategies or means for the accomplishment of some task. It is difficult to trace the origin of this idea to any single author, but the groundwork for such a concept is clearly evident in the work of Klüver (62), Kennard (61), and Hebb (49), among others. Probably because of its apparent simplicity and explanatory appeal, "substitution theory," as it is called, is often mentioned in the contemporary literature (28,78,96,119).

"Substitution theory" has not been formulated in very detailed or explicit terms; consequently, it has never been subjected to rigorous experimental examination, although numerous observations may be relevant to it, particularly those relating to experience. It is evident, for example, that experience provided during development could facilitate behavioral recovery in the brain injured by increasing the opportunity for an organism to form new strategies. As mentioned, the limited evidence available, at least from primates, does not actually provide support for such a view. Even if this attractive and simple model were to hold, still we would not have an adequate physiological explanation of recovery. It would be necessary to know in the experiments with monkeys, for example, why those operated as juveniles or young adults fail to benefit from experience to the same extent as those operated as infants, why brief experiences given at early stages of development may be more effective than more extensive experience at a later age, and what the neural basis of nonspecific environmental effects is. Any explanation of the mechanisms by which experience alters an organism's response to brain injury must account for these boundary conditions.

Physiological explanations of behavioral recovery after brain damage often invoke (a) disappearance of metabolic or neuroelectric abnormalities (diaschisis) in anatomically intact tissue, (b) reinnervation of denervated neurons, or (c) increased sensitivity of partially denervated neurons to remaining inputs (denervation supersensitivity). Each class of explanation is briefly decribed below.

Diaschisis

Damage to the central nervous system often results in depressed functioning in otherwise intact neural tissue. This phenomenon was first systematically explored by Sherrington (105) and has been referred to in classical neurology as "diaschisis" (82,86). Although the physiological basis of diaschisis is not understood, the phenomenon has been given empirical grounding in both animal and human studies (25,50,59,77,110), and testable properties of diaschisis have been postulated (68). The disappearance of electrical or metabolic depression in brain tissue could account for some instances of behavioral recovery (e.g., 25), including those hypothetical instances in which recovery is based on new strategies.

Neuronal Reinnervation

Destruction of presynaptic elements is followed, in some cases, by reinnervation of the denervated neurons by regenerating axons or spreading axon collaterals (13,47,69,115). Such reinnervation may result in behavioral recovery (13). However, reinnervation may also have adverse behavioral effects under some circumstances (101,102).

Denervation Supersensitivity

Deafferentation of neurons is sometimes followed by the increased sensitivity of such neurons to remaining inputs or exogenously applied chemicals (104, 113,130). The development of supersensitivity could compensate for the loss of some presynaptic elements and thus lead to behavioral recovery (26).

GENERAL FRAMEWORK: THE TROPHIC RESPONSE

Walsh and Cummins (124) have provided a convincing argument that the biochemical and anatomical changes in the brains of animals reared in stimulus-rich environments (e.g., 93) are a consequence of prolonged neurological arousal. Electrophysiological evidence (not mentioned by Walsh and Cummins) for increased neurological arousal following rich developmental experience has been provided by findings of shorter photic-evoked potential latencies in "enriched" rats (20,73). The neurological arousal response to rich sensorimotor experience, according to Walsh and Cummins, stimulates a variety of metabolic processes in the brain. In fact, considerable evidence has been obtained for increased metabolic activation in the brains of "enriched" rats (21,66,121). The "transduction" of neuroelectric activity to biosynthetic activity has received extensive recent attention. For example, proprioceptive, exteroceptive, or vestibular stimulation has been found to increase the RNA content of Purkinje cells in different cerebellar areas (58). For experimental convenience, the effects of neuronal stimulation on postsynaptic cellular metabolism are usually studied in peripheral systems. The release of acetylcholine with preganglionic nerve stimulation has been found to increase the apparent synthesis of RNA in rat sympathetic ganglia (24). Increased activity of afferent cholinergic axons resulted in enhanced incorporation of ^{3}H-uridine into RNA in rat adrenal medulla preceding the increased incorporation of ^{3}H-leucine into tyrosine hydroxylase (9). The demonstration of transsynaptic induction of a neurotransmitter-synthesizing enzyme has important implications for our understanding of the control of postsynaptic cells by presynaptic activity.

The long-term influences of neurons on their target cells (i.e., regulation of their metabolic activity) have been referred to as *trophic influences* (46,107). The elicitation of trophic responses has been closely scrutinized in a variety of cellular systems, and on the basis of these studies, Russell, Byus, and Manen (98) have proposed a general model of the sequential biochemical events of a trophic response. According to the model, the first event is sustained activation of adenylate cyclase by neurotransmitters, hormones, or drugs, followed by an increase in intracellular concentration of cyclic AMP. Subsequent activation of cyclic AMP-dependent protein kinase(s) results in the phosphorylation of acidic nuclear protein(s), leading to synthesis of new messenger RNA. The messenger RNA for ornithine decarboxylase is among the newly synthesized mRNA species. Ornithine decarboxylase is suggested to directly activate RNA polymerase I (see ref. 75), causing an increased rate of synthesis of ribosomal RNA, and thus, of protein. In addition, the induction of ornithine decarboxylase would increase synthesis of the polyamines (putrescine, spermidine, and spermine). Spermidine has been shown to stimulate RNA polymerase II from brain cell nuclei (106), which should result in enhanced synthesis of mRNA (131). In general, polyamines are potent stimulators of protein synthesis *in vitro* and *in vivo* (117) and appear to have a ubiquitous role in cellular growth and differentiation (97).

The Walsh-Cummins hypothesis may be extended to suggest that *rich or varied experience during development stimulates trophic responses in brain tissue, and further, that these trophic responses form the basis of the physiological events underlying behavioral recovery from early (and perhaps later) brain damage.* With special emphasis on diaschiasis, the following section examines how the stimulation of trophic responses could influence the proposed physiological mechanisms of recovery.

DIASCHISIS AS A LOSS OF TROPHIC INFLUENCES
FROM DESTROYED NEURONS

The loss of trophic influences from destroyed neurons after brain damage could lead to an overall depression, or disorganization, of postsynaptic cellular metabolism. Likewise, the degeneration of some postsynaptic cells could disrupt the ability of a presynaptic neuron to interact with its remaining postsynaptic cells. Both possibilities are exemplified by research with peripheral adrenergic neurons. Destruction of presynaptic cholinergic axons prevents the transsynaptic induction of tyrosine hydroxylase in developing postsynaptic adrenergic neurons in the superior cervical ganglion (2); a similar effect occurs if the target cells of the ganglion are removed (16), indicating the importance of retrograde trophic influences. The elimination of such influences from ganglionic neurons results in depressed synaptic transmission in the affected cells, a condition which can be reversed by intervention with exogenous nerve growth factor (87; see also Purves and Njå, *this volume*), a potent trophic agent (122). Diaschisis, considered as a loss of transsynaptic trophic influences, can also be demonstrated pharmacologically, as prolonged blockade of ganglionic beta-adrenergic receptors has been found to reduce ganglionic activity of tyrosine hydroxylase and dopamine-beta-hydroxylase (88).

The manifestations of hypotrophism discussed above are probably not restricted to peripheral neurons (19). Following brain damage, hypotrophic ("diaschitic") central neurons would function poorly (if at all), and thus contribute to the effective size of the lesion and the associated behavioral deficits. The elicitation of trophic responses (by whatever means) in the hypotrophic neurons would render them functional, and thereby eliminate whatever deficits were secondary to the condition of diaschisis. This outcome could be achieved, for example, by increased production of neurotransmitter-synthesizing enzymes. The trophic agent, nerve growth factor, is known to stimulate the synthesis of tyrosine hydroxylase (84,120), an effect which may be related to the behavioral recovery detected after administration of the protein to brain-damaged animals (67,116).

If enriched experience results in the stimulation of trophic responses in brain tissue (a view consistent with the evidence reviewed on pp. 292–298), the condition of diaschisis after brain damage could be reversed by such experience. Although we favor the reversal of diaschisis as an explanation of behavioral recovery, the possible role of neuronal reinnervation and denervation supersensitivity may also be considered. As discussed before, enriched experience results in enhanced production of dendritic branches and spines. This effect necessarily involves increased synthesis of structural proteins and of receptor proteins, assuming that the dendritic spines are functional. The proliferation of axon collaterals into denervated zones is analogous to dendritic proliferation; both phenomena reflect the outgrowth of neuronal processes. If enriched experience enhances dendritic proliferation, the spread of axon collaterals should also be facilitated.

If the synthesis of receptor proteins was also increased, the development of denervation supersensitivity could be promoted. This proposal follows from the finding that supersensitivity is associated with an increased number of receptor sites (12,112), an event requiring (in muscle) DNA-dependent RNA synthesis and protein synthesis (6,40). The effects of early experience on the density of receptor sites perhaps could be determined by studies of the specific binding of neurotransmitters or certain drugs to membrane preparations, as employed by Snyder (109) and his colleagues.

DEVELOPMENTAL CONSIDERATIONS

Any explanation of the mechanisms by which experience alters an organism's response to brain injury must account for the efficacy of early, as compared to later, experience. An attractive though not exclusive property of the trophic response hypothesis is that it can account for age differences in the effects of experience on behavioral recovery. First, the cyclic nucleotides (the apparent second messengers in the trophic response) exert a profound, age-dependent influence on the development of the nervous system and other tissues (71). Second, younger animals have a higher rate of synthesis of brain RNA (45) and protein (23). The slower rate of RNA synthesis in older animals has been suggested to be due to an age-dependent decrease in brain RNA polymerase activity, in concert with increasing activity of degradative enzymes, the nucleoside phosphorylases (44).

The potency of biosynthetic activity in younger animals may combine with other advantages of the immature to aid recovery of function. We have previously suggested (30) that animals with early lesions may recover functions to a greater extent than those with comparable tissue destruction sustained in adulthood because they might be less vulnerable to the secondary effects of brain injury. According to this view although the actual size of a lesion may be morphologically equivalent in infants and adults, the *effective* size of the lesion may differ substantially in animals of different ages. Accordingly, experience may be more successful in overcoming the effects of brain damage in younger animals because the consequences to be overcome are less severe.

Another more obvious and possibly the most crucial condition of immaturity is that the nervous system is not completely formed, and experience may have a decisive guiding and validating influence on the course of its future development. Timetables of maturation of course differ in different species. With regard to primates, however, although neurogenesis is virtually completed prenatally (89) and major tracts and pathways are well developed at birth (36,38,63), the formation of the neuropil and the elaboration of synaptic connections continue into the postnatal period. It is becoming clear that at birth or shortly after, there may actually be an overabundance of axons in the vicinity of a given target structure. For example, Innocenti et al. (55), using the axonally transported marker, horseradish peroxidase, recently described callosal projections from area 17 in the newborn kitten that are not demonstrable and presumably do not exist in adult cats. It is not known whether the visual cortex of the newborn monkey is similarly oversupplied by callosal connections. However, Goldman and Nauta (37) observed developmental changes in the callosal projections of frontal association cortex in monkeys that are consistent with oversupply. They described a columnar pattern of terminal distribution in these projections in newborn monkeys by the use of autoradiography. Of particular interest in the present context is the finding that the grain density and width of columns observed in autoradiograms appeared to diminish during postnatal development. Rakic (90,91) has recently shown that the central representation of the two eyes initially overlap in the visual cortex of the monkey fetus and only gradually become segregated into independent domains or ocular dominance stripes after birth. If, as all of these examples imply, more axons are directed at a target structure than will establish permanent synaptic linkages with the neurons comprising the structure, it is not unlikely that *activity or experience could regulate the number and stability of developing axons that survive the competition for terminal space.* Indeed, in the visual system it would appear that monocular deprivation does exactly that. Loss of visual input through one eye results in that eye being represented in the primary visual cortex by ocular dominance stripes of lesser width than those representing the experienced eye (53).

As implied by the foregoing discussion, the trophic response hypothesis can easily be extended to account for the impact of experience on the undamaged as well as the damaged brain. While it is beyond the scope of this chapter to develop this concept fully, brief mention should be made of its further applicability to normal development, again using the visual system for illustration. As is well known, one of the physiological consequences of monocular deprivation during sensitive periods of development is that it reduces the population of visual cortical neurons that can be driven binocularly (52). Thus, sensory loss through one eye renders these neurons hypofunctional or depressed in that they no longer respond equally well to stimuli through either eye. Duffy et al. (18) have recently made the intriguing observation that those neurons which are unresponsive to stimuli through the deprived eye could often be activated following intravenous injections of bicuculline, a gamma-aminobutyric acid (GABA)-receptor antagonist. The loss of responsiveness could be due to depressed activity of choline acetyltransferase in the lateral geniculate bodies and superior colliculi (174). The hypotrophic cholinergic neurons would presumably have reduced output of acetylcholine, a putative excitatory transmitter in the visual system (11,114). If the inhibitory (123) effects of GABA were blocked, the *relative* balance between excitation and inhibition might be restored, resulting in a return of visual function. This interpretation is subject to experimental test. For example, the effect of bicuculline on visual cortical neuronal responsivity should be reversed by cholinergic blockade. In any event, there may be an instructive parallel between inhibitory suppression of synaptic processes caused by "environmental deafferentation" and the loss of trophic influences in neuronal circuits caused by surgical deafferentation. With regard to the role of the environment at least, there is ample evidence that some of the effects of selective stimulation and/or deprivation can be reversed by extensive visual experience (8,42,111), just as the effects of lesions can be ameliorated by interaction with the environment. It is just possible, then, that the potent effects of experience and those of drugs like bicuculline are mediated by a common neuronal mechanism.

GENETIC CONSIDERATIONS

To date, species differences have not been given very serious consideration as a factor in the mode of response to central nervous system injury, but such differences may exist. First, there is a growing body of evidence that genetic variables play an important role in the response of the organism to "environmental injury," e.g., to the impact of sensory deprivation (for review, see ref. 41). A powerful illustration comes from studies of primates. Rosenblum and Kaufman (92) studied the reactions of infant monkeys to separation from their mother. In their now classic study of pigtail and bonnet macaques they obtained strong evidence that this form of reactive depression is species-typical and governed by genetic mechanisms. The recent demonstration that female rhesus monkeys exhibit less severe symptoms than do males following extreme or partial social deprivation is an equally compelling illustration of genetic factors at work (99). A second reason why genetic factors should be considered in reactions to brain injury is more direct. Deficits of different severity occur following brain injury in different species or strains of animals (e.g., 83,129) as well as in relation to gender (e.g., 33). Thirdly, thus far virtually all evidence for axonal regrowth after lesions has come from experiments in immature or fully adult small mammals in whom behavioral recovery from the same lesions is often undemonstrated (e.g., 70,115). In contrast, with the possible exception of anatomical changes following prenatal injuries (34), there has been no unequivocal demonstration of rearranged connections in the central nervous system of primates, who exhibit behavioral recovery to an extraordinary degree. It is of course possible that the lack of such evidence is attributable to the paucity of studies designed to show axonal regrowth following brain injury in primates. In this context, it is appropriate to mention that a long-term search for anomalous pathways in the brains of monkeys that recovered cognitive functions following bilateral orbital prefrontal lesions in infancy has so far failed to uncover such connections (Goldman and Tanaka, *in preparation*). The search has employed various methods (e.g., silver degeneration, autoradiography, and retrograde degeneration) and focused on input to structures like the caudate nucleus that are massively deafferented by the frontal cortical lesions.

In summary, the mechanisms by which animals cope with brain injury may manifest in widely different ways in various mammalian species. Just as vertebrates differ from invertebrates in the capacity for regeneration of cut neurons, it is possible that primates may differ from rodents in the capacity for forming collateral sprouts throughout postnatal and adult life. Plasticity in primates may involve neural redundancy and resourceful use of intact structures as implied by the apparently greater dependence of functional restitution upon environmental stimulation in this species. In all of these hypothetical and various species-typical responses to brain injury, perhaps the lowest common denominator for maintaining the structural and functional integrity of the damaged brain is the trophic response. Further investigation of early experience, recovery of function, trophic phenomena, and possible relations between them could reap dividends in producing new therapies for human brain disease, and further, open the path to an understanding of yet unexplored interactions between genetic and environmental determinants of behavior.

REFERENCES

1. Barlow, H. B. (1975): Visual experience and cortical development. *Nature*, 258:199–204.
2. Black, I. B., Hendry, I. A., and Iversen, L. L. (1971): Transsynaptic regulation of growth and development of adrenergic neurons in a mouse sympathetic ganglion. *Brain Res.*, 34:229–240.
3. Blakemore, C. (1974): Developmental factors in the formation of feature extracting neurons. In: *The Neurosciences: Third Study Program*, edited by F. O. Schmitt and F. G. Worden, pp. 105–113. M.I.T. Press, Cambridge, Mass.
4. Blakemore, C., and Van Sluyters, R. C. (1975): Innate and environmental factors in the development of the kitten's visual cortex. *J. Physiol.*, 248:663–716.
5. Bland, B. H., and Cooper, R. M. (1969): Posterior neodecortication in the rat: age at operation and experience. *J. Comp Physiol. Psychol.*, 69:345–354.
6. Chang, C., and Tung, L. (1974): Inhibition by actinomycin D of the generation of acetylcholine receptors induced by denervation in skeletal muscle. *Eur. J. Pharmacol.*, 26:386–388.
7. Chow, K. L., Riesen, A., and Newell, F. W. (1957): Degeneration of retinal ganglion cells in infant chimpanzees reared in darkness. *J. Comp. Neurol.*, 107:27–42.
8. Chow, K. L., and Stewart, D. L. (1972): Reversal of structural and functional effects of long-term visual deprivation in cats. *Exp. Neurol.*, 34:409–433.
9. Chuang, D. M., and Costa, E. (1976): Trans-synaptic regulation of ribonucleic acid biosynthesis in rat adrenal medulla. *Molec. Pharmacol.*, 12:514–518.
10. Cole, D. D., Sullins, W. R., and Isaac, W. (1967): Pharmacological modification of the effects of spaced occipital ablations. *Psychopharmacology*, 11:311–316.
11. Collier, B., and Mitchell, J. F. (1966): The central release of acetylcholine during stimulation of the visual pathway. *J. Physiol.*, 184:239–254.
12. Creese, I., Burt, D. R., and Snyder, S. H. (1977): Dopamine receptor binding enhancement accompanies lesion-induced behavioral supersensitivity. *Science*, 197:596–598.
13. Devor, M. (1975): Neuroplasticity in the sparing or deterioration of function after early olfactory tract lesions. *Science*, 190:998–1000.
14. Diamond, M. C. (1967): Extensive cortical depth measurements and neuron size increases in the cortex of environmentally enriched rats. *J. Comp. Neurol.*, 131:357–364.
15. Diamond, M. C., Krech, D., and Rosenzweig, M. R. (1964): The effects of an enriched environment on the histology of the rat cerebral cortex. *J. Comp. Neurol.*, 123:111–120.
16. Dibner, M. D., and Black, I. B. (1976): The effect of target organ removal on the development of sympathetic neurons. *Brain Res.*, 103:93–102.
17. Donovick, P., Burright, R., and Swidler, M. (1973): Presurgical rearing environment alters exploration, fluid consumption, and learning of septal lesioned and control rats. *Physiol. Behav.*, 11:543–553.
18. Duffy, F. H., Snodgrass, S. R., Burchfiel, J. L., and Conway, J. L. (1976): Bicuculline reversal of deprivation amblyopia in the cat. *Nature*, 260:256–257.
19. Eccles, J. C. (1974): Trophic interactions in mammalian central nervous system. *Ann. N.Y. Acad. Sci.*, 228:406–423.

20. Edwards, H., Barry, W., and Wyspianski, J. (1969): Effect of differential rearing on photic evoked potentials and brightness discrimination in the albino rat. *Dev. Psychobiol.,* 2:133–138.
21. Ferchmin, P. A., Eterovic, V. A., and Caputto, R. (1970): Studies of brain weight and RNA content after short periods of exposure to environmental complexity. *Brain Res.,* 20:49–57.
22. Finger, S., Walbran, B., and Stein, D. G. (1973): Brain damage and behavioral recovery: serial lesion phenomena. *Brain Res.,* 63:1–18.
23. Gilbert, B. E., Grove, B. K., and Johnson, T. C. (1972): Characteristics and products of a cell-free polypeptide synthesizing system from neonatal and adult mouse brain. *J. Neurochem.,* 19:2835–2842.
24. Gisiger, V. (1971): Triggering of RNA synthesis by acetylcholine stimulation of the postsynaptic membrane in a mammalian sympathetic ganglion. *Brain Res.,* 33:139–146.
25. Glassman, R. B. (1971): Recovery following sensorimotor cortical damage: evoked potentials, brain stimulation and motor control. *Exp. Neurol.,* 33:16–29.
26. Glick, S. D. (1974): Changes in drug sensitivity and mechanisms of functional recovery after central nervous system lesions in rats. In: *Plasticity and Recovery of Function in the Central Nervous System,* edited by D. G. Stein, J. J. Rosen, and N. Butters, pp. 339–372. Academic Press, New York.
27. Globus, A., Rosenzweig, M. R., Bennett, E. L., and Diamond, M. C. (1973): Effects of differential experience on dendritic spine counts in rat cerebral cortex. *J. Comp. Physiol. Psychol.,* 82:175–181.
28. Goldberger, M. E. (1974): Recovery of movement after CNS lesions in monkeys. In: *Plasticity and Recovery of Function in the Central Nervous System,* edited by D. G. Stein, J. J. Rosen, and N. Butters, pp. 265–337. Academic Press, New York.
29. Goldman, P. S. (1971): Functional development of the prefrontal cortex in early life and the problem of neuronal plasticity. *Exp. Neurol.,* 32:366–387.
30. Goldman, P. S. (1974): An alternative to developmental plasticity: Heterology of CNS structures in infants and adults. In: *Plasticity and Recovery of Function in the Central Nervous System,* edited by D. G. Stein, J. J. Rosen, and N. Butters, pp. 149–174. Academic Press, New York.
31. Goldman, P. S. (1976*a*): Maturation of the mammalian nervous system and the ontogeny of behavior. In: *Advances in the Study of Behavior, Vol. 7.,* edited by J. A. Rosenblatt, R. A. Hinde, E. Shaw, and C. Beer, pp. 1–90. Academic Press, New York.
32. Goldman, P. S. (1976*b*): The role of experience in recovery of function following orbital prefrontal lesions in infant monkeys. *Neuropsychologia,* 14:401–412.
33. Goldman, P. S., Crawford, H. T., Stokes, L. P., Galkin, T. W., and Rosvold, H. E. (1974): Sex-dependent behavioral effects of cerebral cortical lesions in the developing rhesus monkey. *Science,* 186:540–542.
34. Goldman, P. S., and Galkin, T. W. (1978): Anatomical and behavioral plasticity following prenatal removal of frontal association cortex in the fetal rhesus monkey. *Brain Res. (in press).*
35. Goldman, P. S., and Mendelson, M. J. (1977): Salutary effects of early experience on deficits caused by lesions of frontal association cortex in developing rhesus monkeys. *Exp. Neurol.,* 57:588–602.
36. Goldman, P. S., and Nauta, W. J. H. (1976): Autoradiographic demonstration of a projection from prefrontal association cortex to the superior colliculus in the rhesus monkey. *Brain Res.,* 116:145–149.
37. Goldman, P. S., and Nauta, W. J. H. (1977*a*): An intricately patterned prefronto-caudate projection in the rhesus monkey. *J. Comp. Neurol.* 171:369–386.
38. Goldman, P. S., and Nauta, W. J. H. (1977*b*): Columnar distribution of cortico-cortical fibers in the frontal association, limbic and motor cortex of the developing rhesus monkey. *Brain Res.,* 122:393–413.
39. Goldstein, K. (1939): *The Organism.* Beacon Press, New York.
40. Grampp, W., Harris, J., and Thesleff, S. (1972): Inhibition of denervation changes in skeletal muscle by blockers of protein synthesis. *J. Physiol.,* 221:743–754.
41. Greenough, W. T., Fass, B., and DeVoogd, T. J. (1976): The influence of experience on recovery following brain damage in rodents: Hypotheses based on development research. In: *Environments as Therapy for Brain Dysfunction.* edited by R. N. Walsh and W. T. Greenough, pp. 10–50. Plenum Press, New York.

42. Grobstein, P., and Chow, K. L. (1975): Receptive field development and individual experience. *Science,* 190:352–358.
43. Grouse, L. D., Schrier, B. K., Bennett, E. L., Rosenzweig, M. R., and Nelson, P. G. (1977): Sequence diversity studies of rat brain RNA: effects of environmental complexity on rat brain RNA diversity. *J. Neurochem. (in press).*
44. Guroff, G., and Brodsky, M. (1971): Enzymes of nucleic acid metabolism in the brains of young and adult rats. *J. Neurochem.,* 18:2077–2084.
45. Guroff, G., Hogans, A. F., and Udenfriend, S. (1968): Biosynthesis of ribonucleic acid in rat brain slices. *J. Neurochem.,* 15:489–497.
46. Guth, L. (1969): "Trophic" effects of vertebrate neurons. *Neurosci. Res. Prog. Bull.,* 7:1–73.
47. Guth, L. (1974): Axonal regeneration and functional plasticity in the central nervous system. *Exper. Neurol.,* 45:606–654.
48. Harrell, L. E., Raubeson, R., and Balagura, S. (1974): Acceleration of functional recovery following lateral hypothalamic damage by means of electrical stimulation in the lesioned areas. *Physiol. Behav.,* 12:897–899.
49. Hebb, D. O. (1949): *The Organization of Behavior.* J. Wiley & Sons, Inc. New York.
50. Høedt-Rasmussen, K., and Skinhøj, E. (1964): Transneuronal depression of the cerebral hemispheric metabolism in man. *Acta Neurol. Scand.,* 40:41–46.
51. Holloway, R. L. (1966): Dendritic branching: some preliminary results of training and complexity in rat visual cortex. *Brain Res.,* 2:393–396.
52. Hubel, D. H., and Wiesel, T. N. (1970): The period of susceptibility to the physiological effects of unilateral eye closure in kittens. *J. Physiol.,* 206:419–436.
53. Hubel, D. H., Wiesel, T. N., and LeVay, S. (1977): Plasticity of ocular dominance columns in monkey striate cortex. *Phil. Trans. R. Soc. Lond. B.,* 278:377–410.
54. Hughes, K. R. (1965): Dorsal and ventral hippocampus lesions and maze learning: influence of preoperative environment. *Can. J. Psychol.,* 19:325–332.
55. Innocenti, G. M., Fiore, L., and Caminiti, R. (1977): Exuberant projections into the corpus callosum from the visual cortex of newborn cats. *Neurosci. Lett.,* 4:237–242.
56. Isaac, W. (1964): Role of stimulation and time in the effects of spaced occipital ablations. *Psychol. Rep.,* 14:151–154.
57. Jacobsen, C. F. (1936): Studies of cerebral function in primates. *Comp. Psychol. Monogr.* 13:1–68.
58. Jarlstedt, J. (1966): Functional localization in the cerebellar cortex studied by quantitative determinations of Purkinje cell RNA. I. RNA changes in rat cerebellar Purkinje cells after proprio- and exteroceptive and vestibular stimulation. *Acta Physiol. Scand.,* 67:243–252.
59. Kempinsky, W. H. (1958): Experimental study of distance effects of acute focal brain injury-a study of diaschisis. *Arch. Neurol. Psychiatry,* 79:376–389.
60. Kennard, M. (1940): Relation of age to motor impairment in man and in subhuman primates. *Arch. Neurol. Psychiatry,* 44:377–397.
61. Kennard, M. (1942): Cortical reorganization of motor function: studies on a series of monkeys of various ages from infancy to maturity. *Arch. Neurol. Psychiatry,* 48:227–240.
62. Klüver, H. (1942): Functional significance of the geniculo-striate system. In: *Visual Mechanisms, Vol. 7,* edited by H. Kluver, pp. 253–299. J. Cattell Press, Lancaster, Pa.
63. Kuypers, H. G. J. M. (1962): Corticospinal connections: postnatal development in the rhesus monkey. *Science,* 138:678–680.
64. Lansdell, H. C. (1953): Effect of brain damage on intelligence in rats. *J. Comp. Physiol. Psychol.,* 46:461–464.
65. Lashley, K. S. (1938): Factors limiting recovery after central nervous lesions. *J. Nerv. Ment. Dis.,* 88:733–755.
66. Levitan, I. B., Mushynski, W. E., and Ramirez, G. (1972): Effects of an enriched environment on amino acid incorporation into rat brain subcellular fractions *in vivo. Brain Res.,* 41:498–502.
67. Lewis, M. E. (1977): Nerve growth factor and recovery of function after brain damage. Unpublished Ph.D. Dissertation, Clark University.
68. Lewis, M. E., and Lancione, R. L. (1976): A mathematical model of recovery from brain damage. *Brain Theory Newsletter* 1:65–66.
69. Lynch, G., Deadwyler, S., and Cotman, C. (1973): Postlesion axonal growth produces permanent functional connections. *Science,* 180:1364–1366.

70. Lynch, G., Stanfield, B., and Cotman, C. W. (1973): Developmental differences in postlesion axonal growth in the hippocampus. *Brain Res.,* 59:155–168.
71. McMahon, D. (1974): Chemical messengers in development: a hypothesis. *Science,* 185:1012–1021.
72. Macht, M. B. (1950): Effects of d-amphetamine on hemidecorticate, decorticate, and decerebrate cats. *Fed. Proc.,* 63:731–732.
73. Mailloux, J. G., Edwards, H. P., Barry, W. F., Rowsell, H. C., and Achorn, E. G. (1974): Effects of differential rearing on cortical evoked potentials of the albino rat. *J. Comp. Physiol. Psychol.,* 87:475–480.
74. Maletta, G. J., and Timiras, P. S. (1968): Choline acetyltransferase activity and total protein content in selected optic areas of the rat after complete light-deprivation during CNS development. *J. Neurochem.,* 15:787–793.
75. Manen, C. A., and Russell, D. H. (1977): Ornithine decarboxylase may function as an initiation factor for RNA polymerase I. *Science,* 195:505–506.
76. Meyer, D. R., Isaac, W., and Maher, B. (1958): The role of stimulation in spontaneous reorganization of visual habits. *J. Comp. Physiol. Psychol.,* 51:546–548.
77. Meyers, J. S., Shinohara, Y., Kanda, T., Fukuuchi, Y., Ericsson, A. D., and Kok, N. K. (1970): Diaschisis resulting from acute unilateral cerebral infarction: quantitative evidence for man. *Arch. Neurol.,* 23:241–247.
78. Meyer, P. M. (1973): Recovery from neocortical damage. In: *Cortical Functioning in Behavior,* edited by G. M. French, pp. 115–138. Scott, Foresman and Co., Palo Alto.
79. Meyer, P. M., Horel, J. A., and Meyer, D. R. (1963): Effects of dl-amphetamine upon placing responses in neodecorticate cats. *J. Comp. Physiol. Psychol.,* 56:402–404.
80. Mishkin, M. (1964): Perseveration of central sets after frontal lesions in monkeys. In: *The Frontal Granular Cortex and Behavior,* edited by J. M. Warren and K. Akert, pp. 219–237. McGraw-Hill, New York.
81. Mistretta, C., and Bradley, R. (1978): Effects of early sensory experience on brain and behavioral development. In: *Studies on Development of Behavior and the Nervous System, Vol. IV: Early influences,* edited by Gilbert Gottlieb, Academic Press *(in press).*
82. Monakow, C. von (1914): *Die Lokalisation in Grosshirnrinde und der Abbau der Funktion durch Korticale Herde.* J. F. Bergmann, Wiesbaden.
83. Murphy, E. H., and Stewart, D. L. (1974): Effects of neonatal and adult striate lesions on visual discrimination in the rabbit. *Exp. Neurol.,* 42:89–96.
84. Nagaiah, K., MacDonnell, P., and Guroff, G. (1977): Induction of tyrosine hydroxylase synthesis in rat superior cervical ganglia *in vitro* by nerve growth factor and dexamethasone. *Biochem. Biophys. Res. Comm.,* 75:832–837.
85. Pettigrew, J. D. (1974): The effect of visual experience on the development of stimulus specificity by kitten cortical neurones. *J. Physiol.,* 237:49–74.
86. Prince, M. (1910): Cerebral localization from the point of view of function and symptoms—with special reference to von Monakow's theory of diaschisis. *J. Nerv. Ment Dis.,* 37:337–354.
87. Purves, D., and Njå, A. (1976): Effect of nerve growth factor on synaptic depression after axotomy. *Nature,* 260:535–536.
88. Raine, A. E. G., and Chubb, I. W. (1977): Long term β-adrenergic blockade reduces tyrosine hydroxylase and dopamine β-hydroxylase activities in sympathetic ganglia. *Nature,* 267:265–267.
89. Rakic, P. (1975): Timing of major ontogenetic events in the visual cortex of the rhesus monkey. In: *Brain Mechanisms in Mental Retardation,* edited by N. A. Buchwald and M. A. Brazier, pp. 3–40. Academic Press, New York.
90. Rakic, P. (1976): Prenatal genesis of connections subserving ocular dominance in the rhesus monkey. *Nature,* 261:467–471.
91. Rakic, P. (1977): Prenatal development of the visual system in rhesus monkey. *Phil. Trans. R. Soc. Lond. B.,* 278:245–260.
92. Rosenblum, L. A., and Kaufman, I. C. (1967): Laboratory observations of early mother-infant relations in pigtail and bonnet macaques. In: *Social Communication Among Primates,* edited by S. A. Altmann. University of Chicago Press, Chicago.
93. Rosenzweig, M. R. (1971): Effects of environment on development of brain and behavior. In: *The Biopsychology of Development,* edited by E. Tobach, L. Aronson, and E. Shaw, pp. 303–342. Academic Press, New York.

94. Rosenzweig, M. R., Bennett, E. L., and Diamond, M. C. (1972): Chemical and anatomical plasticity of brain: Replications and extensions. In: *Macromolecules and Behavior, 2nd Ed.,* edited by J. Gaito, pp. 205–277. Appleton-Century-Crofts, New York.
95. Rosenzweig, M. R., Krech, D., Bennett, E. L., and Diamond, M. C. (1962): Effects of environmental complexity and training on brain chemistry and anatomy. *J. Comp. Physiol. Psychol.,* 55:429–437.
96. Rosner, B. S. (1974): Recovery of function and localization of function in historical perspective. In: *Plasticity and Recovery of Function in the Central Nervous System,* edited by D. G. Stein, J. J. Rosen, and N. Butters, pp. 1–29. Academic Press, New York.
97. Russell, D. H., (Ed.) (1973): *Polyamines in Normal and Neoplastic Growth.* Raven Press, New York.
98. Russell, D. H., Byus, C. V., and Manen, C. A. (1976): Proposed model of major sequential biochemical events of a trophic response. *Life Sci.,* 19:1297–1306.
99. Sackett, G. P., Holm, R. A., Ruppenthal, G. C., and Farhrenbruch, C. E. (1976): The effects of total social isolation rearing on behavior of rhesus and pigtail macaques. In: *Environments as Therapy For Brain Dysfunction,* edited by R. N. Walsh and W. T. Greenough, pp. 115–131. Plenum Press, New York.
100. Schapiro, S., and Vukovich, K. R. (1970): Early experience effects upon cortical dendrites: a proposed model for development. *Science,* 167:292–294.
101. Schneider, G. E. (1970): Mechanisms of functional recovery following lesions of visual cortex or superior colliculus in neonate and adult hamsters. *Brain Behav. Evol.,* 3:295–323.
102. Schneider, G. E. (1973): Early lesions of superior colliculus: factors affecting the formation of abnormal retinal projections. *Brain Behav. Evol.,* 8:73–109.
103. Schwartz, S. (1964): Effects of neonatal cortical lesions and early environmental factors on adult rat behavior. *J. Comp. Physiol. Psychol.,* 57:72–77.
104. Sharpless, S. K. (1975): Disuse supersensitivity. In: *The Developmental Neuropsychology of Sensory Deprivation,* edited by A. H. Riesen, pp. 125–152. Academic Press, New York.
105. Sherrington, C. S. (1906): *The Integrative Action of the Nervous System.* Charles Scribner's Sons, New York.
106. Singh, V. K., and Sung, S. C. (1972): Effect of spermidine on DNA-dependent RNA polymerases from brain cell nuclei. *J. Neurochem.,* 19:2885–2888.
107. Smith, B. H., and Kreutzberg, G. W. (1976): Neuron-target cell interactions. *Neurosci. Res. Prog. Bull.,* 14:211–453.
108. Smith, C. J. (1959): Mass action and early environment in the rat. *J. Comp. Physiol. Psychol.,* 52:154–156.
109. Snyder, S. H. (1975): Neurotransmitter and drug receptors in the brain. *Biochem. Pharmacol.,* 24:1371–1374.
110. Spehlmann, R., and Stahl, S. M. (1974): Neuronal hyposensitivity to dopamine in the caudate nucleus depleted of biogenic amines by tegmental lesions. *Exp. Neurol.,* 42:703–706.
111. Spinelli, D. N., Hirsch, H. V. B., Phelps, R. W., and Metzler, J. (1972): Visual experience as a determinant of the response characteristics of cortical receptive fields in cats. *Exp. Brain Res.,* 15:289–304.
112. Sporn, J. R., Harden, T. K., Wolfe, B. B., and Molinoff, P. B. (1976): β-adrenergic receptor involvement in 6-hydroxydopamine-induced supersensitivity in rat cerebral cortex. *Science,* 194:624–626.
113. Stavraky, G. W. (1961): *Supersensitivity Following Lesions of the Nervous System.* University of Toronto Press, Toronto.
114. Steiner, F. A. (1968): Influence of microelectrophoretically applied acetylcholine on the responsiveness of hippocampal and lateral geniculate neurons. *Pflügers Arch.,* 303:173–180.
115. Stenevi, U., Björklund, A., and Moore, R. Y. (1973): Morphological plasticity of central adrenergic neurons. *Brain Behav. Evol.,* 8:110–134.
116. Stricker, E. M., and Zigmond, M. J. (1976): Recovery of function after damage to central catecholamine-containing neurons: a neurochemical model for the lateral hypothalamic syndrome. *Progress in Psychobiology and Physiological Psychology, Vol. 6,* edited by J. M. Sprague and A. N. Epstein, pp. 121–188. Academic Press, New York.
117. Tabor, C. W., and Tabor, H. (1976): 1,4-diaminobutane (putrescine), spermidine, and spermine. *Ann. Rev. Biochem.,* 45:285–306.
118. Tees, R. C. (1975): The effects of neonatal striate lesions and visual experience on form discrimination in the rat. *Can. J. Psychol.,* 29:66–85.

119. Teuber, H. L. (1974): Recovery of function after lesions of the central nervous system: history and prospects. *Neurosci. Res. Prog. Bull.,* 12:197–209.
120. Thoenen, H., Angeletti, P. V., Levi-Montalcini, R., and Kettler, R. (1971): Selective induction by nerve growth factor of tyrosine hydroxylase and dopamine-β-hydroxylase in the rat superior cervical ganglion. *Proc. Natl. Acad. Sci. USA,* 68:1598–1602.
121. Uphouse, L. L., and Bonner, J. (1975): Preliminary evidence for the effects of environmental complexity on hybridization of rat brain RNA to rat unique DNA. *Dev. Psychobiol.,* 8:171–178.
122. Varon, S. (1975): Nerve growth factor and its mode of action. *Exp. Neurol.* 48:75–92.
123. Wallingford, E., Ostdahl, R., Zarzecki, P., Kaufman, P., and Somjan, G. (1973): Optical and pharmacological stimulation of visual and cortical neurons. *Nature [New Biol.],* 242:210–212.
124. Walsh, R. N., and Cummins, R. A. (1975): Mechanisms mediating the production of environmentally induced brain changes. *Psychol. Bull.* 82:986–1000.
125. Walsh, R. N., and Greenough, W. T. (1976): *Environments as Therapy for Brain Dysfunction.* Plenum Press, New York.
126. Ward, A. A., and Kennard, M. A. (1942): Effect of cholinergic drugs on recovery of function following lesions of the central nervous system. *Yale J. Biol. Med.,* 15:189–228.
127. Will, B. E., Rosenzweig, M. R., and Bennett, E. L. (1976): Effects of differential environments on recovery from neonatal brain lesions, measured by problem-solving scores. *Physiol. Behav.,* 16:603–611.
128. Will, B. E., Rosenzweig, M. R., Bennett, E. L., Herbert, M., and Morimoto, H. (1977): Relatively brief environmental enrichment aids recovery of learning capacity and alters brain measures after postweaning brain lesions in rats. *J. Comp. Physiol. Psychol.,* 91:33–50.
129. Woodruff, M. L., Baisden, R. H., and Isaacson, R. L. (1973): Deficient brightness discrimination in hooded but not albino rats given neocortical ablations. *Physiol. Behav.,* 10:165–169.
130. Yarborough, G. G., and Phillis, J. W. (1975): Supersensitivity of central neurons—a brief review of an emerging concept. *Can. J. Neurol. Sci.,* 2:147–152.
131. Zylber, E. A., and Penman, S. (1971): Products of RNA polymerase in HeLa cell nuclei. *Proc. Natl. Acad. Sci. USA,* 68:2861–2865.

Neuronal Plasticity, edited by
Carl W. Cotman.
Raven Press, New York © 1978.

The Paradox of the Critical Period for Striate Cortex

John D. Pettigrew

Beckman Laboratories of Behavioral Biology, California Institute of Technology, Pasadena, California 91125

Hubel and Wiesel's discovery of a critical period for the development of visual cortical neurons in cat and monkey (24) was recently capped by the demonstration and delineation of a critical period for human binocular vision in two independent studies (2,22). A hitherto puzzling clinical phenomenon "meridional amblyopia" (44) was also provided with an explanation by the demonstration of a critical period for cortical orientation selectivity in the visual cortex of the kitten (5,6,19,20). These two examples provide unusual vindication for the value of basic research to our understanding of human problems, but I should hasten to add that this same line of basic research presents us with a difficult paradox. The paradox is that the same techniques, which demonstrate a remarkable sensitivity to visual experience for a variety of single neuron properties, also appear to demonstrate that these properties are present in adult form in young animals prior to any visual experience at all (e.g., 25,61). Since very short periods of abnormal experience can have permanent effects in both animals and humans (e.g., 1,28), the paradox concerns the role played by a period of plasticity with a great potential for handicap but little apparent potential benefit.

I intend to devote this chapter to a consideration of this paradox and the lines of investigation which may help to resolve it in the future. Since the account will no doubt reflect my prejudices, it may help if I state these clearly at the outset.

I believe that the critical period for primary visual cortex is not merely a potential handicap for the developing organism. Rather it may be a time when neural activity brings about the fine tuning of a cortical organization which is not complete prior to the animal's first experience. This view immediately calls into question one of the sources of the paradox; namely, the stress that has been laid upon innate "prewiring" in the cortex. I shall therefore examine the increasing evidence that this stress has been inappropriate. Further, I consider that the remarkable changes in connectivity within cortex which follow abnormal early experience should not be regarded as pathological or degenerative, but rather as extreme cases of the normal processes by which visual experience exerts its effects upon cortical function during development. If this view is correct, developing visual cortex, along with the song-learning circuit now being defined in birds (see 47), may represent our most promising model for understanding how brain function is altered by experience. I believe that a complete solution of the paradox will require three advances to be made: (a) a better understanding of normal function within visual cortex; (b) other approaches to the conceptual and technical difficulties inherent in study of the cortical function of inexperienced animals at the height of critical period plasticity; and finally, (c) a broader look at the evolutionary context within which the critical period phenomenon arose.

THE CONTROVERSY OVER THE PLASTICITY OF ORIENTATION SELECTIVITY

Before dealing with the implications of critical period plasticity, I wish to speak to some of the current doubts that plasticity exists at all for one aspect of cortical functioning, viz., orientational selectivity. The ocular dominance assay for the effects of neonatal eye occlusion has received much attention, no doubt because of the ease with which both the early manipulation and the assay can be performed. In addition, ocular dominance distributions determined physiologically have a striking anatomical correlate which can be demonstrated with a variety of techniques (38,72). Although the stimulus parameter of orientation is as important in the cortex for neuronal response properties as is ocular dominance, a role for orientation during the critical period has been less clear. There is no *a priori* reason to expect a basic difference between the neural connections whose combination subserves an eye preference in one case, and those which, in a different combination, might subserve orientation preference. Recent demonstrations (M. P. Stryker, *personal communication*) of eye, orientation, and direction subregions with the deoxyglucose technique (35) support this view. One might therefore expect that a larger subregion of cortex would be devoted to neurons preferring a given orientation in animals whose earlier experience had been confined to that orientation, just as eye preference regions are broader for the nondeprived eye following early monocular deprivation. Although a number of studies tend to confirm this expectation (e.g., 6,54), one careful study failed to find any evidence whatever for plasticity of orientational preference after using the rearing technique of Blakemore and Cooper (6). The study attributed failure to the three new recording techniques used (viz., "blind" experimental design, random sampling from cortical regions, and computerized stimulus presentation/recording), although evidence for plasticity *was* obtained with these techniques from the cortex of kittens if the orientation of exposure was different for each eye (67). Rearing in the latter condition was accomplished with the goggle technique introduced by Hirsch (19). Since the Hirsch technique provides independent control of the early input to each eye, one might have attributed the difference in results obtained with the two techniques to the fact that in the "successful" case different orientations were seen by the two eyes. However, rivalrous input does not appear to be the crucial factor since Stryker and Sherk have now reported examples of cortical orientation plasticity following exposure of each eye to the same orientation with Hirsch goggles (66,67).

We are therefore led to conclude that the failure by Stryker and Sherk (67) to demonstrate orientation plasticity in the first instance lies more with the technique of rearing than with the special precautions taken during recording. This conclusion is strengthened by a recent quantitative study which also took precautions to insure impartiality but which did succeed in replicating the phenomenon (8).

The source of the controversy seems therefore likely to be attributable to the difficulties of controlling the orientation of contours on the developing kitten's retina. A glance at figures in the literature will be enough to convince the reader that the "Blakemore tube" is not an ideal way to limit a kitten's early experience to a single orientation because of problems like head-tilt and the extraneous contours formed by the platform on which the kitten stands. The method of choice for workers in the field is now therefore Hirsch's goggle technique. To give credit where it is due, Hirsch had come to all these conclusions about the problems of rearing with control over stimulus orientation while working on his thesis in the 1960s.

THE CONTROVERSY OVER RECEPTIVE FIELD PROPERTIES IN THE VISUAL CORTEX OF YOUNG VISUALLY-INEXPERIENCED KITTEN: HEISENBERGIAN DIFFICULTIES?

The paradox I have proposed hinges somewhat upon one's conception of the state of the visual cortex in early development prior to the first visual experience. The paradox should be the most puzzling to those who conceive of a high degree of adult-like selectivity at this stage and should be a straw-man to those who conceive of an initial broad selectivity which is subsequently narrowed by experience. Two such disparate conceptions might be thought to be unviable in the face of the constant research going on in this area. The fact is, that in spite of much work on the problem, there is still not a universally accepted conclusion of what the cortex *does* look like at this stage. This absence of a clear picture of early cortical function has led to difficulties in interpreting the effects of selected visual experience on cortical development.

Take as an example the number of possible interpretations of the observation that the ocular dominance columns corresponding to the open eye are wider than those for the closed eye in the visual cortex of a monkey which has undergone monocular deprivation since birth. One early interpretation, that there had been sprouting of the geniculocortical terminals for one eye to occupy territory normally occupied by the other eye's terminals, clearly required the existence of well-defined ocular dominance column boundaries prior to lid suture (71). This interpretation has had to be modified in the light of subsequent work showing poor differentiation of the ocular dominance column system at birth. At this time there is only partial segregation of terminals for each eye, and physiological recording reveals large numbers of binocular neurons in IVcβ, the layer characterized in the mature cortex by alternating bands of monocular neurons (31). This puzzling finding of an undifferentiated ocular dominance system at birth deserves close scrutiny because it does not agree with the view that there is a high degree of innate specificity prior to visual experience. The subdivision of geniculate inputs into ocular dominance columns could be regarded as a rather low-level problem in cortical circuitry alongside problems like the development of a binocular neuron whose tightly tuned orientation and directional selectivity is identical on each retina, so it is rather surprising to find this subdivision virtually absent at birth. It is true that Rakic's evidence suggests the *beginnings* of segregation into ocular dominance columns prior to birth, but we should keep in mind the procedure by which this evidence was obtained. Rakic (56) used a fetal eye injection, a manipulation that may be difficult to perform without producing some imbalance in the relative activities emanating from each eye. Such an imbalance might result in a prenatal acceleration of the differentiation process which normally occurs substantially after birth, if this process is affected by activity, as seems likely. Similar caution should be exercised in accepting the view that normal ocular dominance column differentiation is unrelated to visual input because it appears to take place in lid-sutured or dark-raised monkeys. Suture of the thin lids of a monkey provides a limited kind of alteration to a monkey's visual input since light is attenuated by only 0.5 log units (73), and complete dark-rearing is an ideal which is only rarely achieved with young primates. Even should this ideal be reached, it would have to be borne in mind that the cortex is continually being bombarded, total darkness notwithstanding, by spontaneous activity from both retinas via the lateral geniculate nucleus (LGN). Some degree of asynchrony in the activity from the two retinas will be inevitable, since they are independent channels with limited interaction (at the LGN level). This asynchrony could be enough, given time, to bring about an activity-dependent synaptic retraction of the kind required for differentiation of the ocular dominance columns. Since experiments with early embryonic eye removal give very similar results in the LGN to those obtained in the cortical ocular dominance columns following later manipulation (57), a similar mechanism might also apply to the formation of its laminae. These effects occur at an earlier stage in embryonic development, but one where spontaneous activity is doubtless also present. The width of ocular dominance bands is rather similar to the width of geniculate laminae, the surprising constancy of which has been pointed out (33). The common factor here might be the size of the terminal field of an intrinsic inhibitory neuron, whose orientation would determine the pattern of activity and therefore the pattern of final segregation; interneurons oriented along projection lines would result in LGN-type lamination, and interneurons oriented tangentially would result in ocular dominance bands.

The foregoing discussion presupposes that neural activity during development will affect differentiation. A principle which is bound to be important for the developing nervous system is activity-dependent synaptic segregation (12) of which postnatal critical periods can be regarded as the special case (where the activity is more directly linked with the environment).

Let us return to the problem of young, inexperienced cortex. To decide just how much visual experience contributes to normal development of visual cortex, in addition to interpreting the effects of unusual early experience, it is of considerable importance that we have a clear picture of cortical functioning at the outset. The problem is that five different teams have attempted to define the properties of visual cortex prior to any visual experience and arrived at five different conclusions, with only limited agreement. If these studies were to be listed with increasing emphasis on innate factors and decreasing emphasis on experiential ones, the order would read something like this: 4,49,7,10,61,25. All of these workers attempted to establish baseline properties of single cortical neurons at the height of the critical period in kittens (3 to 4 weeks postnatally) but prior to any visual experience. At this time optical imperfections are still found in the ocular media in cats (9) (in contradistinction to the monkey which has clear ocular media at birth), and synaptogenesis is occurring at a high rate (13). The studies of these five teams are so disparate in their emphases, data, and interpretations that it is very difficult to attempt a resolution, but I shall proceed on the basis that (a) some common ground will be found which appears to be universally acceptable, and (b) that there is some plausible basis for the extreme divergence of opinion that has prevailed in this area.

There is general agreement that there are a proportion of neurons in the visual cortex of young, visually inexperienced kittens which are *orientation selective* by most of the strict criteria which should now be insisted upon if a neuron is to be given such a label (18,49,60). The question of the presence or absence of such neurons prior to visual experience has become something of a *cause célèbre* in the nature-nurture debate over young visual cortex, but there are a number of reasons why the finding of some orientation-selective neurons in very young kittens should not be regarded as a triumph for the nativist point of view. To begin with, one cannot at present rule out the possibility that even these neurons become more selective for orientation as a function of visual experience. The distribution of orientation selectivities of normal cortical neurons covers a wide range (18,58,70), and it is more than likely that the most orientation selective neurons in normal adult cortex (whose width of orientation tuning can be as low as 15 to 20°) develop from the most orientation selective neurons in the young kitten, where the narrowest selectivity is more like 60 to 90°. Secondly, it comes as no surprise that the property of orientation selectivity can develop independently of visual experience, as this has already been demonstrated in the rabbit retina (17). The interesting question is whether orientation selectivity *can* be determined by visual experience, a question many still consider to be open and one which I think will be answered in the affirmative. Thirdly, the orientation selective units of young kittens are not completely adult-like in that they are *monocular*. This third point is consistent with the evidence of all five studies, although attention is drawn to it only by two (7,10). In addition these cells may have preferred orientations confined to horizontal or to vertical. This point is based on the assumption that the orientation selective cells described by Leventhal and Hirsch (38) in older binocularly deprived cats correspond to those seen in young kittens. With the added feature of horizontal or vertical preferences, the description of Leventhal and Hirsch (39) corresponds with that of Buisseret and Imbert (10) and Blakemore and Van Sluyters (7). In addition, the data illustrated by the latter workers are not inconsistent, in that all the examples chosen by both groups happen to be horizontal or vertical. Scrutiny of the data of Sherk and Stryker (61) also reveals that the convincingly orientation selective neurons tend to have horizontal or vertical preferences, and these workers also comment upon reduced binocularity in their preparation.

In summary, then, there appears to be agreement that there is a small group of orientation selective neurons which develop without benefit of visual experience. These are characterized by monocularity and orientations limited to either horizontal or vertical. If we couple this with the universal agreement that binocularity and direction selectivity are also present prior to visual experience (all five studies), then one might be led to ask, what was all the debate about? Aren't binocularity, orientation selectivity, and direction selectivity characteristic attributes of normal adult visual cortex? The answer is yes, of course, but normally these attributes are all present on the same single neuron. The essential attribute of normal visual cortical neurons is the selectivity they show for stimulus attributes on *both* retinas. Neurons have *matched* selectivities for each eye, such that a group of neurons with identical specificity in one eye will have closely similar, but not identical stimulus requirements for the other eye (48). This is because they must be capable of distinguishing between real life targets whose images look identical on one retina but have the small variations on the other retina which result from binocular parallax. Since these variations are tiny, binocular tuning must be exquisite for them to be discriminated, and it is this binocular tuning which is absent from the cortex of visually inexperienced young kittens (49). The developmental task appears to be to build up, from the initial set of monocularly activated orientation selective neurons and the binocularly activated nonspecific neurons, a population of binocular neurons *each* of which has precisely defined selectivity on both retinas.

The identification of some points of agreement among these five groups of workers, as outlined above, does not help us greatly to understand the large divergence of opinion expressed on the topic of young, visually inexperienced cortex, and I should not like to discuss ways in which these differences might be resolved. Some of the differences may be methodological. For example, the lack of standard pharmacology and anesthesia for this preparation makes comparisons difficult, particularly with respect to results obtained under barbiturates, extremely low doses of which enhance the action of the inhibitory transmitter gamma-aminobutyric acid (GABA) and could therefore produce marked alterations in the patterns of selectivity known to be dependent upon inhibitory effects (51,62–64). Barbiturates were used to a varying extent in all studies except those of Barlow and Pettigrew. Another methodological difference concerns the way in which stimulation was achieved. The studies which emphasize selectivity for line stimuli spent much time exploring with the same stimuli (e.g., 24,61). The attempts by Sherk and Stryker to compare responses to lines with those to spots completely miss the point I was trying to make in my study (49), since they used spots which were equalized for *area* with respect to the oriented bars. Such broad spots would certainly give less vigorous responses than the small spots I used to demonstrate the absence of an increase in selectivity when such spots were elongated into lines of various orientations. The point of the experiment is to see if a spot of light produces a response to a suboptimal direction of movement which is as good as that to an oriented bar of light with the same width. A positive result is therefore all the stronger in the face of a small spot area and would tend to be confused by the change to a nonoptimal width introduced by an equalization of areas.

The distinction between direction (or axis) selectivity and orientation selectivity is not a trivial one and has led to revisions in a number of areas besides kitten visual cortex. For example, the visual cortical region called Clare-Bishop area [or lateral syprasylvian (LS)] was first described as containing largely orientation selective neurons (27) but has now been shown to be less concerned with orientation than with direction (65). Similarly the ordered system of "orientation columns" demonstrated in young monkeys could equally well be based upon preferred axes of movement (29). There is yet another way in which differences in methodology might produce differences in results in this area— by bringing about reflecting changes in cortical function. This difficulty, which might be dubbed the "Heisenbergian" problem, has been hinted at in the literature, but there has been no really serious effort to confront it so far. Is it possible that the young, visually inexperienced cortex to a large extent mirrors in responsiveness what each experimenter presents to it during an experiment? This hypothesis would certainly account for the fact that the same preparation has yielded such a large number of different results, which are about as numerous as the experiments carried out. Since we can be fairly sure that the cortex will have some preferred paths of differentiation and that these will be the ones which may show up more readily during the course of an experiment, how can we be sure that a particular state of differentiation existed before we began stimulation? Therefore we may not be entitled to conclude, to take one example, that selectivity for straight lines preexisted, when our experiment could tell us only that such selectivity was capable of being generated. Perhaps the cortex would have generated another if we had done a different experiment, a possibility supported by the "planetarium" and "polka dots" experiments of Pettigrew and Freeman (52) and Van Sluyters and Blakemore (69). These workers found little evidence of conventional orientational selectivity in the cortex of kittens whose visual experience had been confined to small spots. Instead there were a majority of neurons with vigorous responses which appeared to be specifically restricted to small spots and unobtainable from elongated targets (and therefore quite distinct from both the normal kittens whose neurons with few exceptions preferred elongated targets as well as from the control, dark-reared kittens whose responsive cortical neurons were non-selective and could not make a distinction between spots and elongated targets). A planetarium of spots is so different from the prevailing clumped visual environment that these results should give us pause to consider once more the evidence that immature cortex has the same predilection for edges found in the mature cortex. It seems more likely that this attribute exists only in potential form early in development (perhaps as a few edge-selective inputs) and is normally brought out by the profusion of edges encountered in the visual world. As already pointed out, the basic algorithm of cortex appears to be the detection of a pair of similar clusters of events, one cluster on each retina. This algorithm may take on a resemblance to "line detection" only because of the common occurrence of extended edges in the environment.

To try to determine the contribution of visual experience to normal cortical development without confronting the problems inherent in studies of very young kittens, workers have tried to develop other paradigms. The two most used of these are older kittens which have been either dark-raised, or binocularly lid-sutured, to prevent the usual visual experience. There is good agreement that the visual cortices of such animals are far from normal, with high proportions of non-selective or unresponsive neurons and few neurons with normal selectivity.

The absence of a normal cortex in such cases at first sight seems to provide evidence for the empiricists' point of view that visual experience plays an essential role in shaping neuronal response characteristics during development. This evidence is however very much weakened by a number of considerations. The first of these is the possibility raised by the data of Buisseret and Imbert (10) that visual experience is essential for the *maintenance* of preexisting connections, which subsequently degenerate if unstimulated. This possibility also explains the large numbers of non-selective and unresponsive neurons found after dark-rearing, but it should be mentioned in passing that the "maintenance" hypothesis is not as incompatible with a constructive role for visual experience as Buisseret and Imbert maintain. For example, if visual experience "functionally validates" an activated subset of preexisting connections which represent a small fraction of the total on a particular neuron, the resultant narrowing of that neuron's response properties will be indistinguishable from the increased selectivity postulated by others to result from visual experience.

A second consideration is the type of visual stimulation provided through closed eyelids. This factor will be subject to a number of variables, such as the degree of pigmentation of the lids and ambient light levels, but cannot be ruled out as trivial. One might expect this factor to play a greater role in baby monkeys where the lid provides only 0.5 log units of light attenuation (73), and there is indeed evidence that this is so. Hubel, Wiesel and LeVay (29) found a decrease in the binocularity within monkey area 17 which followed lid suture, and they noted that they did not observe such a change in similarly treated kittens. The observed decrease in binocularity is similar to that which follows artificial strabismus and might therefore be attributable to the abnormal visual stimulation the monkey receives through his lids. In any event, this is the explanation put forward by Kratz and Spear (36) who observed the same phenomenon in binocularly lid-sutured, but not dark-reared, kittens. As already suggested, the variability of this phenomenon of reduced binocularity following lid suture in kittens [not seen by Hubel and Wiesel (26); seen by Kratz and Spear (36)] may be related to uncontrolled variables such as ambient light levels and variable lid pigmentation. The possibility that a particular kind of visual stimulation occurs through the lids is supported by the unpublished observations of some of us who have encountered neurons following lid suture which are apparently unresponsive to the usual sorts of stimuli but which do respond to movement of diffuse shadows.

If the binocular lid-suture paradigm is flawed in these ways, the dark-rearing paradigm cannot be considered better. Apart from the first consideration of degeneration mentioned above, which applies equally to dark-reared and lid-sutured kittens, there are a number of further potential and proven problems with dark-rearing. As an example of a potential problem, consider the likely endocrine consequences of removing the developing animal from the visual Zeitgeber for its circadian clock. A number of hormones are known to affect brain development so it is not idle to suggest that this will be altered in ways yet to be determined in dark-raised kittens. A second proven problem, and one perhaps related to the hormonal question just mentioned, is that dark-rearing appears to delay the appearance of critical period plasticity. Quite old kittens (up to at least 1 year) will show plastic changes (after monocular deprivation, for example) which are uncharacteristic of their age, if they are brought out following a long period of dark-rearing which began before normal eye opening (15). In other words, some degree of critical period plasticity may be delayed indefinitely by dark-rearing. This finding is reminiscent of Valverde's observation that a sudden spurt of dendritic spine growth, like that observed in the visual cortex of neonatal mice, can also be observed in older mice just after they have been returned to the light after a period of dark-rearing which began at birth (68). Such a "delayed onset" of the critical period, if valid, is not altogether compatible with the view presented above that dark-rearing produces degeneration and could therefore be used as evidence to support the dark-rearing paradigm to determine the characteristics of "naive" visual cortex. However, if the critical period has merely been delayed, then the Heisenbergian problem has also merely been postponed, and it may be difficult to decide what response properties pre-existed, what properties resulted from stimulation during the experiment, and what properties resulted from the long period of dark exposure.

In the light of the foregoing qualifications and quibbles, the reader may well ask in desperation if there is *any* experimental approach which is capable of clarifying the role played by visual experience in normal development.

Such an approach would clearly require a greater understanding of the under-lying mechanism of critical period plasticity. If this mechanism could be experi-mentally put out of action at precisely defined times during early development, in somewhat similar fashion to the way that nature normally puts it out of action in kittens some time after the twelfth week, it would be possible to compare normally reared cats which differed only in the age at which their visual cortices were rendered insensitive to further visual experience. This experi-ment should enable one to determine whether visual experience is necessary for normal receptive field development and if it should prove to be, to see exactly how it contributes. In addition, if it is found that experience is not necessary for receptive field development, such an experiment should make clear whether there is *any* role for visual experience, for example in adjusting receptive field disparities along with head and eye growth.

It cannot be said with any certainty that such an experiment will ultimately be feasible, but very promising progress is being made in the right direction by work on the role of catecholamines in the control of critical period plasticity (34,52). This work is discussed below and shows promise of providing a way of achieving the experiment outlined above. The findings so far suggest that cortical plasticity can be eliminated at any stage of development by chemical treatment which depletes catecholamines.

If a kitten is subjected to catecholamine depletion early in life (around the second week) and then allowed to grow up before recordings are carried out, its adult visual cortex presents a picture which is reminiscent of that painted for the very young, visually inexperienced kitten's cortex in the previous section. That is, both binocularity and orientation selectivity can be demonstrated in the properties of single cells, *but not in the same cells.* The binocular neurons with vigorous responsiveness from each eye all have receptive fields which are non-selective for orientation. The orientation selective neurons have receptive fields which satisfy all the stringent criteria for orientation selectivity, but such receptive fields are monocular; a given orientation selective neuron is driven only by one eye. In addition, there is a tendency for these monocular, orientation selective neurons to prefer either horizontal or vertical.

If the catecholamine depletion is begun later in life, the numbers of orientation selective binocular neurons tend to increase. Treatment of a five-week-old kitten results in a distribution of orientation selective binocular neurons in its adult cortex which is indistinguishable from a normal adult.

These findings support the view already put forward by Pettigrew (49) and Blakemore and Van Sluyters (7) and dealt with again in this chapter that the role of critical period plasticity is linked to the special demands of wiring up a neural system involved in binocular visual processing. If one accepts for the moment the proposition that catecholamine depletion prevents visual experience from exerting any effect upon visual cortical connectivity, then the visual cortex of an adult cat which had been depleted of catecholamines as a kitten at two weeks should reveal to us in what way visual experience may have been necessary for development subsequent to the age of 2 weeks. The finding in such animals of binocular neurons which are non-selective for orientation and orientation selective neurons which are monocular suggests that visual experience is necessary for the development of the usual binocular neurons each of which has tightly tuned stimulus requirements on *both* retinas.

PARALLEL VISUAL PROCESSING

New concepts which affect our thinking about normal functions in the mature visual system are bound also to affect our view of developmental events. One such concept has slowly emerged and now appears to be taking the form of a minor revolution, if we take into account both its clarifying effects, as well as the amount of new work appearing which utilizes this concept. This is the concept of parallel visual processing, perhaps best illustrated by two rapidly growing areas of research: (a) the study of extrastriate visual pathways, and (b) the application of the W, X, Y functional classification to visual neurons.

Broadly stated, parallel visual processing implies the existence of separate, functionally distinct pathways running in parallel from the retina to the central nervous system. The concept is certainly not a new one since it has long been emphasized by comparative neurologists that both retinogeniculate and retinotectal pathways play important roles in visual processing with the relative contribution of each dependent upon the species. The parallel processing point of view nevertheless received less than its due because of the focus upon the primate visual system where the retinogeniculostriate pathway overshadows all the others. The renaissance of this viewpoint stems from (a) the finding that parallel paths can be demonstrated even within the main retinogeniculostriate pathway of the primate, (b) from technical advances in neuroanatomy which have made possible the tracing of finer axonal pathways than the retinogeniculostriate, and (c) from increasingly sophisticated studies of visual systems in diverse species among which comparison can be facilitated by the use of the parallel processing viewpoint.

An excellent review of the large and rapidly moving area on W/X/Y classification exists (59), so I will limit myself to a brief summary and a figure. Figure

1 indicates how much new information has been added to our picture of the
visual pathway.

W-cells have the slowest conducting axons, and apart from this, have really
only one feature to characterize them—their heterogeneity. Both morphologically and physiologically they are extremely diverse, and it will probably turn

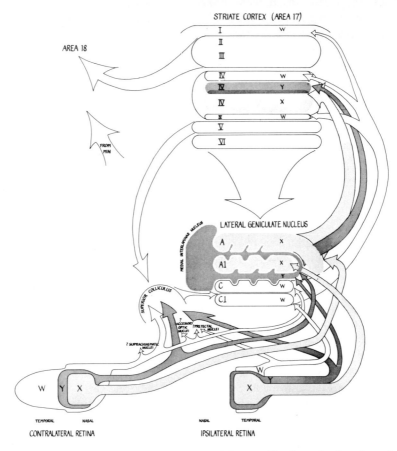

FIG. 1. Connections of the primary visual cortex of the cat. The figure is given to underscore
recent advances in functional classification within the geniculo-striate pathway and to emphasize that the primitive state of present understanding of cortical function does not yet include
the new insights gained from functional classification in the retina and LGN. If there are gaps
in our knowledge about normal cortical function, then it is to be expected that problems may
be encountered in the interpretation of developmental events and the effects of visual experience during the critical period.

The three shades of gray indicate the three broad categories, W, X, and Y (in order of
increasing axonal conduction velocity and size) into which retinal ganglion cells can now be
divided. Lamination in the LGN appears to be related to the tripartite subdivision of ganglion
cells (the Y-cells showing some intermingling, although in the monkey they have very clearly
segregated laminae). A brief description of some of the functional attributes of these three
classes, plus a discussion of their possible relevance to the understanding of puzzles of cortical
development, are given in the text.

out (as I have suggested in Fig. 1) that the destination of their axons will include an equally diverse set of nuclei. Many of them bear resemblances to the highly specialized ganglion cells found in the retina of the rabbit (3,40,67) and the pigeon (43). Their diversity and the technical difficulties of recording from them conspired to ensure that this is the group of which we are presently most ignorant.

X-cells have medium conduction velocity, summate linearly within their receptive fields, project exclusively into the geniculostriate pathway, and largely mediate vision carried out with the fovea, in which area of retina they have a markedly increased density.

Y-cells are rapidly conducting, probably have branched axons, have nonlinear receptive fields, and play a role in visual orientation to, and foveation of, new visual targets. A late-maturing class, they show marked sensitivity to visual deprivation. They project both to LGN and superior colliculus, in each of which structures they contact their own subclass of neurons.

While these functional subgroupings observed at the retinal level are also maintained at the LGN level, not enough work has yet been done at the cortical level with the classificatory scheme in mind. Such work is long overdue. Anatomical studies in monkey visual cortex (41) suggest that laminar organization will be found to be related to functional subgroupings like the W, X, Y system.

A study of development in the kitten LGN has shown the value of functional classifications from the parallel processing approach (46). For example, it is quite clearly shown that, in functional development, X-cells precede the Y-cells, which group still has not attained maturity as late as the fifth week. The study also leaves open the possibility that W-cells mature even earlier than X-cells, since putative W-cells, with highly specialized properties like direction selectivity, are seen as early as the second week of development. The role of these specialized W-cells is a puzzle because they have not been seen at late stages of development, when direction-selective neurons are found in the nucleus of the optic tract (21) but not in the LGN (74). In the light of the foregoing it is clear that current accounts of development of the role of visual experience may be greatly oversimplified and will be modified as more details of the intricacies of *normal* function accumulate. To illustrate the extent to which revisions may be necessary, let me give an example which is altogether improbable but which is nevertheless consistent with all of the available facts. This example concerns the controversial subject of orientational selectivity in young kitten cortex. This example is the subject of the next section.

ORIENTATION SELECTIVE W-CELLS?

The finding of a number of orientationally selective neurons in very young visually inexperienced kittens is a positive one which tends to be more convincing in arguments that early visual experience is unnecessary than the finding of even larger numbers of quite non-selective neurons in the same kittens. It is always easier to make a positive statement about the attributes of something

reach cortex from the misaligned retinal images (26). This interpretation does not hold up if the effect is seen in the total absence of visual experience, and it seems more likely that the explanation lies with an altered proprioceptive input. This possibility is supported further by a corollary experiment in which gross ocular misalignment in kittens is associated with the development of normal binocularity. The misalignment in this case, in contrast to the experiments of Maffei and Bisti (42) and Hubel and Wiesel (26) where a single eye muscle was cut, was brought about by detaching all eye muscles on each globe and then reattaching them with each globe in a slightly different position. In this way, the retinas are grossly misaligned, but the pattern of eye movements is close to normal. In spite of the absence of simultaneous binocular stimulation, many of these animals do not suffer reduced binocularity (14). Is it because they have relatively normal proprioceptive inputs?

TELEOLOGY OF THE CRITICAL PERIOD

Hubel has described neurobiology as a body of knowledge in need of a Copernicus (23). One cannot help but agree that the discipline is sorely in need of some synthesis, but I rather think that the man to achieve it will look more like Charles Darwin. One unifying feature we have to go on is the fact that the brain evolved. It is my own feeling that evolutionary considerations will do much in the future to clarify present enigmas. Thanks to the wide range of powerful neuroanatomical and neurophysiological techniques which are now relatively accessible to all, comparative neurobiology will have to be taken more seriously by chauvinists of favorite, "relevant" species like the macaque. Of course there are tremendous dangers in trying to infer evolutionary sequences based on data which must be largely derived from existing forms. Progress will however be possible along evolutionary lines and may even help in the resolution of the paradox under present consideration—the critical period.

One promising line of investigation concerns the avian visual system. This is a parallel visual system, *par excellence,* since it seems that the peak of its development in the diurnal, hunting birds is characterized by a bifoveate retina, with one fovea for the geniculostriate pathway and the other fovea for the tectofugal pathway (50). Like the geniculostriate pathway of cats and monkeys, the geniculostriate pathway of the owl has critical period plasticity with characteristics which are extremely similar to those found in these two mammals (53). The duration of the critical period in the owl has not yet been determined.

Is it possible to derive any clues about the significance of critical period plasticity from birds which have probably evolved the phenomenon quite independently of mammals? I think the answer is yes, because of the clear separation which appears to be achieved by birds in the initial separation of the two main parallel visual pathways. The geniculostriate pathway in birds is concerned with binocular vision. Very little representation is given to nonbinocular areas within it, and its output neurons appear to be primarily concerned with the binocular visual processing required for depth judgments. In other words the geniculostriate pathway of birds may have evolved primarily for binocular vision at close quarters. This provides independent evidence that the need for critical period plasticity is linked to the special demands during development of a system involved in stereoscopic depth processing.

It will be of considerable interest in the future to see whether the visual systems of other vertebrate orders with the capability for binocular vision (e.g., teleosts, sharks, frogs, lizards) also have forebrain areas involved in stereoscopic processing which are dependent upon early visual experience.

CONCLUSION

Apart from the evidence already outlined from deprivation and developmental studies, there are a number of considerations which increase the attractiveness of the hypothesis that the development of a stereoscopic visual system requires visual experience.

The first of these is the very subtle calculations required to extract disparity information. This calculation requires that a fine line be drawn between judgments of similarity and judgments of difference, since the measurement of a disparity between the two retinal images requires first that the pairs of parts of the two images be identified—a task requiring some judgment of similarity. The statistics required for this maneuver, of using similarities to identify points of difference, must surely be aided by information from the real world about the variations to be found in the various measurements. This is particularly true for the part of the real world which includes the head and eyes through which the information is being gathered.

A second key point is the astronomical accuracy of stereopsis, whose threshold disparity is around 5 sec arc for the best subjects (including monkeys). This means that the cortex is capable of detecting, in one retinal image relative to the other, a displacement which is a small fraction of the angle subtended by one photoreceptor! This is an astonishing feat which has yet to be accounted for adequately, but one likely requirement of a system with this capability is that it know the exact position of each photoreceptor. Such knowledge would have to be modifiable.

A third point, related to the second, is the possible perturbing effect upon such an accurate system of (a) unpredictable optical abnormalities in the eye, (b) limited and perhaps changing oculomotor control and, (c) changes in eye size and position which occur during development. All of these perturbing influences could be major problems for a delicate system operating routinely to seconds of arc accuracy. The capability to rewire binocular connections may be necessary to adjust for these perturbations which would no doubt be greatest during early development. According to this formulation the critical period should correspond to the period of greatest changes in head and eye size and in the oculomotor system.

ACKNOWLEDGEMENTS

This work was supported by the Spencer Foundation and by NIH Grant MH 25852. Eileen Bagdonas gave invaluable assistance in completing the manuscript.

REFERENCES

1. Awaya, S., Miyake, Y., Imaizaki, Y., Shiose, Y., Kanda, T., and Komuno, K. (1973): Amblyopia in man, suggestive of stimulus deprivation amblyopia. *Jap. J. Ophthalmol.,* 17:69–82.
2. Banks, M. S., Aslin, R. N., and Letson, R. D. (1976): Sensitive period for the development of human binocular vision. *Science,* 190:675–677.
3. Barlow, H. B., Hill, R. M., and Levick, W. R. (1964): Retinal ganglion cells responding selectively to direction and speed of image motion in the rabbit. *J. Physiol.,* 173:377–407.
4. Barlow, H. B., and Pettigrew, J. D. (1971): Lack of specificity of neurones in the visual cortex of young kittens. *J. Physiol.,* 218:98–100P.
5. Blakemore, C. (1974): Development of functional connexions in the mammalian visual system. *Brit. Med. Bull.,* 30:152–157.
6. Blakemore, C., and Cooper, G. F. (1970): Development of the brain depends on the visual environment. *Nature,* 228:477–478.
7. Blakemore, C., and Van Sluyters, R. C. (1975): Innate and environmental factors in the development of the kitten visual cortex. *J. Physiol.,* 248:663–716.
8. Blasdel, G. G., Mitchell, D. E., Muir, D. W., and Pettigrew, J. D. (1977): A physiological and behavioural study in cats of the effect of early visual experience with contours of a single orientation. *J. Physiol.,* 265:615–636.
9. Bonds, A. B., and Freeman, R. D. (1976): Development of optical quality in the kitten eye. *ARVO Abstracts 1976*:45.
10. Buisseret, P., and Imbert, M. (1976): Visual cortical cells: their developmental processes in normal and dark reared kittens. *J. Physiol.,* 255:511–525.
11. Buisseret, P., and Maffei, L. (1977): Extraocular proprioceptive projections to the visual cortex. *Exp. Brain Res.,* 28:421–426.
12. Changeux, J. P., and Danchin, A. (1976): Selective stabilisation of developing synapses as a mechanism for the specification of neuronal networks. *Nature,* 264:705–712.
13. Cragg, B. G. (1975): The development of synapses in the visual system of the cat. *J. Comp. Neurol.,* 160:147–166.
14. Crewther, S., and Crewther, D. (1978): A role for extra-ocular afferents in post-critical period reversal of monocular deprivation. *Submitted for publication.*
15. Crewther, S., Crewther, D., and Pettigrew, J. D. (1977): *Manuscript in preparation.*
16. Cynader, M., Berman, N., and Hein, A. (1976): Recovery of function in cat visual cortex following prolonged deprivation. *Exp. Brain Res.,* 25:139–156.
17. Daw, N. W., and Wyatt, H. J. (1974): Raising rabbits in a moving visual environment: an attempt to modify directional sensitivity in the retina. *J. Physiol.,* 240:309–330.
18. Henry, G. H., Dreher, B., and Bishop, P. O. (1973): Orientation specificity and response variability of cells in striate cortex. *Vision Res.,* 13:1771–1779.
19. Hirsch, H. V. B. (1971): Modification of the distribution of receptive field orientation in cats by selective visual exposure during development. *Exp. Brain Res.,* 12:509–524.
20. Hirsch, H. V. B., and Spinelli, D. N. (1970): Visual experience modifies distribution of horizontally and vertically oriented receptive fields in cats. *Science,* 168:869–871.
21. Hoffmann, K.-P., Behrend, K., and Schoppma, A. (1976): Direct afferent visual pathway from nucleus of optic tract to inferior olive in cat. *Brain Res.,* 115:150–153.
22. Hohmann, A., and Creutzfeld, O. D. (1976): Squint and the development of binocularity in humans. *Nature,* 254:613–614.
23. Hubel, D. H. (1977): Neurobiology: A science in search of a Copernicus?
24. Hubel, D. H., and Wiesel, T. N. (1963a): Single-cell responses in striate cortex of kittens deprived of vision in one eye. *J. Neurophysiol.,* 26:1003–1017.
25. Hubel, D. H., and Wiesel, T. N. (1963b): Receptive fields of cells in striate cortex of very young, visually inexperienced kittens. *J. Neurophysiol.,* 26:994–1002.

26. Hubel, D. H., and Wiesel, T. N. (1965): Binocular interaction in striate cortex of kittens reared with artificial squint. *J. Neurophysiol.,* 28:1041–1059.
27. Hubel, D. H., and Wiesel, T. N. (1969): Visual area of the lateral suprasylvian gyrus (Clare-Bishop area) of the cat. *J. Physiol.,* 202:251–260.
28. Hubel, D. H., and Wiesel, T. N. (1970): The period of susceptibility to the physiological effects of unilateral eye closure in kittens. *J. Physiol.,* 206:419–436.
29. Hubel, D. H., and Wiesel, T. N. (1974): Ordered arrangement of orientation columns in monkeys lacking visual experience. *J. Comp. Neurol.,* 158:307–318.
30. Hubel, D. H., Wiesel, T. N., and LeVay, S. (1975): Functional architecture in area 17 in normal and monocularly deprived macaque monkeys. *Cold Spring Harbor Symp. Quant. Biol.,* 40:581–589.
31. Hubel, D. H., Wiesel, T. N., and LeVay, S. (1977): Plasticity of ocular dominance columns in monkey striate cortex. *Phil. Trans. Roy. Soc. Lond. B.,* 278:377–410.
32. Imbert, M., and Buisseret, P. (1975): Receptive field characteristics and plastic properties of visual cortical cells in kittens reared with or without visual experience. *Exp. Brain Res.,* 22:25–36.
33. Kaas, J., Guillery, R., and Allman, J. (1972): Some principles of organization in the dorsal lateral geniculate nucleus. *Brain, Behav. Evol.,* 6:253–299.
34. Kasamatsu, T. (1976): Visual cortical neurons influenced by the oculomotor input: characterization of their receptive field properties. *Brain Res.,* 113:271–292.
34a. Kasamatsu, T., and Pettigrew, J. D. (1976): Depletion of brain catecholamines: Failure of ocular dominance shift after monocular occlusion in kittens. *Science,* 194:206–209.
35. Kennedy, C., Derosie, M. H., Sakurada, O., Shinohar, M., Reivich, M., Jehle, J. W., and Sokoloff, L. (1976): Metabolic mapping of primary visual system of monkey by means of autoradiographic [deoxyglucose-C-14] technique. *Proc. Natl. Acad. Sci. USA,* 73:4230–4234.
36. Kratz, K. E., and Spear, P. D. (1976): Effects of visual deprivation and alterations in binocular competition on responses of striate cortex neurons in the cat. *J. Comp. Neurol.,* 170:141–151.
37. Kratz, K. E., Spear, P. D., and Smith, D. C. (1976): Post-critical period reversal of effects of monocular deprivation on striate cortex cells in the cat. *J. Neurophysiol.,* 39:501–511.
38. LeVay, S., Hubel, D. H., and Wiesel, T. N. (1975): The pattern of ocular dominance columns in macaque visual cortex revealed by a reduced silver stain. *J. Comp. Neurol.,* 159:559–575.
39. Leventhal, A. G., and Hirsch, H. V. B. (1977): Effects of early experience upon orientation sensitivity and binocularity of neurons in visual cortex of cats. *Proc. Natl. Acad. Sci. USA,* 74:1272–1276.
40. Levick, W. R. (1967): Receptive fields and trigger features of ganglion cell in the visual streak of the rabbit's retina. *J. Physiol.,* 188:285–307.
41. Lund, J. S., Lund, R. D., Hendrickson, A. E., Bunt, A. H., and Fuchs, A. F. (1975): The origin of efferent pathways from the primary visual cortex, area ly, of the macaque monkey as shown by retrograde transport of horseradish peroxidase. *J. Comp. Neurol.,* 164:287–304.
42. Maffei, L., and Bisti, S. (1976): Binocular interaction in strabismic kittens deprived of vision. *Science,* 191:579–580.
43. Maturana, H. R., and Frenk, S. (1963): Directional movement and horizontal edge detectors in pigeon retina. *Science,* 142:977–979.
44. Mitchell, D. E., Freeman, R. D., Millodot, M., and Haegenstrom, G. (1973): Meridional amblyopia—Evidence for modification of human visual system by early visual experience. *Vision Res.,* 13:535.
45. Mize, R. R., and Murphy, E. H. (1973): Selective visual experience fails to modify receptive field properties of rabbit striate cortex neurons. *Science,* 180:320–333.
46. Norman, J. L., Daniels, J. D., and Pettigrew, J. D. (1977): Development of single neuron responses in the kitten's lateral geniculate nucleus. *Science,* 198:202–204.
47. Nottebohm, F., Stokes, T. M., and Leonard, C. M. (1976): Central control of song in the canary, *Serinus canarius. J. Comp. Neurol.,* 165:457–486.
48. Pettigrew, J. D. (1972): The neurophysiology of binocular vision. *Sci. Amer.,* 227:84–95.
49. Pettigrew, J. D. (1974): The effect of visual experience on the development of stimulus specificity by kitten cortical neurones. *J. Physiol.,* 237:49–74.
50. Pettigrew, J. D. (1978): Co-evolution of nocturnal and binocular vision. In: *Frontiers of Visual Science,* edited by S. J. Cool and E. L. Smith. Springer, New York.
51. Pettigrew, J. D., and Daniels, J. D. (1973): Gamma-aminobutyric acid antagonism in visual cortex: Different effects on simple, complex, and hypercomplex neurons. *Science,* 182:81–83.

52. Pettigrew, J. D., and Freeman, R. D. (1973): Visual experience without lines: effect on developing cortical neurons. *Science,* 182:599–601.
52a. Pettigrew, J. D., and Kasamatsu, T. (1978): Local perfusion of noradrenaline maintains visual cortical plasticity. *Nature (Lond.) (in press).*
53. Pettigrew, J. D., and Konishi, M. (1976): Effects of monocular deprivation on binocular neurones in the owl's visual Wulst. *Nature,* 264:753–754.
54. Pettigrew, J. D., Olson, C., and Hirsch, H. V. B. (1973): Cortical effect of selective visual experience: degeneration or reorganization? *Brain Res.,* 54:345–351.
55. Pettigrew, J. D., Olson, C., and Barlow, H. B. (1973): Kitten visual cortex: short-term, stimulus-induced changes in connectivity. *Science,* 180:1202–1203.
56. Rakic, P. (1976): Prenatal genesis of connections subserving ocular dominance in the rhesus monkey. *Nature (Lond.),* 261:467–471.
57. Rakic, P. (1977): Prenatal development of the visual system in rhesus monkey. *Phil. Trans. Roy. Soc. Lond. B.,* 278:245–260.
58. Rose, D., and Blakemore, C. (1974): An analysis of orientation selectivity in the cat's visual cortex. *Exp. Brain Res.,* 20:1–17.
59. Rowe, M. H., and Stone, J. (1977): Naming of neurones. Classification and naming of cat retinal ganglion cells. *Brain, Behav. Evol.,* 14:185–216.
60. Schiller, P. H., Finlay, B. L., and Volman, S. F. (1976): Quantitative studies of single-cell properties in monkey striate cortex: II. Orientation specificity and ocular dominance. *J. Neurophysiol.,* 39:1320–1333.
61. Sherk, H., and Stryker, M. P. (1976): Quantitative study of cortical orientation selectivity in visually inexperienced kitten. *J. Neurophysiol.,* 39:63–70.
62. Sillito, A. M. (1974a): Modification of receptive field properties of neurons in visual cortex by bicuculline, a GABA antagonist. *J. Physiol.,* 239:P36–P37.
63. Sillito, A. M. (1974b): Effects of iontophoretic application of bicuculline on receptive-field properties of simple cells in visual cortex of cat. *J. Physiol.,* 242:P127–P128.
64. Sillito, A. M. (1975): Contribution of inhibitory mechanisms to receptive field properties of neurons in striate cortex of cat. *J. Physiol.,* 250:305–329.
65. Spear, P. D., and Baumann, T. P. (1975): Receptive-field characteristics of single neurons in lateral suprasylvian visual area of cat. *J. Neurophysiol.,* 38:1403–1420.
66. Stryker, M. P., Hirsch, H. V. B., Sherk, H., and Leventhal, A. G. (1976): Orientation selectivity in cat visual cortex following selective orientation deprivation using goggles. *ARVO Abst. 1976*:69.
67. Stryker, M. P., and Sherk, H. (1975): Modification of cortical orientation selectivity in the cat by restricted visual experience: a reexamination. *Science,* 190:904–906.
68. Valverde, F. (1967): Apical dendritic spines of the visual cortex and light deprivation in the mouse. *Exp. Brain Res.,* 3:337–352.
69. Van Sluyters, R. C., and Blakemore, C. (1973): Experimental creation of unusual neuronal properties in visual cortex of kitten. *Nature,* 246:506–508.
70. Watkins, D. W., and Berkeley, M. A. (1974): Orientation selectivity of single neurons in cat striate cortex. *Exp. Brain Res.,* 19:433–446.
71. Wiesel, T. N., and Hubel, D. H. (1974): Reorganization of ocular dominance colums in monkey striate cortex. *Soc. Neurosci.* (4th Ann. Meeting Abstr.) 740.
72. Wiesel, T. N., Hubel, D. H., and Lam, D. (1974): Autoradiographic demonstration of ocular dominance columns in the monkey striate cortex by means of transsynaptic transport. *Brain Res.,* 79:273–279.
73. Wiesel, T. N., and Raviola, E. (1977): Myopia and eye enlargement after neonatal lid fusion in monkeys. *Nature,* 266:66–68.
74. Wilson, P. D., Rowe, M. H., and Stone, J. (1976): Properties of relay cells in the cat's lateral geniculate nucleus. A comparison of W-cells with X- and Y-cells. *J. Neurophysiol.,* 39:1193–1219.

Subject Index

A

ACTH, effects on spinal cord regeneration, 54-55

Amino acids, incorporation into protein of, in spinal cord regeneration, 65-68

Axonal sprouting and regeneration
in adults, 74-75
after locus ceruleus injury, 211-212
alteration as result of prior injury, 178-181
axonally transported materials in, 184-185
changes occurring with, 165-170, 173-174
chromatolysis in, 183-184
in damaged nervous tissue, 1-25
initiation of, mechanisms involved in, 175-176
of intact afferents, role in neuronal plasticity, 104-108
movement recovery and, 73-96
nerve cell body in, 155-195
olfactory system as model for, 131-153
postsynaptic potentials in studies of, 114-118
of preganglionic axons, 13-17
after partial denervation, 8-13
rate of, factors affecting, 176-177
RNA changes after, 158-159, 185-186

rules for, 89-92
without axotomy, 170-171

Axons
breakage of, reactions to, in maturity, 30-31
effects of cortical denervation on, 273-289
elongation of, cell body changes with, 171-173
in olfactory bulb, degeneration and regeneration in, 139-148
preganglionic, sprouting and regeneration of, 13-17

Azathioprine, effects on spinal cord regeneration, 58

Axotomy
axonal transport after, 160-162
nerve cell body changes after, 155-195
nerve growth factor, effects after, 39-41
protein changes after, 159-160
initiation, 169
reactions to, 30-31
RNA changes after, 158-159
initiation of changes by, 167-169
synaptic depression after, 32-33
causes of, 34-37

B

Boutons, preganglionic, light microscopy of, 7-8